Evidence-based Clinical Chinese Medicine

Volume 21

Type 2 Diabetes Mellitus

Evidence-based Clinical Chinese Medicine

Print ISSN: 2529-7562
Online ISSN: 2529-7554

Series Co Editors-in-Chief

Charlie Changli Xue *(RMIT University, Australia)*
Chuanjian Lu *(Guangdong Provincial Hospital of Chinese Medicine, China)*

Published

More information on this series can also be found at https://www.worldscientific.com/series/ebccm

(Continued at end of book)

Evidence-based Clinical Chinese Medicine

Co Editors-in-Chief

Charlie Changli Xue
RMIT University, Australia

Chuanjian Lu
Guangdong Provincial Hospital of Chinese Medicine, China

Volume 21
Type 2 Diabetes Mellitus

Lead Authors

Yuan Ming Di
RMIT University, Australia

Lu Sun
Guangdong Provincial Hospital of Chinese Medicine, China

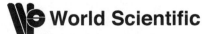 **World Scientific**

NEW JERSEY · LONDON · SINGAPORE · BEIJING · SHANGHAI · HONG KONG · TAIPEI · CHENNAI · TOKYO

Published by

World Scientific Publishing Co. Pte. Ltd.

5 Toh Tuck Link, Singapore 596224

USA office: 27 Warren Street, Suite 401-402, Hackensack, NJ 07601

UK office: 57 Shelton Street, Covent Garden, London WC2H 9HE

Library of Congress Cataloging-in-Publication Data

Names: Xue, Charlie Changli, author. | Lu, Chuan-jian, 1964– author.

Title: Evidence-based clinical Chinese medicine / Charlie Changli Xue, Chuanjian Lu.

Description: New Jersey : World Scientific, 2016. | Includes bibliographical references and index.

Identifiers: LCCN 2015030389| ISBN 9789814723084 (v. 1 : hardcover : alk. paper) |
 ISBN 9789814723091 (v. 1 : paperback : alk. paper) |
 ISBN 9789814723121 (v. 2 : hardcover : alk. paper) |
 ISBN 9789814723138 (v. 2 : paperback : alk. paper) |
 ISBN 9789814759045 (v. 3 : hardcover : alk. paper) |
 ISBN 9789814759052 (v. 3 : paperback : alk. paper)

Subjects: | MESH: Medicine, Chinese Traditional--methods. | Clinical Medicine--methods. |
 Evidence-Based Medicine--methods. | Psoriasis. | Pulmonary Disease, Chronic Obstructive.

Classification: LCC RC81 | NLM WB 55.C4 | DDC 616--dc23

LC record available at http://lccn.loc.gov/2015030389

Volume 21: Type 2 Diabetes Mellitus

ISBN 978-981-126-033-9 (hardcover)

ISBN 978-981-126-034-6 (ebook for institutions)

ISBN 978-981-126-035-3 (ebook for individuals)

British Library Cataloguing-in-Publication Data

A catalogue record for this book is available from the British Library.

For any available supplementary material, please visit
https://www.worldscientific.com/worldscibooks/10.1142/12965#t=suppl

Disclaimer

The information in this monograph is based on systematic analyses of the best available evidence for Chinese medicine interventions, both historical and contemporary. Every effort has been made to ensure the accuracy and completeness of the data in this publication. This book is intended for clinicians, researchers and educators. The practice of evidence-based medicine takes into consideration the best available evidence, clinical experiences and judgement of practitioners, and patient preferences, though not all interventions are acceptable in all countries. It is important to note that some of the substances mentioned in this book may no longer be in use, may be toxic, or are prohibited or restricted under the provisions of the Convention on International Trade in Endangered Species of Wild Fauna and Flora (CITES). Practitioners, researchers and educators are advised to comply with the relevant regulations in their country and restrictions on the trade of species included in CITES appendices I, II and III. This book is not intended as a guide for self-medication. Patients should seek professional advice from qualified Chinese medicine practitioners.

Foreword

Since the late 20th century, Chinese medicine, including acupuncture and herbal medicine, has been increasingly used throughout the world. The parallel development and spread of evidence-based medicine have provided challenges and opportunities for Chinese medicine.

The opportunities have been evidence-based medicine's emphasis on the effective use of the best available clinical evidence and incorporating the clinical experience of clinicians, subject to patients' preferences. Such practices have a patient focus, which reflects the historical nature of Chinese medicine practice. However, the challenges are also significant due to the fact that, despite the long-term development and very rich literature accumulated over 2,000 years, there is an overall lack of high-level clinical evidence for many of the interventions used in Chinese medicine.

To address this knowledge gap, we need to generate clinical evidence through high-quality clinical studies and evaluate evidence to enable the effective use of such available evidence to promote evidence-based Chinese medicine practice.

Modern Chinese medicine is rooted in its classical literature and the legacies of ancient doctors, grounded in the practice of expert clinicians and increasingly informed by clinical and experimental research efforts. In recognition of the unique features of Chinese medicine, a "Whole Evidence" approach is used for each of the conditions in this series to provide a synthesis of the different types and levels of evidence to enable practitioners to make clinical decisions informed by the current best evidence.

There are four main components of this "Whole Evidence" approach. Firstly, we present the current approaches to the diagnosis, differentiation and treatment of each condition based on expert consensus in published textbooks and clinical guidelines. This provides an overview of how the condition is currently managed. The second section provides an analysis of the condition in historical context based on systematic searches of the *Zhong Hua Yi Dian*, which includes the full texts of more than 1,000 classical medical books. These analyses provide objective views on how the condition has been treated over two millennia, reveal the continuities and discontinuities between traditional and modern practice, and suggest avenues for future research.

The third component is the assessment of evidence derived from modern clinical studies of Chinese medicine interventions. The methods established by the *Cochrane Collaboration* are used as the basis for conducting systematic reviews and undertaking meta-analyses of outcome data for randomised controlled trials (RCTs). In addition, the clinical relevance of meta-analysis data is enhanced by examining the herbal formulae, individual herbs and acupuncture treatments assessed in the RCTs, and the evidence base is broadened by the inclusion of data from controlled clinical trials and non-controlled studies. The fourth component is to determine how herbal medicine interventions may achieve the effects indicated by the clinical trials. Thus for each of the most frequently used herbs, we provide reviews of their effects in pre-clinical models and their likely mechanisms of action.

For each condition, this "Whole Evidence" approach links clinical expertise, historical precedent, clinical research data and experimental research to provide the reader with assessments of the current state of the evidence of efficacy and safety for Chinese medicine interventions using herbal medicines, acupuncture and moxibustion and other health care practices such as *tuina*.

Since these books are available in Chinese and English, they can benefit patients, practitioners and educators internationally and enable practitioners to make clinical decisions informed by the current best evidence.

These publications represent a major milestone in Chinese medicine development and make a significant contribution to the development of evidence-based Chinese medicine globally.

Co-Editors-in-Chief
Distinguished Professor Charlie Changli Xue,
RMIT University, Australia

Professor Chuanjian Lu, Guangdong Provincial Hospital of
Chinese Medicine, China

Purpose of the Monograph

This book is intended for clinicians, researchers and educators. It can be used to inform tertiary education and clinical practice by providing systematic, multi-dimensional assessments of the best available evidence for using Chinese medicine to manage each common clinical condition.

How to Use This Monograph

Some Definitions

A glossary is included, containing terms and definitions that frequently appear in the book. It also describes the definitions of statistical tests, methodological terms, evaluation tools and interventions. For example, in this book, Integrative Medicine refers to the combined use of a Chinese medicine treatment with conventional medical management, and Combination Therapies refers to two or more Chinese medicines from different therapy groups (Chinese herbal medicine, acupuncture or other Chinese medicine therapies) administered together. The terminology used throughout the monograph is based where possible or from cited references of the World Health Organization's *Standard Terminologies on Traditional Medicine in the Western Pacific Region* (2007).

Data Analysis and Interpretation of Results

In order to synthesise the clinical evidence, a range of statistical analysis approaches are used. In general, the effect size for dichotomous data is reported as a risk ratio (RR) with 95% confidence intervals (CI), and for continuous data, they are reported as mean difference (MD) with 95% CI. Statistically significant effects are indicated with an asterisk. Readers should note that statistical significance does not necessarily correspond with a clinically important effect. Interpretation of results should take into consideration the clinical significance, quality of studies (expressed as high, low or unclear risk of bias in this book) and heterogeneity amongst the studies. Tests for heterogeneity are conducted using the I^2 statistic. An I^2 score greater than 50% may indicate substantial heterogeneity.

Use of Evidence in Practice

The Grading of Recommendations, Assessment, Development and Evaluation (GRADE) approach was used to summarise the quality of evidence and results of the strength of evidence for critical and important comparisons and outcomes. Due to the diverse nature of Chinese medicine practice, treatment recommendations are not included with the summary of findings tables. Therefore, readers will need to interpret the evidence with reference to the local practice environment.

Limitations

Readers should note some of the methodological limitations on classical literature and clinical evidence.

- Search terms used to search the *Zhong Hua Yi Dian* database may not include all the terms that have been used for the condition, which may alter the findings.
- The Chinese language has changed over time. Citations have been interpreted for analysis, and such interpretations may be subject to disagreement.
- Chinese medicine theory has evolved over time. As such, concepts described in classical Chinese medical literature may no longer be found in contemporary works.

- Symptoms described in citations may be common to many conditions, and judgement was required to determine the likelihood of the citation being related to the condition. This may have introduced some bias due to the subjective nature of the judgement.
- The vast majority of the clinical evidence for Chinese medicine treatments has come from China. The applicability of the findings to other populations and countries requires further assessment.
- Many studies included participants with varying disease severity. Where possible, subgroup analyses were undertaken to examine the effects in different sub-populations. As this was not always possible, the findings may be limited to the population included and not to sub-populations.
- The potential risk of bias found in many included studies suggested methodological limitations. The findings for GRADE assessments based on studies of very low to moderate quality evidence should be interpreted accordingly.
- Nine major English and Chinese language databases were searched to identify clinical studies, in addition to clinical trial registers. Other studies may exist that were not identified through searches and which may alter the findings.
- The calculation of the frequency of herbal formulae use was based on formula names only. It is possible that studies evaluated herbal treatments with the same or similar herb ingredients but were given different formula names. Due to the complexity of herbal formulae, it was considered not appropriate to make a judgement as to the similarity of formulae for analysis. As such, the frequency of formulae reported in Chapter 5 may be underestimated.
- The most frequently utilised herbs that may have contributed to the treatment effect have been described in Chapter 5. These herbs may provide leads for further exploration. Calculation of the herbs with potential effect is based on the frequency of formulae reported in the studies and does not take into consideration the clinical implications and functions of every herb in a formula.

Authors and Contributors

CO-EDITORS-IN-CHIEF
Distinguished Prof. Charlie Changli Xue (*RMIT University, Australia*)
Prof. Chuanjian Lu (*Guangdong Provincial Hospital of Chinese Medicine, China*)

CO-DEPUTY EDITORS-IN-CHIEF
Prof. Anthony Lin Zhang (*RMIT University, Australia*)
Dr. Brian H May (*RMIT University, Australia*)
Prof. Xinfeng Guo (*Guangdong Provincial Hospital of Chinese Medicine, China*)
Prof. Zehuai Wen (*Guangdong Provincial Hospital of Chinese Medicine, China*)

LEAD AUTHORS
Dr. Yuan Ming Di (*RMIT University, Australia*)
Dr. Lu Sun (*Guangdong Provincial Hospital of Chinese Medicine, China*)

CO-AUTHORS:
RMIT University (Australia):
Dr. Kai Yi Wang
Dr. Mary Zhang
Prof. Anthony Lin Zhang
Distinguished Prof. Charlie Changli Xue

Guangdong Provincial Hospital of Chinese Medicine (China):
Prof. Guanjie Fan
Prof. Chuanjian Lu
Prof. Xinfeng Guo
Prof. Xianyu Tang

Member of Advisory Committee and Panel

Co-Chairs of Project Planning Committee
Prof. Peter J Coloe (*RMIT University, Australia*)
Prof. Yubo Lyu (*Guangdong Provincial Hospital of Chinese Medicine, China*)
Prof. Dacan Chen (*Guangdong Provincial Hospital of Chinese Medicine, China*)

Centre Advisory Committee (Alphabetical order)
Prof. Keji Chen (*The Chinese Academy of Sciences, China*)
Prof. Aiping Lu (*Hong Kong Baptist University, China*)
Prof. Caroline Smith (*Western Sydney University, Australia*)
Prof. David F Story (*RMIT University, Australia*)

Methodology Expert Advisory Panel (Alphabetical order)
Prof. Zhaoxiang Bian (*Hong Kong Baptist University, China*)
Prof. Lixing Lao (*The University of Hong Kong, China*)
The Late Prof. George Lewith (*University of Southampton, United Kingdom*)
Prof. Jianping Liu (*Beijing University of Chinese Medicine, China*)
Prof. Frank Thien (*Monash University, Australia*)
Prof. Jialiang Wang (*Sichuan University, China*)

Content Expert Advisory Panel (Alphabetical order)
Prof. Yiming Mu (*General Hospital of People's Liberation Army, China*)
Prof. Dalong Zhu (*Nanjing Drum Tower Hospital, China*)

Distinguished Professor
Charlie Changli Xue, Ph.D.

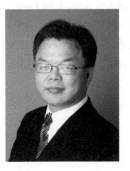

Distinguished Professor Charlie Changli Xue holds a Bachelor of Medicine (majoring in Chinese Medicine) from Guangzhou University of Chinese Medicine, China (1987), and a PhD from RMIT University, Australia (2000). He has been an academic, researcher, regulator, and practitioner for over three decades. Distinguished Professor Xue has made significant contributions to evidence-based educational development, clinical research, regulatory framework and policy development, and provision of high-quality clinical care to the community. Distinguished Professor Xue is recognised internationally as an expert in evidence-based traditional medicine and integrative healthcare.

Distinguished Professor Xue was appointed by the Australian Health Workforce Ministerial Council in 2011 as the Inaugural National Chair of the Chinese Medicine Board of Australia, and he was reappointed in 2014 and 2017 for second and third terms. Since 2007, he has been a Member of the World Health Organization's (WHO) Expert Advisory Panel for Traditional and Complementary Medicine, Geneva. Distinguished Professor Xue is also an Honorary Senior Principal Research Fellow at the Guangdong Provincial Academy of Chinese Medical Sciences, China.

At RMIT, Distinguished Professor Xue is an Associate Deputy Vice-Chancellor (International). He is also the Director of WHO's Collaborating Centre for Traditional Medicine.

Between 1995 and 2010, Distinguished Professor Xue was Discipline Head of Chinese Medicine at RMIT University. He leads the development of five successful undergraduate and postgraduate degree programs in Chinese Medicine at RMIT University, which is now a global leader in Chinese medicine education and research.

Distinguished Professor Xue's research has been supported by over AU$15 million in research grants, including six project grants from the Australian Government's National Health and Medical Research Council (NHMRC) and two Australian Research Council (ARC) grants. He has contributed over 200 publications and has been frequently invited as keynote speaker for numerous national and international conferences. Distinguished Professor Xue has contributed to over 300 media interviews on issues related to complementary medicine education, research, regulation, and practice.

Professor Chuanjian Lu, M.D.

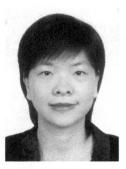 Professor Chuanjian Lu, Doctor of Medicine, is the Vice President of Guangdong Provincial Hospital of Chinese Medicine (Guangdong Provincial Academy of Chinese Medical Sciences, Second Clinical Medical College of Guangzhou University of Chinese Medicine). She also is the chair of the Guangdong Traditional Chinese Medicine (TCM) Standardization Technical Committee and the vice-chair of the Immunity Specialty Committee of the World Federation of Chinese Medicine Societies (WFCMS).

Professor Lu has engaged in scientific research into TCM, clinical practice and teaching for some 25 years. Her research has been devoted to integrated traditional and western medicine. She has edited and published 12 monographs and 120 academic research articles as the first author and corresponding author, with over 30 articles being included in SCI journals.

She has received widespread recognition for her achievements with awards for "Excellent Teacher of South China", "National Outstanding Women TCM Doctor", and "National Outstanding Young Doctor of TCM". She also received "The Science and Technology Star of the Association of Chinese Medicine", "National Excellent Science and Technology Workers of China Award" and "Five-Continent Women's Scientific Awards of China Medical Women's Association".

Professor Lu has won the Award of Science and Technology Progress over 10 times from Guangdong Provincial Government, China Association of Chinese Medicine and Chinese Hospital Association.

Acknowledgements

The authors and contributors would like to acknowledge the valuable contributions of the following people who assisted with database searches, data extraction, data screening, data assessment, translation of documents, editing and/or administrative tasks: Edward Caruso, Zenan Fang, Chunyi Zhao and Jing Chen.

Contents

Contents

Contents

List of Figures

List of Tables

1

Introduction to Type 2 Diabetes Mellitus

OVERVIEW

Type 2 diabetes mellitus is the most common form of diabetes mellitus and affects millions of people worldwide, although many people are often undiagnosed. People with type 2 diabetes may present with characteristic symptoms such as thirst, polyuria and weight loss. Type 2 diabetes mellitus causes a huge burden on the global health expenditure, disability-adjusted life-years, and mortality rates. The exact cause of Type 2 diabetes is unknown; however, genetic and metabolic factors determine the risk of developing the condition. Treatments include lifestyle management, anti-glycaemics and insulin therapy. This chapter describes the definition, risk factors, epidemiological profile, pathological processes, diagnosis and treatment of type 2 diabetes mellitus.

Definition of Type 2 Diabetes Mellitus

Diabetes mellitus describes a metabolic disorder characterised by chronic hyperglycaemia with disturbances of carbohydrate, fat and protein metabolism resulting from defects in insulin secretion or insulin action, or both.[1-3] Type 2 diabetes mellitus (T2DM) is the most common form of diabetes mellitus and is characterised by insulin secretion defects and peripheral insulin resistance.[1-3] It accounts for approximately 90–95% of diabetes mellitus and was previously known as "noninsulin-dependent diabetes" or "adult-onset diabetes".[1,3]

Clinical Presentation

People with T2DM may present with characteristic symptoms such as thirst, polyuria, blurring of vision and weight loss.[1] In its most severe forms, ketoacidosis or a non-ketotic hyperosmolar state may develop and lead to stupor, coma and, in the absence of effective treatment, death.[1]

However, T2DM is often undiagnosed for many years because hyperglycaemia develops over time and is not severe enough at earlier stages to present the classic symptoms.[3] The proportion of those undiagnosed varies widely — a recent review of data from seven countries found that between 24% and 62% of people with diabetes were undiagnosed and untreated.[4] Even in high-income countries, the proportion of undiagnosed diabetes can be as high as 30–50%.[5]

Epidemiology

Types of diabetes mellitus are often not distinguished in population-level estimates; therefore, the term diabetes mellitus in this section refers to all types of diabetes mellitus unless T2DM is specified. Globally, the number of adults with diabetes has risen from 108 million (4.7%) in 1980 to 422 million (8.5%) in 2014.[6] With the increasing trend of diabetes, it is estimated that 629 million people aged 20–79 years will have diabetes (9.9% of the global population) in 221 countries and territories by 2045.[7] In the United States (US), an estimated 30.3 million people of all ages had diabetes in 2015 (9.4% of the population), of which 30.2 million were adults aged 18 years or older (12.2% of all US adults).[8] Only about 5% of those with diabetes were Type 1 diabetes. Diabetes was diagnosed in 23.1 million people and 23.8% of these were unaware or did not report having diabetes (7.2 million).[8]

Based on self-reported data, an estimated 1 million (5%) Australian adults had T2DM in 2014–2015.[9] The number of T2DM is similar among men and women (6% and 5%), though the rates for males were higher than females from age 55 years onward.[9] When socioeconomic groups are compared, the rate of T2DM in the lowest socioeconomic group (8%) is more than two times higher than that in the highest socioeconomic group (3%).[9]

In Europe, 7% of adults across European countries in 2014 reported to have diabetes.[10] Diabetes prevalence ranged from less than 5% in Lithuania, Denmark, Latvia, Romania, Sweden and Austria, to over 9% in Greece, Portugal and France.[10] People with the lowest level of education are more than twice as likely to report having diabetes as those with the highest level on average.[10] Almost 3.7 million people have been diagnosed with diabetes in the United Kingdom (UK); around 90% have T2DM.[11] Data also showed that 12.3 million people are at risk of T2DM and there are currently 4.6 million people living with diabetes in the UK.[11]

In the south-east Asia region, 10.1% of the population (aged 20–79) have diabetes.[7] In 2017, China (114.4 million) and India (72.9 million) were the top two countries in this region with the most number of people with diabetes and are projected to remain there even in 2045.[7] It has been estimated that 47.2 million people are living with undiagnosed diabetes in south-east Asia.[7] No country has diagnosed every person as having diabetes or no diabetes.[7] In Africa, where many low-income countries with wide rural areas are located, the proportion of undiagnosed diabetes is 69.2%, likely due to limited resources and low prioritisation of diabetes screening.[7] Even in high-income countries, 37.3% of people with diabetes have not been diagnosed.[7]

Burden

Diabetes imposes a large economic burden on the global healthcare system and the wider global economy.[6] This burden can be measured through direct medical costs, indirect costs associated with productivity loss, premature mortality, and the negative impact of diabetes on nations' gross domestic product.[6] The global healthcare expenditures for diabetes were USD 727 billion in 2017; this is an 8% increase compared to the 2015 estimate.[7] Moreover, with the increased ageing population and prevalence, the global health expenditure for diabetes is projected to be USD 776 billion by 2045.[7]

Of the seven International Diabetes Federation regions, the North American and Caribbean region has the highest expenditure on diabetes — international dollar (ID) 383 billion (20–79 years), which corresponds to 52% of the total amount spent globally in 2017.[7] The second highest expenditure on diabetes is the European region (ID 181 billion), followed by the Western Pacific (ID 179 billion). This corresponds to 23% and 17%, respectively, of the total global spending.[7] On a country level, the highest expenditures on diabetes were observed in the US (ID 348 billion), followed by China (ID 110 billion), and then Germany (ID 42 billion).[7]

Globally, the burden of health loss due to diabetes measured by the all age disability-adjusted life-years (DALYs) in 2016 was 57,233.7 (thousands).[12] Diabetes is the fourth leading cause of US DALYs and increased by 11% from 1990 to 2016.[13] In Australia, diabetes was among the top 15 causes of total burden measured by DALY in 2011 (101,653) and is 2.3% of the total DALYs.[14]

In 2002, diabetes was ranked the 11th leading cause of death globally;[15] in 2013 it was identified as the ninth major cause of reduced life expectancy.[16] According to projections, it will be the seventh cause of death by the year 2030.[15] In 2010, it was estimated that diabetes mellitus caused 3.96 million deaths in adults aged 20–79 years during that year (6.8% of global mortality).[17] This estimate was raised to between 3.2 and 5.0 million deaths due to diabetes mellitus, which is equivalent to one death every eight seconds, in the IDF 2017 report.[7] In Australia, diabetes contributed to over 16,400 deaths or 10% of all deaths in 2015 — about 9,000 deaths were caused by T2DM — when it is listed as the underlying and/or cause of death.[9] Taken together, diabetes causes a huge burden on the global health expenditure, DALYs and mortality rates.

Risk Factors

The risk of T2DM is determined by genetic and metabolic factors; these include: ethnicity, family history of diabetes, women with prior gestational diabetes, older age, overweight and obesity, an unhealthy diet, physical inactivity, smoking, and individuals with hypertension or dyslipidaemia.[3,18]

Table 1.1. Criteria for Defining Prediabetes (adapted from the American Diabetes Association)[3]

FPG 100 mg/dL (5.6 mmol/L) to 125 mg/dL (6.9 mmol/L) (IFG)

OR

2-h PG in the 75-g OGTT 140 mg/dL (7.8 mmol/L) to 199 mg/dL (11.0 mmol/L) (IGT)

OR

A1C 5.72–6.4% (39–47 mmol/mol)

*For all three tests, risk is continuous, extending below the lower limit of the range and becoming disproportionately greater at the higher end of the range.

Abbreviations: A1C, glycated haemoglobin; FPG, fasting plasma glucose; IFG, impaired fasting glycaemia; OGTT, oral glucose tolerance test; PG, postprandial glucose.

Another group of people who have a high risk of developing diabetes are pre-diabetes people whose glucose levels do not meet the criteria for diabetes, yet are higher than those who are considered normal.[3,19,20] Diagnostic testing levels that define impaired fasting glucose (IFG) or impaired glucose tolerance (IGT) are summarised in Table 1.1.

Furthermore, pre-diabetes is associated with abdominal obesity, dyslipidaemia and hypertension, which are also risk factors of T2DM. Therefore, screening for pre-diabetes is an essential step in identifying risk patients. However, not all patients will present with diabetic symptoms. Table 1.2 presents an informal assessment of risk factors for diabetes or pre-diabetes in asymptomatic adults.

Pathological Processes

T2DM is a condition of multiple aetiology, but the specific reason for disease onset is unknown.[1,21] In T2DM, patients' beta cells are not destroyed due to autoimmunity, and this is not caused by other causes such as diseases of the exocrine pancreas, endocrinopathies, drug-or-chemical impairment of insulin secretion or infections.[22] The pathogenesis of T2DM is complex and involves the interaction of genetic and environmental factors.[23,24] It is a progressive and complex metabolic disorder characterised by coexisting defects of multiple organ sites, including insulin resistance in muscle and

Table 1.2.   Criteria for Testing for Diabetes or Prediabetes in Asymptomatic Adults (adapted from the American Diabetes Association)[3]

1. Testing should be considered in overweight or obese (BMI ≥ 25 kg/m² or >23 kg/m² in Asian Americans) adults who have one or more of the following risk factors:
   - A1C ≥ 5.7% (39 mmol/mol), IGT, or IFG on previous testing,
   - First-degree relative with diabetes,
   - High-risk race/ethnicity (e.g., African American, Latino, Native American, Asian American, Pacific Islander),
   - History of cardiovascular disease,
   - Hypertension (>140/90 mmHg or on therapy for hypertension),
   - High-density lipoprotein cholesterol level <35 mg/dL (0.90 mmol/L) and/or a triglyceride level >250 mg/dL (2.82 mmol/L),
   - Women with polycystic ovary syndrome,
   - Physical inactivity, and
   - Other clinical conditions associated with insulin resistance (e.g., severe obesity, acanthosis nigricans).
2. Patients with prediabetes (A1C ≥ 5.7% [39 mmol/mol], IGT or IFG) should be tested yearly.
3. Women who were diagnosed with gestational diabetes mellitus should have lifelong testing at least every three years.
4. For all other patients, testing should begin at age 45 years.
5. If results are normal, testing should be repeated at a minimum of 3-year intervals, with a consideration for more frequent testing depending on initial results (e.g., those with pre-diabetes should be tested yearly) and risk status.

Abbreviations: A1C, glycated haemoglobin; BMI, body mass index; IFG, impaired fasting glycaemia; IGT, impaired glucose tolerance.

adipose tissue, a progressive decline in pancreatic insulin secretion, uncontrolled hepatic glucose production, and other hormonal deficiencies.[25] The key pathological processes of T2DM are summarised here.

Beta Cell Dysfunction, Insulin Resistance

Insulin is a vital hormone produced by the pancreas that allows blood glucose passage into the body's cells, providing fuel for the body's systems. Insulin maintains normal blood glucose levels by facilitating cellular glucose uptake and regulates carbohydrate, lipid and protein metabolism. Without insulin, excess glucose will build up in the bloodstream leading to hyperglycaemia, a hallmark metabolic abnormality associated with T2DM.[1]

Normal regulation of glucose metabolism is determined by a feedback loop involving the islet β-cell and insulin-sensitive tissues such as muscle, liver and adipose tissue.[26] Tissue sensitivity to insulin determines the magnitude of the β-cell response and insulin release. Insulin released in response to β-cell stimulation mediates the uptake of glucose, amino acids and fatty acids by insulin-sensitive tissues. These tissues provide the islet cell with information on their need for insulin.

Insulin resistance suggests an impaired biological response to insulin and is characterised by reduced transport and metabolism of insulin-stimulated glucose in adipocytes and skeletal muscles, and impaired suppression of hepatic glucose production.[24] The β-cell retains normal glucose tolerance by increasing insulin production when the β-cell is unable to release enough insulin in the presence of insulin resistance. As a result, the glucose levels rise.[26]

Insulin resistance can be broadly defined as a decrease in tissue response to insulin or an increase in insulin levels with normal plasma glucose.[23] Insulin resistance can be measured directly by the ability of a fixed dose of insulin to promote total glucose disposal or indirectly by measuring fasting insulin levels.[27] Insulin action can be affected by the abnormalities of insulin receptor concentration or affinity, or both. However, clinically insulin resistance is a common result of defects in the post-receptor intracellular signalling pathways.[23]

Although most people with T2DM have insulin resistance, most people with insulin resistance do not have diabetes because their islet β-cells compensate for decreased insulin sensitivity by increasing insulin secretion.[23,27] Among susceptible individuals with obesity, β-cell loss may be accelerated by ectopic fat deposition in the islets, local obesity-induced inflammation in the islets, and local and circulating adipokines and inflammatory cytokines. As β-cell failure progresses, levels of glucose and free fatty acids start to rise, which may, in turn, cause further β-cell toxicity. Increased demand on a decreased β-cell mass may cause further damage through endoplasmic reticulum stress and the increased formation of toxic islet amyloid polypeptide oligomers. Then once diabetes is established, all of these mechanisms may further contribute to the progressive decline in β-cell function that characterise T2DM.[23] As the disease progresses, β-cell decompensation with impaired insulin secretion follows and insulin sensitivity continues to decrease.[27]

Most patients with T2DM are obese, and obesity itself causes some degree of insulin resistance. Those who are not obese by the traditional weight criteria may have an increased percentage of body fat distributed predominantly in the abdominal region.[21] Increases in visceral adiposity also correlate with increased insulin resistance.[23]

The disposal of glucose after meals depends on the ability of insulin to increase peripheral glucose uptake and at the same time decrease endogenous glucose production. In insulin resistance, insulin has reduced ability to suppress lipolysis in adipose tissue, and glucagon secretion by alpha cells in the islet results in increased gluconeogenesis and thus increases glucose output. In addition, insulin inhibition of glycogenolysis is also impaired. Therefore, both hepatic and peripheral insulin resistance result in abnormal glucose production by the liver,[24] contributing further to the impaired glucose metabolism.

Genes

T2DM has a strong genetic link — most individuals with T2DM have other family members with the same condition and multiple genes contribute to this disease. Positive family history confers a 2.4-fold increased risk for T2DM.[28] Identified genes that contribute to T2DM are mostly involved in β-cell function and turnover. Efforts to identify the genes involved in polygenic T2DM have focused on two approaches: candidate gene testing and genome-wide association study. Using the candidate gene approach, *PPARγ* was the first gene identified.[29] Since then, more than 50 gene loci have been linked to T2DM using genome-wide association studies, and 19 mutations of the *insulin* gene and subunits of the ATP-sensitive potassium channel have also been associated with T2DM.[30] Other genetic defects in the pancreatic β-cells, including mutations in several genes causing autosomal recessive syndromes with defects in β-cell functions, have been identified. Mitochondrial DNA mutations that impair the transfer of leucine into mitochondrial proteins have now been described in a large number of families and result from impaired β-cell function.[23]

Diet and Obesity

Increased caloric intake and decreased energy expenditure contribute to the development of obesity and T2DM. Diet and nutrition play an important part in the development of T2DM, specifically increased amounts of dietary fat and saturated fat are important in determining the development of obesity, insulin resistance, β-cell dysfunction and glucose intolerance.[31]

Most patients with this form of diabetes are obese, and obesity itself causes some degree of insulin resistance.[32] Patients who are not obese by the traditional weight criteria may have an increased percentage of body fat distributed predominantly in the abdominal region.[32] Most people with T2DM have excess adiposity, although the prevalence of obesity in association with T2DM varies among different racial groups, with higher incidence in North Americans, Europeans and Africans (60–80%), and lower percentages in Chinese and Japanese people (30%).[23]

A number of circulating hormones, cytokines and metabolic fuels, such as non-esterified (free) fatty acids (NEFA) originate in the adipocyte and modulate insulin action.[28] An increased mass of stored triglyceride, especially in visceral or deep subcutaneous adipose depots, leads to large adipocytes that are themselves resistant to the ability of insulin to suppress lipolysis.[28] This results in increased release and circulating levels of NEFA and glycerol; both aggravate insulin resistance in skeletal muscle and the liver.[33] Furthermore, insulin resistance is strongly associated with obesity and increased visceral adiposity.[23,28]

Importance of Intestine

Incretins glucagon-like peptide 1 (GLP-1) and glucose-dependent insulinotropic polypeptide (GIP) are intestinal peptide hormones released in response to food ingestion.[34] They enhance meal-related insulin secretion and promote glucose tolerance, a phenomenon called the incretin effect. In T2DM patients, the incretin effect is reduced. Besides insulin secretion enhancement, GLP-1 also suppresses glucagon secretion from the pancreatic alpha cells in a glucose-dependent matter; glucagon secretion is inhibited under hyperglycaemic conditions and even increased under hypoglycaemia.

Systemic Inflammation

Adipose tissue can affect the insulin sensitivity of other tissues through the secretion of signalling molecules called adipokines. It inhibits (TNF-α, IL-6, leptin, resistin and others) or enhances (adiponectin) insulin signalling locally or in distal target tissues.[23] The release of fatty acids by the engorged adipocytes, especially visceral adipocytes, from which fatty acids are more readily mobilised, may play a role in the development of insulin resistance. Oxidation of fatty acids by muscle and other tissues could inhibit glycolysis and reduce insulin-stimulated glucose removal.[23] In addition to adipocytes, adipose tissue contains a variety of other cell types, including inflammatory/immune cells, such as macrophages and lymphocytes; these cells implicate obesity-induced insulin resistance. The activated macrophages then release a variety of molecules that decrease the insulin sensitivity of the adipocytes and further increase their release of proinflammatory cytokines, and along with the increased release of free fatty acids and development of ectopic lipid accumulation, promotes the development of inflammation and insulin resistance in other key insulin-target tissues, such as muscles and the liver.[23]

In summary, several pathogenic processes are involved in the development of T2DM. Fundamental abnormalities include:[1,24]

- Defect in the β-cell of the pancreas with consequent defective insulin secretion and insulin deficiency, particularly in response to a glucose stimulus,
- Resistance to the action of insulin in peripheral tissues, particularly muscles and fats, but also the liver, and
- Increased glucose production by the liver.

Screening

Due to the compensatory mechanism of β-cells producing more insulin in insulin-resistant people, there is a long pre-symptomatic phase before the diagnosis of T2DM, so screening for pre-diabetes and T2DM using an assessment of risk factors is recommended.[3] Screening for pre-diabetes is an essential step in identifying risk patients. However, not all patients will present with diabetic symptoms, informal assessment of risk factors for diabetes or prediabetes in asymptomatic adults is presented in Table 1.2.

Assessment tools are available to screen for diabetes, such as the ADA risk test and AUSDRISK.[2,3] For all patients, testing should begin at age 45. In the US, testing for diabetes is considered for overweight or obese children and young adults with two or more additional risk factors for diabetes as outlined in Table 1.2.[2,3] In Australia, testing begins at 40 years of age, or even at 18 years of age for Aboriginals and Torres Strait Islanders.[2] If their results are normal, testing should be repeated at 3-year intervals, with consideration for more frequent testing depending on initial results (e.g., those with pre-diabetes should be tested yearly) and risk status.

There is an increase in the incidence and prevalence of T2DM in adolescents over the last decade, and this continues to rise.[35–37] In the US, incidence rates of T2DM in youths who were 10–19 years of age increased by 7.1% annually (from 9.0 cases per 100,000 youths per year in 2002–2003 to 12.5 cases per 100,000 youths per year in 2011–2012).[36] The American Diabetes Association recommended criteria and risk factors for the screening of pre-diabetes and T2DM are outlined in Table 1.3.[3]

Table 1.3. Testing for Type 2 diabetes or Pre-diabetes in Asymptomatic Children and Adolescents in a Clinical Setting (adapted from the American Diabetes Association)[3]

Testing should be considered in youths* who are overweight (≥ 85% percentile) or obese (≥ 95 percentile) with one or more additional risk factors based on the strength of their association with diabetes:

- Maternal history of diabetes or gestational diabetes mellitus during the child's gestation,
- Family history of T2DM in first- or second-degree relatives, and
- Race/ethnicity (Native American, African American, Latino, Asian American, Pacific Islander).

Signs of insulin resistance or conditions associated with insulin resistance (acanthosis nigricans, hypertension, dyslipidaemia, polycystic ovary syndrome, or small-for-gestational-age birth weight).

*After the onset of puberty or after 10 years of age, whichever occurs earlier. If tests are normal, repeat testing at a minimum of 3-year intervals, or more frequently if the body mass index is increasing, is recommended.

Diagnosis

T2DM is often undiagnosed for many years because the hyperglycaemia develops over time and at earlier stages are not severe enough to present the classic symptoms of diabetes.[3] Diabetes may be identified in low-risk individuals who by chance have a glucose testing, in individuals tested based on diabetes risk assessment, and in symptomatic patients.[3]

Diagnosis of diabetes may be based on plasma glucose criteria using three types of biochemical analyses: either the fasting plasma glucose (FGP) or the 2-h plasma glucose (2-h PG) value after a 75-g oral glucose tolerance test (OGTT) or glycated haemoglobin (A1C) criteria (Table 1.4).[2,3,18,32,38] These tests are equally appropriate for diagnostic testing for diabetes, but it does not necessarily mean that the tests will detect diabetes in the same individual.[3]

The International Expert Committee recommends the use of A1C to diagnose diabetes.[38] Those with A1C levels above the laboratory "normal" range but below the diagnostic cut point for diabetes (6.0 to <6.5%) are at very high risk of developing diabetes — the risk is more than 10 times than those with lower levels.[39–42] However,

Table 1.4. Criteria for the Diagnosis of Diabetes (adapted from American Diabetes Association)[3]

FPG ≥ 126 mg/dL (7.0 mmol/L). Fasting is defined as no caloric intake for at least 8 h.*
OR
2-h PG ≥ 200 mg/dL (11.1 mmol/L) during an OGTT. The test should be performed as described by the WHO, using a glucose load containing the equivalent of 75 g anhydrous glucose dissolved in water.*
OR
A1C ≥ 6.5% (48 mmol/mol). The test should be performed in a laboratory using a method that is NGSP certified and standardised to the DCCT assay.*
In a patient with classic symptoms of hyperglycaemia or hyperglycaemic crisis, a random plasma glucose ≥200 mg/dL (11.1 mmol/L).
*In the absence of unequivocal hyperglycaemia, results should be confirmed by repeat testing.

Abbreviations: A1C, glycated haemoglobin; DCCT, Diabetes Control and Complications Trial; FPG, fasting plasma glucose; NGSP, National Glycohemoglobin Standardization Program; OGTT, oral glucose tolerance test; PG, postprandial glucose; WHO, World Health Organization.

the 6.0–6.56 range failed to identify a substantial number of patients who have IFG and/or IGT.

In asymptomatic patients, a second test is required to confirm a T2DM diagnosis. It is recommended that the same test be repeated without delay by using a new blood sample for confirmation because there will be a greater likelihood of concurrence.[21] For example, if the A1C is 7.0% (53 mmol/mol) and a repeat result is 6.8% (51 mmol/mol), the diagnosis of diabetes is confirmed. If two different tests (such as A1C and FPG) are both above the diagnostic threshold, this also confirms the diagnosis.

When results from two different tests are conflicting, then the test result that is above the diagnostic cut point should be repeated. The diagnosis is made on the basis of the confirmed test. For example, if a patient meets the diabetes criterion of the A1C (two results ≥ 6.5% [48 mmol/mol]) but not the FPG (126 mg/dL [7.0 mmol/L]), then that person should still be considered to have diabetes. If patients have test results near the margins of the diagnostic threshold, the health care professional should follow the patient closely and repeat the test in 3–6 months.

Management

The management of diabetes can be achieved through preventative measures before the disease is established. Once T2DM is established, management can occur using pharmacological therapies or non-pharmacological interventions, as discussed below.

Prevention

T2DM is a progressive medical condition and is preventable.[2] Through the screening process, those who are determined to be at high risk for T2DM — including people with A1C 5.7–6.4% (39–47mmol/mol), impaired glucose tolerance, or impaired fasting glucose — are ideal candidates for diabetes prevention efforts, and annual monitoring for the development of diabetes is recommended.[3]

There are effective interventions that prevent the progression from pre-diabetes to diabetes through structured lifestyle intervention. Working towards a goal of increasing physical activity and producing 5–10% loss of body weight have shown to prevent or delay the development of diabetes in people with insulin glucose tolerance.[3] The Diabetes Prevention Program have two major goals: achieve and maintain a minimum of 7% weight loss, and 150 minutes of physical activity per week, which should be similar in intensity to brisk walking. This includes aerobic dancing, bicycle riding, skating and swimming,[43] all of which could reduce the incidence of T2DM by 58% over three years,[44] result in a sustained reduction in the rate of conversion to T2DM,[43,45,46] and improve insulin sensitivity and reduce abdominal fat in obese children and young adults.[47,48] Resistance training can also be introduced to individuals at risk of T2DM;[44] combined aerobics training and resistance training may produce a greater decrease in total body fat and waist circumference in obese adolescents.[49]

Other features of the intensive lifestyle intervention include: (1) case managers or "lifestyle coaches" to deliver the intervention, (2) frequent contact and ongoing intervention throughout the trial to help participants achieve and maintain the weight and physical activity goals, (3) "toolbox" strategies to tailor the intervention to the individual participant, (4) intervention materials and strategies to address the needs of an ethnically diverse population, and (5) an extensive local and national network that provides training, feedback and clinical support for the interventionists.[43] Reducing caloric intake is also very important for those at high risk of developing T2DM; overall healthy low-calorie eating patterns should be encouraged.[3]

Pharmacologic agents have shown to decrease incident diabetes to various degrees in those with pre-diabetes; these include metformin, α-glucosidase inhibitors, orlistat, glucagon-like peptide 1 receptor agonists, and thiazolidinediones.[3] The ADA recommends that metformin should be considered in pre-diabetic individuals with a BMI ≥ 35 kg/m², aged <60 years, are women with prior gestational diabetes mellitus, and/or those with rising A1C despite lifestyle intervention.[3] Metformin has demonstrated long-term safety as a preventative therapy for diabetes.[50] Furthermore, diabetes self-management education and support programs may be appropriate venues for people with pre-diabetes to receive education and support to develop and maintain behaviours that can prevent or delay the development of diabetes.[3]

Pharmacological Treatment

The pharmacological treatment goal for T2DM is to reduce hyperglycaemia and reach the target blood glucose level.[51] This can be accomplished via addressing different pathophysiologic mechanisms that contribute to the development of T2DM. Current oral antihyperglycaemic agents can reduce blood glucose levels either through the promotion of insulin levels in the body or an increase of insulin sensitivity of target cells (peripheral tissues and liver) or via other glucose metabolism-associated pathways. These therapeutic effects can be achieved through insulin sensitisers (e.g., biguanides), insulin secretagogues (e.g., sulfonylureas and meglitinides) and external insulin delivery (insulin analogues).

Biguanides are insulin sensitisers with predominant action in the liver; they do not increase insulin levels and are therefore not associated with a significant risk of hypoglycaemia.[24] Metformin is the most commonly used biguanide, but the precise mechanism of action of metformin is unknown.[24]

Thiazolidinedione is a class of drugs that are insulin sensitisers with predominant action in peripheral insulin-sensitive tissues. These agents work through binding and modulation of the activity of a family of nuclear transcription factors peroxisome proliferator-activated receptors (PPARs).[24] Thiazolidinediones include pioglitazone and rosiglitazone.

Insulin secretagogues agents bind to the sulfonylurea receptor (SUR1), a subunit of the K_{ATP} potassium channel on the plasma membrane of pancreatic beta cells. The SUR1 subunit regulates the activity of the channel and also binds ATP and ADP, effectively functioning as a glucose sensor and trigger for insulin secretion.[24] Insulin secretagogues include sulfonylureas (glimepiride, glipizide, glyburide) and meglitinides (repaglinide and nateglinide).

α-glucosidase inhibitors work to inhibit the terminal step of carbohydrate digestion at the brush border of the intestinal epithelium. As a result, carbohydrate absorption is shifted more distally in the intestine and is delayed, allowing the sluggish insulin secretory dynamics characteristic of T2DM to catch up with carbohydrate absorption.[24] α-glucosidase inhibitors include acarbose and miglitol.

Dipeptidyl peptidase-4 (DPP-4) inhibitors prevent the inactivation of glucagon-like peptide 1 (GLP-1), which increases levels of active GLP-1. This increases insulin secretion and reduces glucagon secretion, thereby lowering glucose levels.[52]

GLP-1 receptor agonists are exogenous analogues promoting the incretin effect that is normally diminished in patients with T2DM. Short-acting GLP-1 receptor agonists (such as exenatide and lixisenatide) lower postprandial glucose levels and insulin concentrations via retardation of gastric emptying.[53] Long-acting GLP-1 receptor agonists (such as albiglutide, dulaglutide, exenatide long-acting release and liraglutide) lower blood glucose levels through the stimulation of insulin secretion and reduction of glucagon levels.[53]

The kidney plays a role in regulating glucose levels by medicating the reabsorption of glucose back into the plasma following filtration of the blood. Sodium-glucose co-transporters (SGLT2) inhibitors inhibit renal glucose reabsorption.[54]

There are other agents that are associated with improvements in glycaemic control in T2DM, such as bile acid sequestrant colesevelam, which is used primarily for dyslipidaemia, or dopamine-2 receptor agonist bromocriptine, which is historically used for treating Parkinson's disease. Their exact mechanism of action on glycaemic control is unknown.[55]

Metformin is considered the first-line therapy for T2DM. It is effective, safe, inexpensive, and may reduce the risk of cardiovascular events and death.[56] For most patients, metformin will be a monotherapy in combination with lifestyle modifications.[57] In patients with metformin contraindications or intolerance, a "dual therapy" of metformin and an initial drug from another class can be considered.[58] A meta-analysis suggests that most 2-noninsulin agent combinations similarly reduce A1C levels; each new class of agents added to the initial therapy generally lowers A1C approximately by 0.7–1.0%.[59] If the A1C target is not achieved after approximately three months and the patient does not have atherosclerotic cardiovascular disease or chronic kidney disease, consider a combination of metformin and one of the six available treatment options: sulfonylurea, thiazolidinedione, DPP-4 inhibitor, SGLT2 inhibitor, GLP-1 receptor agonist or basal insulin. The selection of the agent depends on drug-specific effects and patient factors.[58] If the A1C target is still not achieved after three months of dual therapy, proceed to a 3-drug combination. Again, if the A1C target is not achieved even after three months of triple therapy, proceed to combination injectable therapy.

Insulin has the advantage of being effective when other agents are not and should be considered as part of any combination regimen when hyperglycaemia is severe, especially when weight loss, hypertriglyceridemia and ketosis are present.[58] When A1C is ≥10% (86 mmol/mol), or blood glucose is ≥300 mg/dL (16.7 mmol/L), or when symptoms of hyperglycaemia are present, insulin injectable therapy should be considered.[58] When the patient's glucose toxicity resolves and A1C levels are closer to target levels, the regimen may be simplified and possibly changing to oral agents.[58]

The choice of hypoglycaemics agent is based on patient preference, as well as patient comorbidity and drug characteristics, with the goal of reducing blood glucose levels while minimising side effects, especially hypoglycaemia. Different classes of oral hypoglycaemics drugs and possible side effects to consider are presented in Table 1.5.[58]

Table 1.5. Glucose-lowering Agents and Drug-specific Factors to Consider when Selecting Antihyperglycaemic Treatment in Adults with Type 2 Diabetes (adapted from the American Diabetes Association, 2019)

Class	Compound(s)	Efficacy	Hypoglycaemia	Additional Consideration
Biguanides	Metformin	High	No	• Gastrointestinal side effects common (diarrhoea, nausea) • Potential for B12 deficiency
Sulfonylureas (2nd generation)	• Glimepiride • Glipizide • Glyburide	High	Yes	• FDA Special Warning on increased risk of cardiovascular mortality based on studies of an older sulfonylurea (tolbutamide)
Thiazolidinediones	• Pioglitazone • Rosiglitazone	High	No	• FDA Black box: Congestive heart failure (pioglitazone, rosiglitazone)

Table 1.5. (*Continued*)

Class	Compound(s)	Efficacy	Hypoglycaemia	Additional Consideration
				• Fluid retention (oedema, heart failure) • Benefit in NASH • Risk of bone fracture • Bladder cancer (pioglitazone) • Increases LDL cholesterol (rosiglitazone)
α-Glucosidase inhibitors	• Acarbose • Miglitol			
Meglitinides (glinides)	• Nateglinide • Repaglinide			
DPP-4 inhibitors	• Alogliptin • Saxagliptin • Linagliptin • Sitagliptin	Intermediate	No	• Potential risk of acute pancreatitis • Joint pain
SGLT2 inhibitors	• Ertugliflozin • Dapagliflozin • Canagliflozin • Empagliflozin	Intermediate	No	• FDA Black Box: Risk of amputation (canagliflozin) • Risk of bone fractures (canagliflozin) • DKA risk (all agents, rare in T2DM) • Genitourinary infections • Risk of volume depletion, hypotension • Increases LDL cholesterol (rosiglitazone) • Risk of Fournier's gangrene

(*Continued*)

Table 1.5. (*Continued*)

Class	Compound(s)	Efficacy	Hypoglycaemia	Additional Consideration
GLP-1 receptor agonists	• Exenatide (extended release) • Exenatide • Dulaglutide • Semaglutide • Liraglutide	High	No	• FDA Black Box: Risk of thyroid C-cell tumours (liraglutide, albiglutide, dulaglutide, exenatide extended release) • Gastrointestinal side effects common (nausea, vomiting, diarrhea) • Injection site reactions • Acute pancreatitis risk
Bile acid sequestrants	• Colesevelam			• Constipation
Dopamine-2 agonists	• Bromocriptine			
Amylin mimetics	• Pramlintide			

Abbreviations: DPP-4 inhibitors, dipeptidyl peptidase-4 inhibitors; FDA, Food and Drug Administration; GLP-1, glucagon-like peptide 1; LDL, low density lipoprotein; NASH, non-alcoholic steatohepatitis; SGLT-2, sodium-glucose cotransporter-2.

Non-pharmacological Treatment

Lifestyle management is a fundamental part of managing T2DM and plays an important role in glycaemic control and cardiovascular risk management.[2] Lifestyle management of diabetes includes diabetes self-management education (DSME), diabetes self-management support (DSMS), nutrition therapy, physical activity, smoking cessation and psychosocial care.[2,60] DSME is the process where diabetic patients are equipped with the knowledge, skill and ability necessary for diabetes self-care.[61] DSMS refers to the support needed for applying coping skills and behaviours required to self-manage diabetes on an ongoing basis.[61] The objectives of DSME are to support informed decision-making, self-care behaviours, problem-solving, and active collaboration with the health care team to improve clinical outcomes, health status and quality of life.[62] Diabetic patients are at the centre of the diabetes education and support process, and need to manage the condition on a daily basis, and the educators' role is to make the work easier.[62]

Nutrition therapy is another important part of lifestyle management for people with diabetes.[60] Individuals with diabetes are advised to adopt an individualised eating plan, as there is no one-size-fits-all food plan or eating pattern that would suit everybody.

Physical activity includes body movements that increase energy expenditure. It has been shown that participating in regular physical activity improves blood glucose control and can prevent or delay T2DM; in addition, physical activity has a positive impact on the measures of lipids, blood pressure, cardiovascular events, mortality and quality of life.[63] Exercise is a structured physical activity that improves physical fitness. Structured exercise intervention has been shown to lower A1C by an average of 0.66% in people with T2DM.[64] If the patient is physically capable, it is recommended that people with T2DM should do at least two weekly sessions of resistance exercise (exercise with free weights or weight machines), with each session consisting of at least one set (group of consecutive repetitive exercise motions) of five or more different resistance exercises involving the large muscle groups.[63] Furthermore, they are advised to aim for a minimum of 210 minutes per week of moderate-intensity exercise or 125 minutes per week of vigorous-intensity exercise.[65] This total amount of exercise should consist of a combination of aerobic and resistance training, and exercise should be done at least three days each week with no more than two consecutive days without training.[65]

Smoking cessation is another part of T2DM management. It has been shown in clinical and experimental studies that there is a significant association between cigarette smoking and the development of impaired glycaemic control and diabetic complications.[66,67] Furthermore, smoking increases cardiovascular risks, which are complications of T2DM. Therefore, smoking cessation is critical to support glycaemic control and prevents the development of diabetic complications.[66]

T2DM patients and their families face many challenges when integrating diabetes management into their daily lives. Therefore, it is important to integrate psychosocial care with patient-centred medical care.[68] Providers should consider an assessment of symptoms of diabetes distress, depression, anxiety, and disordered eating and cognitive capacities using patient-appropriate standardised/validated tools at the initial visit, at periodic intervals, and when there is a change in disease, treatment or life circumstance.[68] Caregivers and family members are also recommended to consider this assessment.[68]

With patient-centred care plans — a combination of hypoglycaemics agents, education and management programs, diet therapy, exercise therapy and looking after one's psychological well-being — it is possible to promote optimal medical outcomes and psychological well-being.

Prognosis

With the combination of patient-centred pharmacological and non-pharmacological management for T2DM, it is possible to reach and maintain target glycaemic levels. However, current T2DM treatment approaches do not prevent or slow the loss of beta cell function.[26] T2DM is a lifelong disease and therefore requires lifelong management and monitoring of patients' blood glucose levels.

Over time, people with diabetes have an increased risk of developing complications; these include the progressive development of specific complications of retinopathy with potential blindness, nephropathy that may lead to renal failure and/or potential foot ulcers, limb amputations, Charcot joints, and features of autonomic dysfunction, including sexual dysfunction.[1,22] If left undiagnosed or poorly managed, T2DM can lead to coronary artery disease, a stroke, kidney failure, limb amputation and blindness.[2]

References

1. World Health Organization. (1999) Definition, diagnosis and classification of diabetes mellitus and its complications: Report of a WHO consultation. Part 1, Diagnosis and classification of diabetes mellitus. Geneva, Switzerland.
2. The Royal Australian College of General Practitioners. (2016) General practice management of Type 2 diabetes. 2016–18. RACGP, East Melbourne, VIC.
3. American Diabetes Association. (2019) 2. Classification and diagnosis of diabetes: Standards of medical care in diabetes — 2019. *Diabetes Care* **42**(Supplement 1): S13.
4. Gakidou E, Mallinger L, Abbott-Klafter J, *et al.* (2011) Management of diabetes and associated cardiovascular risk factors in seven countries: A comparison of data from national health examination surveys. *Bull World Health Organ* **89**(3): 172–183.
5. Beagley J, Guariguata L, Weil C, Motala AA. (2014) Global estimates of undiagnosed diabetes in adults. *Diabetes Res Clin Pract* **103**(2): 150–160.
6. World Health Organization. (2016) Global report on diabetes.
7. International Diabetes Federation. (2017) *IDF Diabetes Atlas.* 8th edition. Available from: https://diabetesatlas.org/en/
8. Centers for Disease Control and Prevention. (2017) National Diabetes Statistics Report, 2017 Estimates of diabetes and its burden in the United States. Available from: https://dev.diabetes.org/sites/default/files/2019-06/cdc-statistics-report-2017.pdf
9. Australian Institute of Health and Welfare. (2017) *Diabetes Compendium.*
10. Organization for Economic Cooperation and Development Europe. (2016) *Health at a Glance: Europe 2016 — State of Health in the EU cycle.* OECD Publishing, Paris.
11. Diabetes UK. (2017) Diabetes prevalence 2017. Available from: https://www.diabetes.org.uk/professionals/position-statements-reports/statistics/diabetes-prevalence-2017
12. GBD 2016 DALYs and HALE Collaborators. (2017) Global, regional, and national disability-adjusted life-years (DALYs) for 333 diseases and injuries and healthy life expectancy (HALE) for 195 countries and

territories, 1990–2016: A systematic analysis for the Global Burden of Disease Study 2016. *Lancet* **390**(10100): 1260–1344.

13. Mokdad AH, Ballestros K, Echko M, *et al.* (2018) The state of US health, 1990–2016: Burden of diseases, injuries, and risk factors among US states. *JAMA* **319**(14): 1444–1472.

14. Australian Institute of Health and Welfare. (2011) Australian Burden of Disease Study: Impact and causes of illness and death in Australia 2011. Australian Burden of Disease Study series no. 3. BOD 4. Australian Institute of Health and Welfare, Canberra, Australia.

15. Mathers CD, Loncar D. (2006) Projections of global mortality and burden of disease from 2002 to 2030. *PLoS Med* **3**(11): e442.

16. GBD 2013 Mortality and Causes of Death Collaborators. (2015) Global, regional, and national age-sex specific all-cause and cause-specific mortality for 240 causes of death, 1990–2013: A systematic analysis for the Global Burden of Disease Study 2013. *Lancet* **385**(9963): 117–171.

17. Roglic G, Unwin N. (2010) Mortality attributable to diabetes: Estimates for the year 2010. *Diabetes Res Clin Pract* **87**(1): 15–19.

18. World Health Organization. (2011) WHO Guidelines approved by the Guidelines Review Committee. Use of glycated haemoglobin (HbA1c) in the diagnosis of diabetes mellitus: Abbreviated report of a WHO consultation. Geneva, Switzerland.

19. Genuth S, Alberti KG, Bennett P, *et al.* (2003) Follow-up report on the diagnosis of diabetes mellitus. *Diabetes Care* **26**(11): 3160–3167.

20. Expert Committee on the Diagnosis and Classification of Diabetes Mellitus. (1997) Report of the Expert Committee on the diagnosis and classification of diabetes mellitus. *Diabetes Care* **20**(7): 1183–1197.

21. American Diabetes Association. (2017) 2. Classification and diagnosis of diabetes. *Diabetes Care* **40**(Supplement 1): S11–S24.

22. American Diabetes Association. (2010) 2. Diagnosis and classification of diabetes mellitus. *Diabetes Care* **33**(Supplement 1): S62–S69.

23. Gardner DG, Shoback D. (2018) *Greenspan's Basic and Clinical Endocrinology.* 10th edition. McGraw-Hill Education.

24. Melmed S, Polonsky KS, Larsen PR, Kronenberg HM. (2011) *Williams Textbook of Endocrinology*, 12th edition. Elsevier Sauders, Philadelphia USA.

25. Handelsman Y, Mechanick J, Blonde L, *et al.* (2011) American Association of Clinical Endocrinologists medical guidelines for clinical practice for developing a diabetes mellitus comprehensive care plan: Executive summary. *Endocr Pract* **17**(2): 287–302.

26. Kahn SE, Cooper ME, Del Prato S. (2014) Pathophysiology and treatment of Type 2 diabetes: Perspectives on the past, present, and future. *Lancet* **383**(9922): 1068–1083.

27. Rosak C. (2002) The pathophysiologic basis of efficacy and clinical experience with the new oral antidiabetic agents. *J Diabetes Complications* **16**(1): 123–132.

28. Stumvoll M, Goldstein BJ, van Haeften TW. (2005) Type 2 diabetes: Principles of pathogenesis and therapy. *Lancet* **365**(9467): 1333–1346.

29. Deeb SS, Fajas L, Nemoto M, *et al.* (1998) A Pro12Ala substitution in PPARgamma2 associated with decreased receptor activity, lower body mass index and improved insulin sensitivity. *Nat Genet* **20**(3): 284–287.

30. Morris AP, Voight BF, Teslovich TM, *et al.* (2012) Large-scale association analysis provides insights into the genetic architecture and pathophysiology of Type 2 diabetes. *Nat Genet* **44**(9): 981–990.

31. Hu FB, van Dam RM, Liu S. (2001) Diet and risk of Type II diabetes: The role of types of fat and carbohydrate. *Diabetologia* **44**(7): 805–817.

32. American Diabetes Association. (2014) Diagnosis and classification of diabetes mellitus. *Diabetes Care* **37**(Supplement 1): S81–S90.

33. Boden G. (1997) Role of fatty acids in the pathogenesis of insulin resistance and NIDDM. *Diabetes* **46**(1): 3–10.

34. Holst JJ. (2007) The physiology of glucagon-like peptide 1. *Physiol Rev* **87**(4): 1409–1439.

35. Fagot-Campagna A, Pettitt DJ, Engelgau MM, *et al.* (2000) Type 2 diabetes among North American children and adolescents: An epidemiologic review and a public health perspective. *J Pediatr* **136**(5): 664–672.

36. Mayer-Davis EJ, Lawrence JM, Dabelea D, *et al.* (2017) Incidence trends of Type 1 and Type 2 diabetes among youths, 2002–2012. *N Engl J Med* **376**(15): 1419–1429.

37. American Diabetes Association. (2000) Type 2 diabetes in children and adolescents. *Pediatrics* **105**(3 Pt 1): 671–680.

38. International Expert Committee. (2009) International Expert Committee Report on the role of the A1C assay in the diagnosis of diabetes. *Diabetes Care* **32**(7): 1327–1334.

39. Edelman D, Olsen MK, Dudley TK, *et al.* (2004) Utility of hemoglobin A1C in predicting diabetes risk. *J Gen Intern Med* **19**(12): 1175–1180.

40. Pradhan AD, Rifai N, Buring JE, Ridker PM. (2007) Hemoglobin A1C predicts diabetes but not cardiovascular disease in nondiabetic women. *Am J Med* **120**(8): 720–727.

41. Sato KK, Hayashi T, Harita N, *et al.* (2009) Combined measurement of fasting plasma glucose and A1C is effective for the prediction of Type 2 diabetes: The Kansai Healthcare Study. *Diabetes Care* **32**(4): 644–646.
42. Shimazaki T, Kadowaki T, Ohyama Y, *et al.* (2007) Hemoglobin A1C (HbA1c) predicts future drug treatment for diabetes mellitus: A follow-up study using routine clinical data in a Japanese university hospital. *Transl Res* **149**(4): 196–204.
43. The Diabetes Prevention Program Research Group. (2002) The Diabetes Prevention Program (DPP): Description of lifestyle intervention. *Diabetes Care* **25**(12): 2165–2171.
44. Lindstrom J, Ilanne-Parikka P, Peltonen M, *et al.* (2006) Sustained reduction in the incidence of Type 2 diabetes by lifestyle intervention: Follow-up of the Finnish Diabetes Prevention Study. *Lancet* **368**(9548): 1673–1679.
45. Diabetes Prevention Program Research Group, Knowler WC, Fowler SE, *et al.* (2009) 10-year follow-up of diabetes incidence and weight loss in the Diabetes Prevention Program Outcomes Study. *Lancet* **374**(9702): 1677–1686.
46. Li G, Zhang P, Wang J, *et al.* (2008) The long-term effect of lifestyle interventions to prevent diabetes in the China Da Qing Diabetes Prevention Study: A 20-year follow-up study. *Lancet* **371**(9626): 1783–1789.
47. Davis CL, Pollock NK, Waller JL, *et al.* (2012) Exercise dose and diabetes risk in overweight and obese children: A randomized controlled trial. *JAMA* **308**(11): 1103–1112.
48. Fedewa MV, Gist NH, Evans EM, Dishman RK. (2014) Exercise and insulin resistance in youth: A meta-analysis. *Pediatrics* **133**(1): e163–e174.
49. Sigal RJ, Alberga AS, Goldfield GS, *et al.* (2014) Effects of aerobic training, resistance training, or both on percentage body fat and cardiometabolic risk markers in obese adolescents: The healthy eating aerobic and resistance training in youth randomized clinical trial. *JAMA Pediatr* **168**(11): 1006–1014.
50. Diabetes Prevention Program Research Group. (2012) Long-term safety, tolerability, and weight loss associated with metformin in the Diabetes Prevention Program Outcomes Study. *Diabetes Care* **33**(4): 731–737.
51. Ahrén B. (2010) Use of DPP-4 inhibitors in Type 2 diabetes: Focus on sitagliptin. *Diabetes Metab Syndr Obes: Targets Ther* **3**: 31–41.

52. Ahrén B. (2007) DPP-4 inhibitors. *Best Pract Res Cl En* **21**(4): 517–533.
53. Meier JJ. (2012) GLP-1 receptor agonists for individualized treatment of Type 2 diabetes mellitus. *Nat Rev* **8**(12): 728–742.
54. Chao EC, Henry RR. (2010) SGLT2 inhibition — a novel strategy for diabetes treatment. *Nature Reviews Drug Discovery* **9**: 551.
55. Irons BK, Minze MG. (2014) Drug treatment of Type 2 diabetes mellitus in patients for whom metformin is contraindicated. *Diabetes Metab Syndr Obes: Targets Ther* **7**: 15–24.
56. Holman RR, Paul SK, Bethel MA, *et al.* (2008) 10-year follow-up of intensive glucose control in Type 2 diabetes. *N Engl J Med* **359**(15): 1577–1589.
57. American Diabetes Association. (2018) 8. Pharmacologic approaches to glycaemic treatment: Standards of medical care in diabetes — 2018. *Diabetes Care* **41**(Supplement 1): S73.
58. American Diabetes Association. (2019) 9. Pharmacologic approaches to glycaemic treatment: Standards of medical care in diabetes — 2019. *Diabetes Care* **42**(Supplement 1): S90.
59. Bennett WL, Maruthur NM, Singh S, *et al.* (2011) Comparative effectiveness and safety of medications for Type 2 diabetes: An update including new drugs and 2-drug combinations. *Ann Intern Med* **154**(9): 602–613.
60. American Diabetes Association. (2019) 5. Lifestyle management: Standards of medical care in diabetes — 2019. *Diabetes Care* **42**(Supplement 1): S46.
61. Powers MA, Bardsley J, Cypress M, *et al.* (2017) Diabetes self-management education and support in Type 2 diabetes. *Diabetes Educ* **43**(1): 40–53.
62. Haas L, Maryniuk M, Beck J, *et al.* (2012) National standards for diabetes self-management education and support. *Diabetes Care* **35**(11): 2393–2401.
63. Colberg SR, Sigal RJ, Fernhall B, *et al.* (2010) Exercise and Type 2 diabetes: The American College of Sports Medicine and the American Diabetes Association: Joint position statement executive summary. *Diabetes Care* **33**(12): 2692–2696.
64. Boule NG, Haddad E, Kenny GP, *et al.* (2001) Effects of exercise on glycaemic control and body mass in Type 2 diabetes mellitus: A meta-analysis of controlled clinical trials. *JAMA* **286**(10): 1218–1227.
65. Hordern MD, Dunstan DW, Prins JB, *et al.* (2012) Exercise prescription for patients with Type 2 diabetes and pre-diabetes: A position statement from Exercise and Sport Science Australia. *J Sci Med Sport* **15**(1): 25–31.

66. Centers for Disease Control and Prevention. (n.d.) About underlying cause of death 1999–2017. CDC WONDER Database. Accessed 1 June 2018. Available from: http://wonder.cdc.gov/ucd-icd10.html

67. Willi C, Bodenmann P, Ghali WA, *et al.* (2007) Active smoking and the risk of Type 2 diabetes: A systematic review and meta-analysis. *JAMA* **298**(22): 2654–2664.

68. Young-Hyman D, de Groot M, Hill-Briggs F, *et al.* (2016) Psychosocial care for people with diabetes: A position statement of the American Diabetes Association. *Diabetes Care* **39**(12): 2126.

2

Type 2 Diabetes Mellitus in Chinese Medicine

OVERVIEW

In Chinese medicine (CM), Type 2 diabetes mellitus (T2DM) disease and treatment records can be found under CM terms such as *xiao ke* 消渴, *xiao dan* 消瘅 and *san xiao* 三消. Contemporary CM literature describes T2DM as a disease of deficiency and excess syndromes. The disease location is in the five *zang* organs, mainly the Spleen (Stomach), Liver and Kidney. Based on CM guidelines and textbooks for T2DM, this chapter introduces the CM names, aetiology, pathogenesis, syndrome differentiation and T2DM treatments. T2DM treatments using Chinese herbal medicine, acupuncture and other Chinese medicine therapies will also be presented. Furthermore, preventive care from a CM perspective will be discussed.

Introduction

In Chinese medicine (CM) classical texts, there is no record of the disease "Type 2 diabetes mellitus" (T2DM). However, common symptoms of T2DM such as polydipsia, polyphagia, polyuria and weight loss were often described by CM practitioners in the past, seen throughout various stages of the CM medical history. Records of T2DM symptoms can be found in well-known CM medical books, such as the *Huang Di Nei Jing* 黄帝内经, *Shang Han Za Bing Lun* 伤寒杂病论, *Xiao Pin Fang* 小平方, *Zhu Bing Yuan Hou Lun* 诸病源侯论,

Qian Jin Fang 千金方, *Dan Xi Xin Fa* 丹溪心法, *Jing Yue Quan Shu* 景岳全书, *Ming Yi Lei An* 名医类案 and contemporary CM textbooks.

CM scholars today, through medical analysis, comparison of herb use and statistical analysis, have explored the similarities and differences of ancient T2DM terms. They concluded that although T2DM disease in CM can be named through different methods, they all still essentially describe T2DM. If the name is according to the location of the disease plus its main symptom, their names can be *pi dan* 脾瘅, *shang xiao* 上消, *zhong xiao* 中消, *xiao zhong* 消中, *xia xiao* 下消, *ge xiao* 膈消, *fei xiao* 肺消 and *xiao shen* 消肾. If the name is according to the nature of the disease plus its main symptom, their names can be *wei re ke* 胃热渴, *re ke* 热渴, *xu ke* 虚渴 and *feng xiao* 风消. The name can also be based on the presenting symptoms and course of the disease, such as chronic excessive thirst, *jiu ke* 久渴. Finally, the disease name can be in the form of the main symptoms, such as *xiao ke* 消渴, *xiao dan* 消瘅, *xiao ke fan zao* 消渴烦躁, *fan ke* 烦渴, *xiao ke kou she gan zao* 消渴口舌干燥, *ke li* 渴利 and *xiao shen* 消肾.

In the period of the *Huang Di Nei Jing* 黄帝内经 (BCE 618), T2DM symptoms were called *xiao dan* 消瘅, but after the Jin (c. 1115–1271 CE) and Yuan (c. 1272–1368 CE) dynasties, it was changed to the unified name of *xiao ke* 消渴.

Different CM disease names can also represent different T2DM symptoms. For example, *ge xiao* 膈消, *ge xiao* 鬲消, *shang xiao* 上消 and *xiao* 痟 generally refer to polydipsia; *xiao li* 消利, *ke li* 渴利, *nei xiao* 内消, *xia xiao* 下消, *xiao shen* 消肾 and *shen xiao* 肾消 refer to polyuria and turbid urine; *feng xiao* 风消 and *shen xiao* 肾消 represent weight loss; and *xiao ke* 消渴, *xiao dan* 消瘅 and *san xiao* 三消 generally refer to polydipsia, polyuria, polyphagia and weight loss symptoms. These names often appear in the description of a disease, involving the occurrence, development and transformation of the disease.

Currently, *xiao ke* 消渴 is the most recognised CM name for T2DM. Professor Renhe Lv, a Chinese medicine master, believes that T2DM belongs to the category of "*xiao ke bing* 消渴病", in which *xiao ke* 消渴 corresponds to modern diabetes.[1] However, *xiao ke* 消渴 can be divided broadly or on a more specific level. *Xiao ke* 消渴 can broadly refer to a class of diseases characterised by "thirst, polydipsia, polyuria and polyphagia", which is comparable to diabetes mellitus, diabetes insipidus, psychogenic polydipsia, hyperthyroidism and other diseases in modern medicine. More specifically, *xiao ke* 消渴 refers to the disease characterised by "polydipsia, polydipsia, polyuria, emaciation and sweet urine". The broad sense of *xiao ke* 消渴 is that it is not the same as diabetes, and the narrow sense of *xiao ke* 消渴 summarises some cases of diabetes. Thus, although there is a cross-relationship between *xiao ke* 消渴 and T2DM, these are two different concepts.

Therefore, when identifying "*xiao ke* 消渴", "*xiao dan* 消瘅", "*san xiao* 三消" and other CM disease names, it is necessary to make a specific analysis and judgement based on the modern definition of T2DM, the differential diagnosis of T2DM, and the background of ancient texts of CM in order to get an accurate understanding of T2DM.

Aetiology and Pathogenesis

As early as in the *Huang Di Nei Jing* 黄帝内经 (BCE 618), it has been proposed that constitutional deficiency, the five *zang* 五脏 organ deficiency, emotional upsets, overeating of sweet and fatty foods, and obesity are closely related to the development of diabetes. Thereafter, generations of CM practitioners have continued to develop and enrich the theory of aetiology and pathogenesis of diabetes.

Aetiology

In the Chinese medicine theory, the aetiology of T2DM involves deficiencies of *yin* and the five *zang* 五脏 organs, an unhealthy diet, obesity, emotional imbalance or the invasion of external pathogenic factors, which will be discussed here.[2-5] *Yin* deficiency and weak five *zang* 五脏 organs may be due to congenital deficiency, weak five *zang* organs 五脏, or are a result of deficient *yin* and body fluid. Among them, ancient CM practitioners emphasised the importance of the deficiency of the Kidney and Spleen at the onset of diabetes.

Unhealthy diets and obesity are recognised as an aetiology of T2DM in CM. Long-term consumption of fatty and sweet foods and obesity damage the Spleen and Stomach, which fails to transport and transform, resulting in internal heat accumulation that injures the body fluids and *yin,* leading to diabetes. Long-term alcohol consumption also injures the Spleen and Stomach, creating internal heat that turns into fire that will damage the *jin* 津. Excessive sexual activities deplete the Kidney essence, resulting in deficient fire, damaging the *yin* and *jin* 津 fluids. This can also cause diabetes.

Long-term emotional upsets resulting in sadness or anger cause Liver *qi* stagnation, which over time transforms into Liver fire, that can travel upwards to consume Stomach *yin* and *jin* 津 or downwards and consume Kidney *jin* 津. Worrying and overthinking will cause Heart *qi* stagnation, which will turn into hyperactive Heart fire, consuming the Heart and Spleen *jin* 津 and damaging the Stomach and Kidney *yin* fluids. These can all lead to diabetes.

In ancient China, after the Sui (c. 581–618 CE) and Tang (c. 618–907 CE) dynasties, people often took medicine made of mineral drugs for enhancing sexual performance or prolonging longevity. However, these medicines also created endogenous dryness and heat and depleted *yin* and body fluids, leading to diabetes.

Invasion of external pathogenic factors such as dryness, wind and heat evils can invade the *zang* and *fu* organs; the heat can injure the body fluids, which can also cause diabetes.

Pathogenesis

The pathogenesis of diabetes will be discussed based on different stages of the disease.[2–6] During the early stages of diabetes, deficiency of *yin* and *jin* 津 fluids is the underlying cause of excess dryness and heat; however, the heat will further deplete *yin* and *jin* 津 fluids, creating a vicious cycle. Although all five *zang* organs are affected in diabetes, the main viscera affected are the Lung, Spleen (Stomach) and Kidney. Furthermore, these three *zang* organs are closely related and affect each other's functions. For instance, when dryness in the Lungs is present, *jin* 津 fluids fail to be dispersed, therefore the Spleen cannot be nourished, and Kidney essence is not supported. If there is heat in the Stomach and Spleen, the heat can travel upwards to consume the Lung fluids and downwards to consume Kidney *yin*. When Kidney essence is deficient, leading to *yin* deficiency heat, it can travel upwards to damage the Lung and Stomach. In the end, Lung dryness, Stomach heat, Spleen deficiency and Kidney deficiency will coexist. The symptoms of polydipsia, polyphagia and polyuria can often be seen at the same time.

During the middle stage of diabetes, the disease will have been present for a while — both *qi* and *yin* are damaged — and there is stagnation in the meridians and collaterals. If diabetes is not treated timely with appropriate treatments in the early stage, the disease duration will be prolonged, dryness heat will consume the *yin* and lead to both *qi* and *yin* deficiency. At the same time, an imbalance of the *zang fu* organs will occur, failing to distribute and disperse body fluids. This will block *qi* and Blood movements, leading to phlegm dampness and Blood stagnation, causing stagnation in the collaterals, in turn leading to malnourishment of the *zang fu* organs, resulting in diabetes complications.

During the late stage of the disease, both *yin* and *yang* are impaired and deficient. The *yin* and *yang* of the body are mutually important to one another and are interdependent. *Xiao ke* 消渴 is fundamentally a disease of *yin* deficiency. However, when the disease duration is prolonged, a deficiency in *yin* will affect the *yang*, or due to improper treatment, excessive use of bitter cold herb products will damage the *yang* and eventually lead to both *yin* and *yang* deficiency. When Spleen *yang* is deficient, Kidney *yang* can also be damaged; damp retention caused by Spleen *yang* will lead to turbidity stagnation, obstructing the Triple Energiser, resulting in symptoms such as systemic oedema, cold limbs, dementia, vomiting, nausea, a pale complexion and oliguria. When the Heart and Kidney *yang* fails to transform the *yin*, dampness and turbidity will travel upwards and damage the Lung and the Heart, leading to chest tightness, palpitations, oedema, asthma, being unable to lie on one's back, and even the sudden emergence of critical conditions such as breathlessness, sweating, limb convulsions and a faint pulse. If the Liver and Kidney *yin* is exhausted, the *qi* of the five *zang* will be weak, the *yang* will escape and there will be *yin–yang* separation presenting in symptoms such as sudden fainting spells, delirium, eyes closed but with the mouth open, faint breathing, cold hands and feet, and incontinence.

In addition, some *xiao ke* 消渴 patients have a sudden onset and serious downturn of the condition. This quickly leads to extreme loss of *yin* and body fluid. The *yin* cannot restrain the *yang*, leading to the latter escaping to the body surface, which presents with irritability, a red face, headaches and vomiting, dry skin, sunken eyes, dry lips and tongue, deep breathing, and breath smelling of rotten apples. If not rescued in time, the *yin* and *yang* will be exhausted, resulting in coma and death.

Syndrome Differentiation and Treatments

The treatment of T2DM should focus on both the root cause (*Ben* 本) and manifestation syndromes (*Biao* 表). The root cause (*Ben* 本) is *qi* and *yin* deficiency and its manifestation (*Biao* 表) syndromes are dryness and heat, Blood stasis, phlegm turbidity, Liver *qi* stagnation, damp-heat retention, and phlegm and dampness retention. Deficiencies in diabetes can be related to different viscera and can be presented concurrently, therefore clinical manifestations are complex and diverse.

Several references can be used that describe CM syndrome differentiation for T2DM. *Internal Medicine of Chinese Medicine*, a national higher education textbook of Chinese Medicine,[3] provides comprehensive information on the syndrome differentiation of T2DM. Guidelines developed by the China Association of Chinese Medicine and the Chinese Diabetes Society have a focus on the prevention and treatment of diabetes in traditional Chinese Medicine.[4,7] The State Administration of Traditional Chinese Medicine developed the *Criteria for the Diagnosis and Curative Effect of CM Syndromes* 中医病证诊断疗效标准,[2] with a focus on standards of syndrome differentiation and recommended treatments. *Clinical Diagnosis and Treatment for Endocrinology and Rheumatism in Chinse Medicine* 专科专病中医临床诊治丛书 — 内分泌科专病与风湿病中医临床诊治 was developed on expert consensus.[6] These guidelines are the main reference for CM practitioners in China, in terms of syndrome differentiation and treatment for T2DM.

Oral Chinese Medicine Herbal Medicine Treatment Based on Syndrome Differentiation

Dryness-Heat Damaging the *jin* 热盛伤津

Clinical manifestations: The main symptoms are thirst and dry stools; other presenting symptoms include dry mouth, increased appetite, irritability, hot or yellowish-red urine, hot hands and feet, a red tongue, yellow and dry tongue coating, and a large and rapid pulse.

Treatment principle: Clear heat and dryness, nourish *yin* and generate body fluids.

Formula: Modified *Bai hu jia ren shen tang* 白虎加人参汤加减 or Modified *Xiao ke fang* 消渴方加减.[3–5]

Herbs: *Tian hua fen* 天花粉, *shi gao* 石膏, *huang lian* 黄连, *sheng di huang* 生地黄, *tai zi shen* 太子参, *ge gen* 葛根, *mai men dong* 麦门冬, *ou zhi* 藕汁 and *gan cao* 甘草.

Main actions of herbs: *Shi gao* clears internal heat; *sheng di huang, mai men dong, tian hua fen* and *tai zi shen* nourish the *yin* and generate fluids; *huang lian* clears heat and dries dampness; *ge gen* and *ou zhi* generates fluids and stops thirst, *gao cao* harmonises all herbs.

Modifications: If the dryness heat is severe and the patient is presenting with difficulty in passing stools or constipation in severe cases, mix *mang xiao* 芒硝 with water and drink the solution, and add *fan xie ye* 番泻叶 to assist *da huang* 大黄 and *zhi shi* 枳实 to clear heat and dryness; if the dryness heat causes upward rebellious *qi*, presenting with a cough or hoarse voice, add *zhi zi* 栀子 and *ju hua* 菊花 to clear the heat and disperse Lung *qi*; during the mid- to late stages of diabetes mellitus, the patient presents with intermittent dry stools, or alternate with diarrhoea and constipation, along with irritability and a dry mouth, then focus on nourishing the *yin* and generate fluids, and tonify *qi* and move the Blood, using *huang qi* 黄芪, *xuan shen* 玄参,

mai men dong 麦门冬, *shu di huang* 熟地黄, *chuan xiong* 川芎, *tao ren* 桃仁 and *dang gui* 当归.

Spleen *Qi* Deficiency and Damp Retention 脾虚湿滞

Clinical manifestations: The main symptoms are abdominal fullness and a thick tongue coating. Other symptoms include nausea, vomiting, fatigue, loss of appetite, dizziness, a pale and enlarged tongue body, thick tongue coating at the middle and edge of the tongue (like tofu residues), and a weak and sluggish pulse.

Treatment principle: Strengthen the Spleen and tonify the *qi*, and transform and transport dampness.

Formula: Modified *Huo pu xia ling tang* 藿朴夏苓汤加减.[6]

Herbs: *Huo xiang* 藿香, *hou pu* 厚朴, *fa ban xia* 法半夏, *yi yi ren* 薏苡仁, *cang zhu* 苍术, *fu ling* 茯苓, *chai hu* 柴胡, *xiang fu* 香附 and *gan cao* 甘草.

Main actions of herbs: *Huo xiang*, *cang zhu* and *fu ling* tonify the Spleen and remove dampness; *hou pu* and *fa ban xia* invigorate *qi* and transform dampness; *yi yi ren* tonifies the Spleen by removing damp-heat; *chai hu* and *xiang fu* drains the heat and regulates *qi*; and *gao cao* harmonises all herbs.

Modifications: To tonify severe Spleen *qi* deficiency, add *dang shen* 党参 and *bai zhu* 白术; if there is a lack of appetite and abdominal fullness, add *shan zha* 山楂, *mai ya* 麦芽 and *shen qu* 神曲 to tonify the Spleen and increase one's appetite; if damp retention is severe and the tongue coating is thick and greasy, add *cao dou kou* 草豆蔻, *bai dou kou* 白豆蔻, *cao guo* 草果 and *sha ren* 砂仁 to reinforce the function of eliminating dampness and removing stagnation.

Liver *Qi* Stagnation 肝郁气滞

Clinical manifestations: Main symptoms are chest fullness, chest tightness, and sighing. Other symptoms are hypochondriac pain, a bitter taste in the mouth, a dry mouth and throat, impatient, being irritable, pink tongue with thin white coating, and a wiry pulse. Women may present with breast distension, breast pain and irregular menstruation.

Treatment principle: Sooth the Liver, regulate *qi*, and harmonise the Liver and Spleen.

Formula: Modified *Si ni san* 四逆散加减.[6]

Herbs: *Chai hu* 柴胡, *zhi ke* 枳壳, *bai shao* 白芍, *zhi shi* 枳实, *chi shao* 赤芍, *chuan xiong* 川芎, *fu ling* 茯苓, *bai zhu* 白术 and *gan cao* 甘草.

Main actions of herbs: *Chai hu* raises *yang qi*, regulates the Liver and removes stagnation; *zhi shi* and *zhi qiao* guide *qi* downwards and break stagnation, and work in partnership with *chai hu* to regulate *qi*; *bai shao* restrains *yin*, nourishes the Blood and softens Liver *qi* stagnation, and prevents potential damage to the *yin* by using *chai hu*; *chi shao* and *chuan xiong* act on the Liver meridian, invigorate *qi*, remove stagnation and invigorate the Blood; *fu ling* and *bai zhu* strengthen the Spleen and tonify *qi*, to support the transformation and transportation process to produce *qi* and Blood; *gao cao* harmonises all herbs.

Modifications: If Liver stagnation has turned to hyperactive Liver fire, with symptoms such as red, painful swollen eyes and irritability, add *mu dan pi* 牡丹皮 and *zhi zi* 栀子 to reduce the Liver fire; for constipation, add *da huang* 大黄 to drain the heat; for dizziness, headache and insomnia, add *tian ma* 天麻, *gou teng* 钩藤 and *ci ji li* 刺蒺藜 to calm the Liver and pacify the *yang*.

Retention of Dampness 水湿停聚

Clinical manifestations: Oedema is the main symptom. Other symptoms are difficulty urinating, heaviness in the head and body, the sensation of having a towel wrapped around one's head, lack of appetite, pale and enlarged tongue with white thick coating, and a wiry and slippery pulse.

Treatment principle: Transform dampness, invigorate the Spleen and reduce turbidity.

Formula: Modified *Wu ling san* 五苓散加减.[6]

Herbs: *Fu ling* 茯苓, *zhu ling* 猪苓, *ze xie* 泽泻, *bai zhu* 白术, *gui zhi* 桂枝, *bai mao gen* 白茅根, *che qian cao* 车前草, *yu mi xu* 玉米须 and *yi mu cao* 益母草.

Main actions of herbs: *Ze xie* promotes diuresis and removes dampness; *zhu ling* and *fu ling* assist *ze xie* to remove dampness; *bai zhu* tonifies the Spleen to transform dampness; *gui zhi* invigorates Bladder *qi* to transform and assists in removing dampness; *bai mao gen* and *che qian zi* clear heat and promote urination; *yu mi xu* reduces swelling and promotes urination; and *yi mu cao* invigorates Blood, promotes urination and clears heat.

Modifications: If water retention is caused by Spleen *qi* deficiency, add *huang qi* 黄芪 to tonify *qi*; for oedema with purple lips or ecchymosis and a hesitant pulse, add *huai niu xi* 怀牛膝 and *ze lan* 泽兰 to move the Blood, remove stagnation and reduce swelling; for oedema with low back pain, weak and sore knees and back, add *xu duan* 续断, *nv zhen zi* 女贞子 and *han lian cao* 旱莲草 to tonify the Liver and Kidney; for oedema with a cough and shortness of breath, add *qian hu* 前胡 and *xing ren* 杏仁 to stop coughing.

Deficiency of *Qi* and Blood 气血亏虚

Clinical manifestations: The main symptoms are mental exhaustion and sleepiness, pale lips, tongue, nails and eyelids. Other symptoms: the patient prefers to sit down and not move around, speaks with a low voice, and suffers from a lack of concentration, insomnia, a pale tongue, and a fine, weak (*Xi Ruo*) pulse.

Treatment principle: Supplementing *qi* and nourishing the Blood.

Formula: Modified *Dang gui bu xue tang* 当归补血汤加减.[6]

Herbs: *Huang qi* 黄芪, *dang gui* 当归, *dang shen* 党参, *shan yao* 山药, *bai zhu* 白术, *dan shen* 丹参, *e jiao* 阿胶, *wu wei zi* 五味子, *long yan rou* 龙眼肉 and *zhi gan cao* 炙甘草.

Main action of herbs: *Huang qi* tonifies Lung *qi* and Spleen *qi*; *dang gui* nourishes the Blood and harmonises *ying* 营; *dang shen* tonifies the Spleen and Stomach, moistens the Lungs, generates fluids and transports *Zhong* (中) *qi*; *shan yao* tonifies the Spleen and Lung, consolidates the Kidneys and Essence (精); *bai zhu* tonifies the Spleen and benefits *qi*; *dan shen* invigorates the Blood and removes stasis; *e jiao* nourishes the *yin* and Blood; *wu wei zi* astringes and consolidates, tonifies *qi*, generates fluids and tonifies the Kidneys and Heart; *long yan rou* tonifies the Heart and Spleen, nourishes the Blood and calms the Shen (神); *zhi gan cao* nourishes the *yin* and Blood, benefits *qi* and moves the *yang*.

Modifications: If the patient presents with indigestion and no appetite, add *shan zha* 山楂 and *shen qu* 神曲 to tonify the Spleen and aid digestion, and support *qi* and Blood production; for hypochondriac distension and pain, add *mu xiang* 木香 6 g, *qin pi* 青皮 10 g and *chen pi* 陈皮 10 g to free flow *qi*; the Kidney governs the bone and produces bone marrow, which produces essence that translates to *qi* and Blood, therefore herbs such as *gou qi zi* 枸杞子 10 g, *zhi shou wu* 制首乌 15 g and *tu si zi* 菟丝子 10 g can tonify the essence and the Kidneys, in turn tonifying *qi* and the Blood.

Blood Stasis 瘀血阻滞

Clinical manifestations: Main symptoms are dark lips and tongue body and local vein cyanosis. Other presenting symptoms include localised sharp pain, dribbling urine, blood in urine, localised pain that is worse at night, a dark tongue with bruises or ecchymosis, and a choppy (*Se*) or knotted and intermittent (*Jie Dai*) pulse.

Treatment principle: Promote Blood circulation and remove Blood stasis.

Formula: Modified *Tao hong si wu tang* or *Bu yang huan wu tang* 桃红四物汤或补阳还五汤加减.[4,6]

Herbs: *Tao ren* 桃仁, *hong hua* 红花, *xue jie* 血竭, *shui zhi* 水蛭, *chuan xiong* 川芎, *bai shao* 白芍, *gan cao* 甘草, *gui jian yu* 鬼箭羽, *dan shen* 丹参, *huang qi* 黄芪, *di long* 地龙 and *chi shao* 赤芍.

Main actions of herbs: *Huang qi* tonifies Lung *qi* and Spleen *qi* and invigorates *qi* and Blood flow to remove stagnation and free flow the collaterals; *tao ren, hong hua, chuang xiong, chi shao, xue jie* and *dan shen* invigorate the Blood and remove stasis; *shui zhi* and *gui jian yu* break up Blood stasis and remove obstruction in the meridians; *bai shao* tonifies the Blood and harmonises the Liver; *di long* activates the meridians and collaterals to remove stasis; *gan cao* harmonises all herbs.

Modifications: Depending on the location of the Blood stasis, different herbs should be used. If the stasis is in the brain add *huai niu xi* 怀牛膝 15 g to guide the Blood downwards, and add *yu jin* 郁金 10 g and *shi chang pu* 石菖蒲 15 g to open the orifice; for stasis in the Heart, add *xie bai* 薤白 10 g, *quan gua lou* 全瓜蒌 15 g to open the chest and free flow the *yang*; for stasis in the shoulders and back, add *jiang huang* 姜黄 10 g and *gui zhi* 桂枝 6 g; for stasis in the lower limbs, add *huai niu xi* 怀牛膝 15 g and *hai er cha* 孩儿茶 10 g.

Deficiency of Kidney *Yang* 肾阳亏虚

Clinical manifestations: Aversion to the cold, cold limbs and knees, diarrhoea, clear and prolonged urination, frequent nocturnal urine, impotence, sexual dysfunction, a pale tongue with thin white coating, and a fine and thin (*Xi Wei*) pulse.

Treatment principle: Tonify the Kidney and strengthen the *yang*.

Formula: Modified *Jin kui shen qi wan* 金匮肾气丸加减.[3,6]

Herbs: *Gou qi zi* 枸杞子, *sang shen* 桑椹, *rou gui* 肉桂, *shan yao* 山药, *shan zhu yu* 山茱萸, *mu dan pi* 牡丹皮, *ze xie* 泽泻, *tu si zi* 菟丝子, *yin yang huo* 淫羊藿, *zi he che* 紫河车 and *lu jiao jiao* 鹿角胶.

Main action of herbs: *Yin yang huo, rou gui, zi he che* and *lu jiao jiao* warm and tonify Kidney *yang*, enhance *jing* 精 and *marrow* 髓; *gou qi zi, sang shen* and *tu si zi* nourish the Yin, Kidney, Liver and Spleen; *shan yao* and *shan zhu yu* nourish and tonify the Liver and Spleen, and tonify Kidney *yin*; *mu dan pi* and *ze xie* promote diuresis and remove dampness, clearing the Liver and draining fire.

Modifications: For frequent nocturnal urination, clear and prolonged urination, add *fu peng zi* 覆盆子 20 g. If there are no results then add *lu rong fen* 鹿茸粉 0.5 g. *Gan jiang* 干姜 and *xi xin* 细辛 can also be used, but only in small amounts. For male sexual dysfunction, use more *tu si zi* 菟丝子, *yin yang huo* 淫羊藿 and *xiong can er* 雄蚕蛾.

Deficiency of Kidney *Yin* 肾阴亏虚

Clinical manifestations: Irritability, insomnia and dreams, sore, weak knees and lower back, and a fine pulse; other symptoms include heat in the palm and soles, hot flushes and a red face, a light red tongue with little coating, and a fine and rapid (*Xi Shu*) pulse.

Treatment principle: Nourish the Kidney and nourish *yin*.

Formula: Modified *Zuo gui wan* or *Liu wei di huang wan* 左归丸或六味地黄加减.[3,4,6]

Herbs: *Sang shen* 桑椹, *gou qi zi* 枸杞子, *huang jing* 黄精, *zhi shou wu* 制首乌, *nv zhen zi* 女贞子, *han lian cao* 旱莲草, *sang ji sheng* 桑寄生, *xuan shen* 玄参, *huai niu xi* 怀牛膝, *tu si zi* 菟丝子, *sheng di huang* 生地黄, *shan zhu yu* 山茱萸 and *gan cao* 甘草.

Main actions of herbs: *Sheng di huang* nourishes the *yin* and generates body fluids; *sang shen*, *gou qi zi* and *tu si zi* nourish the *yin*, tonify the Kidney, Liver and Spleen; *huang jing* tonifies *qi*, nourishes the *yin* and tonifies the Spleen and Kidney; *shan zhu yu*, *nv zhen zi* and *han lian cao* tonify the Liver and Kidney, and tonify Kidney *yin*; *zhi shou wu* nourishes Liver Blood and benefits Kidney *jing* (精); *sang ji sheng* and *huai niu xi* tonify the Liver and Kidney, and strengthen bones and tendons; *xuan shen* nourishes the *yin* and cools the Blood; *gan cao* harmonises all herbs.

Modifications: For deficient heat add *zhi mu* 知母 10 g, *huang bai* 黄柏 10 g, *gui jia* 12 g and *mu dan pi* 10 g to tonify the *yin* and clear the heat; for *yin* and *yang* deficiency, use modified *Zuo gui wan* plus *Jin gui shen qi wan* to tonify Kidney *yang*; for sore, weak knees and lower back, add *du zhong* 12 g, *xu duan* 10 g, *mu gua* 15 g and *du huo* (10 g) to tonify the Kidney and strengthen the knees and lower back.

Damp-Heat in the Liver and Gallbladder 肝胆湿热

Clinical manifestations: Fullness in the chest, abdominal distension, distension after meals, hypochondriac distension and pain, nausea and bitter taste in the mouth. Also seen are heaviness in the limbs and sore muscles, or yellowish colour in the sclera, nails and skin, yellow urine, a red tongue with thick and greasy coating, and a slippery and rapid (*Hua Shu*) pulse.

Treatment principle: Clear damp and heat in the Liver and Gallbladder.

Formula: Modified *Yin chen hao tang* or *Da chai hu tang* 茵陈蒿汤或大柴胡汤加减.[6,7]

Herbs: *Da huang* 大黄 (add later), *yin chen hao* 茵陈蒿, *shan zhi zi* 山栀子, *huang qin* 黄芩, *huang lian* 黄连, *cang zhu* 苍术, *chai hu* 柴胡, *zhi shi* 枳实, *bai shao* 白芍 and *gan cao* 甘草.

Main action of herbs: *Yin chen hao* removes dampness; *shan zhi zi* clears the *San Jiao* 三焦 and guides damp-heat downwards; *da huang* and *zhi shi* drain heat and remove stasis; *chai hu* releases the exterior and clears heat; *huang qin* and *huang lian* clear heat and resolve dampness, drain fire and remove toxins; *bai shao* nourishes the Blood, harmonises the Liver, and calms Liver *yang*; *gan cao* harmonises all herbs.

Modifications: For fatigue and a lack of appetite, add *fu ling* 茯苓 15 g, *bai zhu* 白术 10 g, *dang shen* 党参 15 g and *chen pi* 陈皮 10 g to tonify *qi* and the Spleen; for distension after meals, add *mu xiang* 木香 6 g and *xiang fu* 香附 10 g to regulate *qi* and aid digestion; for severe hypochondriac pain, add *chuan xiong* 川芎 12 g, *yu jin* 郁金 10 g and *zhi ke* 枳壳 10 g to regulate the Liver, remove stagnation and stop pain.

Damp-Heat in the Lower-*jiao* 湿热下注

Clinical manifestations: Abdominal distension, distension after meal intake, frequent, urgent and painful urination, or diarrhoea, a burning feeling in the anus and bowel passing that is not smooth. Also seen: heaviness in the limbs, muscle soreness, a red tongue body with thick and greasy coating towards the back, and a slippery and rapid (*Hua Shu*) pulse.

Treatment principle: Clear damp-heat from the lower-*jiao* 下焦.

Formula: Modified *Si miao san* or *Ge gen qin lian tang* 四妙散或葛根芩连汤加减.[6,7]

Herbs: *Huang bai* 黄柏, *cang zhu* 苍术, *che qian cao* 车前草, *yi yi ren* 薏苡仁, *huang qin* 黄芩, *huang lian* 黄连, *huai niu xi* 怀牛膝 and *ge gen* 葛根.

Main actions of herbs: *Huang bai* and *cang zhu* clear heat and remove dampness; *ge gen* clears heats and raises clear *yang qi* (阳气); *huang lian* and *huang qin* clear heat in the Stomach and intestines; *che qian cao* and *yi yi ren* promote urination and clear heat; *huai niu xi* guides all herbs to the lower-*jiao* (焦).

Modifications: If the Kidney and Bladder are affected, add *shi wei* shiwei 20 g, *lian qiao* 15 g, *tu fu ling* 15 g and *sheng gan cao* 3 g to clear damp heat; if the Large Intestine is affected, add *mu xiang* 6 g (later) and *jiao bing lang* 10 g to regulate the Large Intestine; for itchiness in the genitalia, add *ku shen* 10 g, *chuan bie xie* 12 g and *lian qiao* 15 g to clear heat and stop the itching; for leg cramps caused by damp heat, add *mu guan* 15 g, *du huo* 10 g and *da qing ye* 15 g to clear damp *bi* 痹.

The above syndromes can be seen independently or simultaneously. Therefore, they need to be handled with flexibility according to the specific conditions and with reference to the above syndromes. In advanced diabetic patients, the condition is complex and cannot be simply classified as a certain syndrome type or a certain type of treatment. A summary of the syndromes and formulae is presented in Table 2.1.

Table 2.1. Summary of Chinese Herbal Medicines for Diabetes Mellitus

Syndrome Differentiation	Treatment Principle	Formula
Dryness-heat 燥热内盛	Clear heat and dryness, nourish *yin* and generate body fluids.	Modified *Zeng ye cheng qi tang* 增液承气汤加减.[3–5]
Spleen *qi* deficiency and damp retention 脾虚湿滞	Strengthen the Spleen and tonify *qi*, and transform and transport dampness.	Modified *Huo pu xia ling tang* 藿朴夏苓汤加减.[6]
Liver *qi* stagnation 肝郁气滞	Sooth the Liver, regulate *qi*, and harmonise the Liver and Spleen.	Modified *Si ni san* 四逆散加减.[6]
Retention of dampness 水湿停聚	Transform dampness, invigorate the Spleen and reduce turbidity.	Modified *Wu ling san* 五苓散加减.[6]
Deficiency of *qi* and Blood 气血亏虚	Supplement *qi* and nourish the Blood.	Modified *Dang gui bu xue tang* 当归补血汤加减.[6]
Blood stasis 瘀血阻滞	Promote Blood circulation and remove Blood stasis.	Modified *Tao hong si wu tang* or *Bu yang huan wu tang* 桃红四物汤或补阳还五汤加减.[4,6]
Deficiency of Kidney *yang* 肾阳亏虚	Tonify the Kidney and strengthen the *yang*	Modified *Jin kui shen qi wan* 金匮肾气丸加减[3,6]
Deficiency of Kidney *yin* 肾阴亏虚	Nourish Kidney and nourish *yin*.	Modified *Zuo gui wan* or *Liu wei di huang wan* 左归丸或六味地黄加减.[3,4,6]
Damp-heat in the Liver and Gallbladder 肝胆湿热	Clear damp and heat in the Liver and Gallbladder.	Modified *Yin chen hao tang* or *Da chai hu tang* 茵陈蒿汤或大柴胡汤加减.[6,7]
Damp-heat in the lower-*jiao* 湿热下注	Clear damp-heat from the lower-*jiao*.	Modified *Si miao san* or *Ge gen qin lian tang* 四妙散或葛根芩连汤加减.[6,7]

Other Herbal Formula

The following formula or diet therapy recipes are based on a collection of clinical expertise.[6]

- This formula is suitable for T2DM with a deficiency of both *qi* and *yin*. Herbal ingredients are: *Huang qi* 黄芪, *dang shen* 党参, *mai men dong* 麦门冬, *fu ling* 茯苓, *sang piao qiao* 桑螵蛸, *yuan zhi* 远志, *wu wei zi* 五味子, *xuan shen* 玄参, *lv dou yi* 绿豆衣, *tian hua fen* 天花粉, *sheng di huang* 生地黄, *shan zhu yu* 山茱萸, *he shou wu* 何首乌, *shan yao* 山药 and *wu mei* 乌梅.

- This formula clears heat and nourishes the *yin* and body fluids to stop thirst. *Zhu du wan fang* 猪肚丸方 includes *zhu du* 猪肚, *huang lian* 黄连, *xiao mai* 小麦, *tian hua fen* 天花粉 and *fu ling* 茯苓. Medicines are ground into fine powder, sewed into the pork stomach, cooked and then made into pills. Take 70 pills at a time together with rice soup.

- Black beans and wheat bran, 500 g each. Grind into powder, roll into a round dough and then steam. Consume three times a day.

- Boil Mung beans (120 g) with water until they are cooked. Then, drink the soup and eat the beans.

- *Sheng di huang* 生地黄, *shu di huang* 熟地黄, *tu si zi* 菟丝子, *huang lian* 黄连, *tian men dong* 天门冬, *mai men dong* 麦门冬, *xian shen* 玄参, *da fu pi* 大腹皮, *fu ling* 茯苓, *zhi mu* 知母, *wu wei zi* 五味子, *shan zhu yu* 山茱萸, *dang shen* 党参, *huang qi* 黄芪 and *sheng shi gao* 生石膏. The above herbs are boiled down into a concentrated mixture (containing 1 g of crude drugs per millilitre). Take three times a day, 50 to 80 mL each time.

- *Zhu ye shi gao tang* 竹叶石膏汤, *zhu ye* 竹叶, *sheng shi gao* 生石膏, *fa ban xia* 法半夏, *mai men tong* 麦门冬, *ren shen* 人参, *gan cao* 甘草 and *jing mi* 粳米. Decoct one bag of herbs per day with water before consuming it twice a day. The decoction is suitable for diabetic patients with symptoms of thirst and excessive drinking, a dry mouth and throat, a red tongue with little coating, breathlessness and nausea, thin body stature, and a deficient pulse.

Acupuncture and Related Treatments

Acupuncture therapies have been documented since the *Huang Di Nei Jing* 黄帝内经 (BCE 618). Acupuncture may alleviate the symptoms of diabetes. Excess syndromes should be treated with purging methods, while deficiency syndromes should be treated with tonifying methods. Commonly used acupuncture points for common syndromes of diabetes are summarised below.

Body Acupuncture

Body acupuncture can be applied using syndrome differentiation:

1. Lung heat that damages body fluids, Kidney *yin* deficiency[4,6]

Acupoint selection: ST36 *Zusanli* 足三里, SP6 *Sanyinjiao* 三阴交, LI11 *Quchi* 曲池, BL20 *Pishu* 脾俞, BL13 *Feishu* 肺俞, BL23 *Shenshu* 肾俞, TE6 *Zhigou* 支沟 and CV12 *Zhongwan* 中脘.

Manipulation: To tonify deficiency and reduce excess or use a neutral method.

2. Kidney *qi* deficiency[4,6]

Acupoint selection: BL23 *Shenshu* 肾俞, BL20 *Pishu* 脾俞, BL17 *Geshu* 膈俞, ST36 *Zusanli* 足三里, SP6 *Sanyinjiao* 三阴交, CV4 *Guanyuan* 关元 and CV6 *Qihai* 气海.

Manipulation: Neutral tonifying and reducing method.

Auricular Needling

Acupoint selection: CO11 *Yidan* (Pancreas and Gallbladder) 胰胆, CO18 *Neifenmi* (Endocrine) 内分泌, CO17 *Sanjiao* 三焦, R2 *Ermigen* 耳迷根, TF4 *Shenmen* 神门, CO14 *Fei* (Lung) 肺, CO4 *Wei* (Stomach) 胃 and CO10 *Shen* (Kidney) 肾. The method of using ear pellets at ear points are used.

Moxibustion

Moxibustion can also be used for T2DM.[6] CV6 *Qihai* 气海, CV4 *Guanyuan* 关元, SP6 *Sanyinjiao* 三阴交, SP9 *Yinlingquan* 阴陵泉, KI3 *Taixi* 太溪, BL23 *Shenshu* 肾俞, GV4 *Mingmen* 命门, BL20 *Pishu* 脾俞, CV3 *Zhongji* 中极, KI7 *Fuliu* 复溜 and ST36 *Zusanli* 足三里 points had moxibustion five to 10 times at each point, six points at a time, and the above points were used alternately. Treat once a day over 15 days for a course of treatment.

Current studies show that time-selective needling is a major feature of acupuncture treatment for diseases.[8] Acupuncture at the peak of insulin secretion can be selected.[9] The decrease of fasting and a 2-hour postprandial blood sugar concentration in patients is significantly better than that in other times. Moxibustion or ginger-separated moxibustion can also be applied at *bei shu* 背俞穴 and abdominal *mu* 募穴 points.

Precautions need to be taken into consideration when performing acupuncture and moxibustion for T2DM. Acupuncture and moxibustion are mainly used for mild to moderate T2DM and have poor curative effects on severe, long-term T2DM. Acupuncture and moxibustion therapy have the advantages of convenient acupoint selection, safety and cost efficiency. Nevertheless, as adjuvant therapy for diabetes mellitus, they must be combined with hypoglycaemic agents, diet, exercise and other therapies to achieve beneficial glucose metabolism.

Tuina Massage

1. Indications: *yin* deficiency with deficient fire.[5,6]
   a) Massage on the back:
      i) Push along the Governor Vessel (posterior median line) four times, then push along the Bladder meridian on both sides of the spine through the Bladder meridian line (1.5 cun from the posterior median line) four times and the Bladder meridian line (3 cun from the posterior median line) four times, for about four minutes.

   ii) Massage EX-B3 *Yishu* 胰俞 (1.5 cun below the eighth thoracic spinous process) and local *Ashi* points (pain points) and rub both sides of the midline of the lower back for two minutes.

   iii) Rub the Bladder meridian (1.5 cun from the midline) on the back, then horizontally rub the lower back until it is warm.

b) Massage on the hypochondriac and abdomen regions: Press and knead CV12 *Zhongwan* 中脘, ST21 *Liangmen* 梁门, CV6 *Qihai* 气海 and CV4 *Guanyuan* 关元 with the thumb for two minutes at each point. On the CV8 *Shenque* 神阙 point, press down with the palm and use it to vibrate for two minutes, then push on the upper and lower abdomen for about four minutes. Rub the hypochondriac region with both hands until it is warm.

c) Massage the limbs: Knead LI11 *Quchi* 曲池 with fingers for one minute and massage SP6 *Sanyinjiao* 三阴交 for two minutes until the point becomes achy. Massage the arms and legs four times, using the kneading method and pinching method. Rub on the KI11 *Yongquan* 涌泉 acupoint until it is warm. End the massage with gentle drumming.

2. Indications: Deficiency of *qi* and *yin* and Blood stasis.[5,6]

Patients are to lie in a supine position. First, press the patients' cardiac reflex zones to check their physical condition, which will determine the strength of the massage. First, massage the left foot then the right foot. Patients may present with nodules on the inside of the big toe or a nodule cord that runs from the root to the tip of the inside of the big toe. The nodule needs to be gradually massaged until it has softened or disappears. If there are nodules on the heel, the heel also needs to be massaged for five minutes. Finally, push the adrenal gland, kidney, ureter and bladder reflex area on the foot. Drink about 300 mL of warm water within half an hour after the massage. Diabetic patients with ketoacidosis or other serious complications should not be treated with this method. If patients have taken medication before the massage, they should continue to take medication during the massage. At the same time, they should pay close attention to blood glucose and clinical signs, and gradually reduce the dosage according to the degree of alleviation of the disease until the medication is completely discontinued. Treat once a day over 12 days for a course of treatment.

A summary of acupuncture and related therapies for diabetes mellitus is presented in Table 2.2.

Table 2.2. Summary of Acupuncture Therapies for Diabetes Mellitus

Intervention	Acupuncture Points/Body Areas	Treatment Frequency
Body acupuncture	For Lung heat that damages body fluids and Kidney *yin* deficiency: ST36 *Zusanli* 足三里, SP9 *Sanyinjiao* 三阴交, LI11 *Quchi* 曲池, BL20 *Pishu* 脾俞, BL13 *Feishu* 肺俞, BL23 *Shenshu* 肾俞, TE6 *Zhigou* 支沟, CV12 *Zhongwan* 中脘. For Kidney *qi* deficiency: BL23 *Shenshu* 肾俞, BL20 *Pishu* 脾俞, BL17 *Geshu* 膈俞, ST36 *Zusanli* 足三里, SP6 *Sanyinjiao* 三阴交, CV4 *Guanyuan* 关元 and CV6 *Qihai* 气海.	30 minutes treatment daily for six days, then one rest day. Treat for four consecutive weeks (one course).
Auricular acupuncture	CO11 *Yidan* 胰胆, CO18 *Neifenmi* 内分泌, CO17 *Sanjiao* 三焦, R2 *Ermigen* 耳迷根, TF4 *Shenmen* 神门, CO11 *Fei* 肺, CO4 *Wei* 胃 and CO10 *Shen* 肾.	3–4 points daily or on alternate days, retain ear pellets.
Moxibustion	Main points: CV6 *Qihai* 气海, CV4 *Guanyuan* 关元, SP6 *Sanyinjiao* 三阴交, SP9 *Yinlingquan* 阴陵泉, KI3 *Taixi* 太溪, BL23 *Shenshu* 肾俞, GV4 *Mingmen* 命门, BL20 *Pishu* 脾俞, CV3 *Zhongji* 中极, KI7 *Fuliu* 复溜 and ST36 *Zusanli* 足三里.	Use 5–6 points on alternate days; treat once a day, 15 days for a course of treatment.
Tuina massage	For *yin* deficiency with deficient fire: push along the Governor Vessel, Bladder meridian, massage EX-B3 *Yishu* 胰俞, then massage along the abdomen and hypochondriac region, finish with kneading LI11 *Quchi* 曲, SP6 *Sanyinjiao* 三阴交 and KI11 *Yongquan* 涌泉. For deficiency of *qi* and *yin* and Blood stasis, massage the left then right foot, rub out any nodules on the toes, then the heels.	For acupoints, rub for 1 minute each, for the area rub until warm. Once a day, 12 days for a course of treatment.

Other Management Strategies

Prevention

1. Reinforce education and knowledge on diabetes mellitus and highlight the risk factors of diabetes mellitus, such as obesity, lack of physical activity, and an inappropriate diet structure. It is emphasised that diabetes mellitus should be detected, treated and prevented early. Effective measures should be taken to prevent diabetes mellitus in patients with impaired glucose tolerance.[5,6]
2. Increase physical exercise, especially for those over 40 years of age and for those who are gradually gaining weight.
3. People should pay attention to their diets. Try to avoid too much fat and protein, which can lead to weight gain and an increased risk of diabetes mellitus. Therefore, it is of great significance to adjust one's dietary structure to prevent the occurrence of diabetes mellitus.

Rehabilitation

Lifestyle

Take care to adapt to the weather. When a change of season occurs, add or reduce clothing accordingly and actively avoid emotional upsets to prevent the aggravation of T2DM. People with T2DM are also encouraged to stop unhealthy habits, such as smoking and gambling.[5,6]

Dietary

Dietary recommendations should be based on people's needs and their ages, and living conditions should be taken into consideration. Recommendations for children should meet their growth and development needs, while those for pregnant women should meet the needs of foetal growth. Overeating on meat, eggs and fatty foods are also not conducive to treatment. Food that is smoked, pickled and fermented should be avoided or their intake reduced as much as possible.

There are many herbal medicines that can be used as dietary therapy. They should be consumed under the guidance of CM doctors. Otherwise, if someone with a cold syndrome is given food with cold or cooling properties, and someone with heat syndrome is given warm products, this will aggravate the condition.

The following herbs and foods may be used as dietary therapy for *yin* deficiency and dryness-heat type patients: *Bai he* 百合, *chuan bei mu* 川贝母, *mai men dong* 麦门冬, *sheng di huang* 生地黄, *xuan shen* 玄参, *zhi mu* 知母, *sheng shi gao* 生石膏, *tian hua fen* 天花粉, *ge gen* 葛根, *ku gua* 苦瓜, *lv dou* 绿豆, *ya rou* 鸭肉, *shi hu* 石斛, *da huang* 大黄, *bo he* 薄荷 and *dou fu* 豆腐; *qi* and *yin* deficiency patients may choose herbs and foods such as *Huang qi* 黄芪, *xi yang shen* 西洋参, *tai zi shen* 太子参, *hong shen* 红参, *bai zhu* 白术, *shan yao* 山药, *lian zi* 莲子, *yi yi ren* 薏苡仁, *sha shen* 沙参, *gou qi zi* 枸杞子, *gui zhi* 桂枝, *wu wei zi* 五味子, *mai men dong* 麦门冬, *huang jing* 黄精, *shu di huang* 熟地黄, *gan cao* 甘草, *bai shao* 白芍, chicken, pork, *nan gua* 南瓜, fish, *zhu yi* 猪胰, *he tao* 核桃 and *zhi ma* 芝麻.[6]

Patients can also incorporate the following dietary therapy for diabetes mellitus into their daily lives and health care[6]:

(1) Bitter melon tea: Use 30 grams of dried bitter melon, decoct for tea and consume one dose per day. This tea is suitable for T2DM patients with symptoms that include thirst, excessive drinking, irritability, normal or increased appetite, and a red tongue with yellow coating.

(2) *Gou qi zi ju hua* tea: Mix *gou qi zi* 枸杞子 and *ju hua* 菊花 with hot water to make tea. It is suitable for diabetic cataract and blurred vision.

(3) Three beans drink: Use 30 g each of mung beans, red adzuki beans and black soybeans. Decoct the beans in water until they are cooked and the soup is thick; drink once a day. This is suitable for hungry and thirsty people with the syndrome *zhong xiao* 中消.

(4) *Huang qi shan yao* porridge: Use *huang qi* 黄芪 and *shan yao* 山药. First, boil *huang qi* 黄芪 in water, then keep the decoction and remove the residue. Mix the decoction into *shan yao* 山药

powder to form porridge, which is to be taken twice a day. This porridge is suitable for diabetic patients with prolonged Spleen and Kidney deficiency.

(5) Onion soup: Use freshly sliced onions (90 g) and lean pork (60 g). First, cook the pork in water, then add onions, and stew into a soup. Suitable for x*ia xiao* 下消 with symptoms of frequent urine and exhaustion.

(6) Carrot and glutinous rice congee: Use chopped carrots plus glutinous rice (50 g). Cook with water until all ingredients are cooked and softened. Can be taken either in the morning or at night. It is suitable for people with diabetes who are prone to polyphagia, hunger, dizziness and day-by-day wasting.

Mental Health Care

Diabetic patients should be open-minded and avoid emotional irritation. Emotional disorder is also one of the causes of acute complications of diabetes mellitus in the clinic. Therefore, we should try to be happy, take part in social activities, and consult a psychologist when necessary.

References

1. 傅强, 王世东, 肖永华, *et al.* (2017) 吕仁和教授分期辨治糖尿病学术思想探微. 世界中医药 **12**(1): 21–24.
2. 国家中医药管理局. (1994) 中医病证诊断疗效标准. 南京大学出版社, 南京.
3. 吴勉华, 王新月. (2012) 全国中医药行业高等教育 '十二五' 规划教材, 中医内科学. 中国中医药出版社, 北京.
4. 中华中医药学会. (2008) 中医内科常见病诊疗指南: 中医病证部分. 中国中医药出版社, 北京.
5. 中华中医药学会. (2011) 糖尿病中医防治指南. 中国中医药现代远程教育 **9**(4): 148–151.
6. 范冠杰, 邓兆智. (2013) 专科专病中医临床诊治丛书 — 内分泌科专病与风湿病中医临床诊治. 人民卫生出版社, 北京.

7. 中华医学会糖尿病学分会. (2018) 中国 2 型糖尿病防治指南 (2017 年版). 中华糖尿病杂志 **10**(1): 4–67.

8. 王玲玲. (1990) 《内经》择时针灸法初探. 南京中医学院学报 **6**(1): 52–53.

9. 张慧玲, 薄亚丽. (2003) 逢时针灸治疗糖尿病临床观察. 中国针灸 **1**(23): 13–14.

3

Classical Chinese Medicine Literature

OVERVIEW

Classical Chinese medicine (CM) literature has contributed valuable resources to the prevention and management of various health conditions. As an important section of the "whole evidence" approach, this chapter systematically summarises and evaluates the classical CM literature for diabetes in *Zhong Hua Yi Dian* 中华医典, one of the most complete collections of classical CM works. More than 300 citations were identified. Search terms, aetiology and pathogenesis, and CM management for diabetes are described and analysed.

Introduction

Chinese medicine (CM) therapies have been practised for managing various conditions for thousands of years, with the earliest professional practice citation dating back to the late Spring & Autumn (770–476 BCE) or the early Warring States (474–221 BCE) periods.[1] Valuable information and knowledge on the aetiology and pathogenesis, symptoms, syndromes and clinical management of different conditions have been described in-depth in CM classical literature. During this time, ancient CM practitioners accumulated abundant experience in managing diabetes-related symptoms, which continues to guide contemporary practice.

In contemporary CM clinical textbooks and practice guidelines, *xiao ke* 消渴 (emaciation and polydipsia disease) has been typically used in classical literature to describe diabetes.[2,3] In history, *xiao ke* 消渴 was commonly diagnosed according to a cluster of distinctive symptoms such as sweet urine, emaciation, polydipsia, polyphagia and polyuria. These are like the diabetes symptoms that we know today. Contemporary literature suggests that the earliest *xiao ke* 消渴 citation was from the *Huang Di Nei Jing Su Wen* 黄帝内经素问 (c. 762 CE).[4] Various terms related to diabetes were also mentioned in the *Huang Di Nei Jing Su Wen* 黄帝内经素问 according to different aetiology and pathogenesis (e.g., *Fei xiao* 肺消 emaciation of Lung and *ge xiao* 膈消 emaciation of diaphragm) and typical symptoms (e.g., *xiao zhong* 消中 middle emaciation). In this book, the authors also pointed out that the deficiency of the five *zang*, overconsumption of food, and emotional instability were the main pathological factors of *xiao ke* 消渴.

Over a long history of managing diabetes mellitus in CM practice, knowledge on the treatment of diabetes mellitus has been accumulated and described in many of the classical CM texts. To summarise and evaluate the evidence of CM classical literature for diabetes, the *Zhong Hua Yi Dian* (ZHYD) 中华医典 CD-ROM was searched.[5] This collection includes more than 1,000 medical books of classical CM literature. It is currently the largest and representative of other collections of classical and pre-modern CM literature.[6,7] The findings are presented below.

Search Terms

The most commonly used term for diabetes in contemporary CM practice is *xiao ke* 消渴, describing typical clinical manifestations, emaciation and polydipsia. Various terms have also been used to describe diabetes historically, such as *shang xiao* 上消, *zhong xiao* 中消 and *xia xiao* 下消, which are used for classifying diabetes patients' main symptoms as polydipsia, polyphagia and polyuria, respectively.[8] To summarise the classical literature evidence comprehensively, relevant search terms were collected through hand searches from contemporary CM textbooks,[4,8–11] clinical guidelines[12–14] and professional books.[15,16] Identified terms were reviewed by CM specialists and experts, and a total of 19 search terms related to diabetes were included for searching the ZHYD (Table 3.1).

Table 3.1. Terms Used to Identify Classical Literature Citations

Search Terms of Diabetes in Pinyin	Search Terms of Diabetes in Chinese	English Translation[17]
Feng xiao	风消	Wind and emaciation disease
Fei xiao	肺消	Emaciation of Lung
Fei pang	肥胖	Obesity
Ge xiao	鬲消	Emaciation of Diaphragm
Ge xiao	膈消	Emaciation of Diaphragm
Ke li	渴利	Polydipsia and polyuria disease
Nei xiao	内消	Internal emaciation
Pi dan	脾瘅	Heat disease of Spleen
Shen xiao	肾消	Emaciation of Kidney
Shang xiao	上消	Upper emaciation
San xiao	三消	Three (upper, medium and lower) emaciation
Xiao	痟	Emaciation
Xiao shen	消肾	Emaciation of Kidney
Xiao dan	消瘅	Emaciation and Heat disease
Xiao ke	消渴	Emaciation and polydipsia disease
Xiao li	消利	Emaciation and polyuria disease
Xiao zhong	消中	Medium emaciation
Xia xiao	下消	Lower emaciation
Zhong xiao	中消	Medium emaciation

Procedures for Search, Data Coding, Data Analysis

Included search terms were entered in the ZHYD search fields separately. Both headings and full texts searches were conducted for each term, and the search results were exported to Excel spreadsheets for data cleaning and data coding. A "citation" was defined as a distinct passage of text referring to one or more of the search terms. Duplicate citations identified by different search terms were removed from the data set. Citations published after 1949 were not considered classical literature and were removed from the data set.

Citations were coded for the likelihood of being diabetes according to the symptom descriptions. The coding was conducted based

Table 3.2. Symptoms Grading Criteria

Grades	Chinese Terms in Pinyin Referring to Diabetes Symptoms	Translation
A	*Niao tian* 尿甜	Sweet urine
B	*Duo yin* 多饮, *duo niao* 多尿, *duo shi* 多食, *xiao shou* 消瘦	Polydipsia, polyuria, polyphagia, emaciation
C	*Pi juan* 疲倦, *bian mi* 便秘, *yao xi suan ruan* 腰膝酸软, *niao zhuo* 尿浊, *xing ti fei pang* 形体肥胖	Fatigue, constipation, weakness and soreness in the back and knees, turbid urine, obesity
D	*Xiao ke ri jiu* 消渴日久, *xiao ke bing* 消渴并, *xiao/ke hou* 消/渴后, *you er* 幼儿, *fa re* 发热, *jing qian yi ce/liang ce jie kuai zhong da* 颈前一侧或两侧结块肿大, *qing zhi shi tiao* 情志失调	Long-term emaciation and polydipsia and/after emaciation and/or polydipsia, fever, paediatric, unilateral/bilateral anterior swelling nodule of neck, emotional instability

on a symptom grading system (Table 3.2). Symptom description terms were grouped according to the nature of the disease (Grade A: sweet urine 尿甜), typical symptoms of diabetes (Grade B: polydipsia 多饮, polyuria 多尿, polyphagia 多食 and emaciation 消瘦), and other common symptoms of diabetes (Grade C: fatigue 疲倦, constipation 便秘, weakness and soreness in the back and knees 腰膝酸软, turbid urine 尿浊 and obesity 形体肥胖).

It should be noted that this monograph focuses on adult diabetes patients with diabetes as the primary disease. Any citation considered as secondary diabetes, paediatric diabetes, or containing terms referring to other diseases/conditions was excluded from further analysis. A group of condition terms (Grade D) was clustered together for citation exclusion criteria: long-term emaciation and polydipsia disease 消渴日久, and/after emaciation and/or polydipsia disease 消渴并/消/渴后, paediatric 幼儿, fever 发热, unilateral/bilateral anterior swelling nodule of neck 颈前一侧或两侧结块肿大 and emotional instability 情志失调.

Using the symptom grading system, citations were further judged as "most likely" to be diabetes citations, "possible" diabetes citations, and ineligible citations (presented in Table 3.3).

Table 3.3. Citation Judgement Criteria

Citation Judgement	Citation Judgement Criteria
Most likely to be a diabetes citation	1. Contains symptom from Grade A 2. Contains symptom from Grade A with any symptom from Grade B or C
Possible diabetes citation	1. Contains all four symptoms from Grade B 2. Contains any three symptoms from Grade B, with any one symptom from Grade C
Ineligible citation	1. Contains any symptom from Grade D 2. Contains fewer than three symptoms from Grade B and C

- "Most likely" diabetes citations refer to citations that contain the most representative symptoms of diabetes. These citations should contain the symptom of sweet urine 尿甜 (Grade A), with any other symptom from Grade B or C.
- "Possible" diabetes citations refer to the citations judged most likely to be diabetes or citations that contain some of the typical diabetes symptoms, but uncertainty remains. These citations should contain all of the four typical diabetes symptoms (Grade B symptoms) or any three typical symptoms with "other common symptoms of diabetes" (Grade C symptoms).
- "Ineligible citation" means that the citations either contained conditions meeting the exclusion criteria (Grade D conditions/symptoms) or insufficient information to be judged as diabetes (i.e., containing fewer than three symptoms from Grade B and C). Ineligible citations were excluded from further analysis.

All relevant citations were reviewed to identify the best descriptions of diabetes and its aetiology or pathogenesis. Relevant citations that did not include treatment details were excluded from further analyses. The final data set included citations considered to potentially refer to "possible" diabetes, which described CM treatments (Chinese herbal medicine, acupuncture and related therapies, or other CM therapies). When a citation referred to multiple treatments, each treatment was considered as a separate citation for the

calculation of formulae, herbs or acupuncture points. For those identified Chinese herbal formulae with no ingredients, ingredients were
sourced from the same formula in the same book if possible.

Included citations were grouped according to the CM intervention for further analysis. Data were presented for the frequencies of
identified formulae, herbs and acupuncture points for "possible" and
"most likely" diabetes citation data sets, respectively. All formulae
were further reviewed for the similarity of herbal ingredients.
Formulae with similar ingredients but different formula names were
considered to be the same and were combined for frequency
analysis.

Search Results

The search procedure is presented in Figure 3.1.

A total of 12,916 hits (or instances of the search terms) were
obtained through heading and body text search in the ZHYD by the

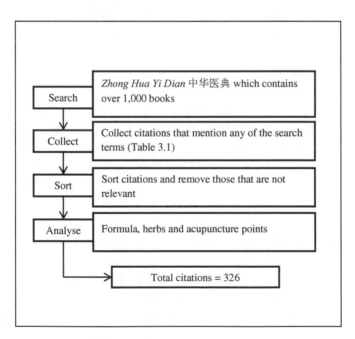

Figure 3.1. Classical literature citations.

Table 3.4. Hit Frequency by Search Term

Pinyin	Chinese Characters	Total Hit Frequency (*n*, %)
Xiao ke	消渴	6220 (48.2)
Nei xiao	内消	1773 (13.7)
San xiao	三消	738 (5.7)
Xiao zhong	消中	624 (4.8)
Xiao dan	消瘅	536 (4.1)
Zhong xiao	中消	498 (3.9)
Xia xiao	下消	425 (3.3)
Shang xiao	上消	303 (2.3)
Feng xiao	风消	292 (2.3)
Shen xiao	肾消	289 (2.2)
Xiao shen	消肾	248 (1.9)
Ge xiao	膈消	239 (1.9)
Fei xiao	肺消	174 (1.3)
Fei pang	肥胖	147 (1.1)
Ke li	渴利	133 (1.0)
Pi dan	脾瘅	132 (1.0)
Xiao	痟	83 (0.6)
Ge xiao	鬲消	39 (0.3)
Xiao li	消利	23 (0.2)

19 search terms (Table 3.4). The term *xiao ke* 消渴, which describes "emaciation and polydipsia" in the Chinese language, produced the highest number of hits (6,220 instances, 48.2%). *Nei xiao* 内消 identified 1,773 (5.8%) hits. Other search terms identified 5% or less of the total hits.

Citations Related to Diabetes

After duplicate removal and exclusions of all "ineligible citations" as above-mentioned, a total of 571 citations met the inclusion criteria and were judged as "possible diabetes" citations. Of these, 245 citations did not describe any CM interventions and were excluded from further analysis.

All included citations were also reviewed to identify and synthesis the aetiology or pathogenesis details of the disease. Citations that described the aetiology or pathogenesis details, or citations with no-treatment details, were also reviewed to identify appropriate explanations of the disease.

Of the 326 "possible diabetes" citations that included details on CM interventions, 316 citations described Chinese Herbal Medicine (CHM) treatments, while 10 citations mentioned acupuncture therapies. Among these, 26 citations contained the most representative symptoms of diabetes and were considered as "most likely" diabetes citations. These all described CHM interventions for diabetes.

Definitions of the Condition and Aetiology

Diabetes was first described as *xiao ke* 消渴 disease in the *Huang Di Nei Jing Su Wen* 黄帝内经素问 (c. 762 CE). Possible pathogenesis, symptoms and CHM treatment of diabetes were described in this citation: diabetes patients over-indulged on greasy and sweet food. The greasiness in the food caused internal heat, while the sweetness caused abdominal distension in people. Consequently, excessive *qi* 气 overflowed upwards and caused emaciation and polydipsia. *Lan* 兰 can be used to treat this disease in resolving the excessive *qi* 气. (... 此人必数食甘美而多肥也, 肥者令人内热, 甘者令人中满, 故其气上溢, 转为消渴. 治之以兰, 除陈气也).

In the long history of managing diabetes, CM practitioners have described its symptoms in detailed texts. According to patients' main symptoms, diabetes was often classified as containing three sub-classes: *shang xiao* 上消, *zhong xiao* 中消 and *xia xiao* 下消. In the *Pu Ji Ben Shi Fang* 普济本事方 (c. 1132) by *Xu Shu Wei* in the Song dynasty, the first instance of the three kinds of *xiao ke* 消渴 was described: "*xiao ke* 消渴 disease was defined as experiencing polydipsia and polyuria with turbid and sweet urine; *xiao zhong* 消中 disease was defined as polyphagia without excessive thirst, with less amount but frequent turbid urine; *shen xiao* 肾消 disease was defined as patients having excessive thirst but were not able to drink much water, oedema of legs but with thin and small feet, erectile dysfunction and polyuria". ('...消渴有三种：一者渴而饮水多, 小便数, 脂似麸片, 甜者消渴病也; 二者吃食多, 不甚渴, 小便少, 似有油而数者, 消中病也; 三者渴饮水不能多, 但腿肿, 脚先瘦小, 阴痿弱, 小便数, 此肾消病也'.)

Wu Qian in the Qing dynasty further clarified the three different kinds of *xiao ke* 消渴 and their characteristic symptoms in the book *Yi Zong Jin Jian• Za Bing Xin Fa Yao Jue* 医宗金鉴• 杂病心法要诀 (c. 1742). This book pointed out that *shang xiao* 上消 was related to the Lung, where patients could have polydipsia but normal urine; *zhong xiao* 中消 was related to the Stomach, where patients could have polydipsia but produced dark yellow and small amounts of urine; *xia xiao* 下消 was related to the Kidney, where patients could have experienced symptoms of polyuria and turbid urine. Three types of *xiao* were all caused by dryness and heat (上消属肺, 饮水多而小便如常; 中消属胃, 饮水多而小便短赤, 下消属肾, 饮水多而小便浑浊, 三消皆燥热病也).

The aetiology and pathogenesis of diabetes were also discussed in various classical citations. Several citations pointed out that the latent heat and deficiency of *zang* 脏 and *fu* 腑 could be two main factors causing diabetes. One typical citation from the *Ren zhai zhi zhi fang lun* 仁斋直指方论 (c. 1264) discussed this in depth: "... The heat *qi* 气 moves upwards and invades into the deficient Heart. The Heart fire permeates and causes chest tightness, a red tongue and lips, thirst and polydipsia, and frequent and small amounts of urine. The disease is in the Upper *jiao* 焦 and it is called *xiao ke* 消渴. The heat accumulates in the Middle *jiao* 焦 and invades into the deficient Spleen. The latent *yang* steams the Stomach and causes polyphagia. However, the muscles are not nourished. The patient feels thirsty and prefers cold drinks. The urine is frequent with a sweet taste. This disease is in the Middle *jiao* 焦 and is called *xiao zhong* 消中. When the heat accumulates in the Lower *jiao* 焦 and invades the Kidney, the patient could have skinny legs and sore joints. The *jing* 精 and *sui* 髓 dissipate, and the patient drinks water to relieve the severe thirst. The patient feels thirsty but drinks a small amount. The patient urinates immediately after drinking, and the urine is large in quantity and turbid in appearance" (热气上腾, 心虚受之, 心火散漫, 不能收敛, 胸中烦躁, 舌赤唇红, 此渴引饮常多, 小便数而少, 病属上焦, 谓之消渴. 热蓄于中, 脾虚受之, 伏阳蒸胃, 消谷善饥, 饮食倍常, 不生肌肉, 此渴亦不甚烦, 但欲饮冷, 小便数而甜, 病属中焦, 谓之消中. 热伏于下, 肾虚受之, 腿膝枯细, 骨节酸痛, 精走髓虚, 引水自救, 此渴水饮不多, 随即溺下, 小便多而浊, 病属下焦, 谓之消肾).

The ancient CM practitioner also recognised that overeating could be a main cause of diabetes. The very first citation related to diabetes from the *Huang Di Nei Jing Su Wen* 黄帝内经素问 (see above translation) described the aetiology of an improper diet. *Wang Huai Yin* also discussed in his book *Tai Ping Sheng Hui Fang* 太平圣惠方 (c. 992) that diabetes patients may have taken mineral drugs with hot properties from a young age, overconsumed liquor, meat and spicy food, and indulgence in sexual activities. These may have caused an exhaustion of body fluids and vitality. The heat toxin could accumulate in the Heart and Lung, and the excessive meat may do harm to the Stomach, inducing diabetes (… 此盖由少年服乳石热药. 耽嗜酒肉荤辛. 热面炙爆. 荒淫色欲. 不能将理. 致使津液耗竭. 元气衰虚. 热毒积聚于心肺. 腥膻并伤于胃腑…).

Chinese Herbal Medicine

The 316 citations describing CHM treatments were identified in 96 books. *Pu Ji Fang* 普济方 (c. 1406) produced a large portion of the included citations. Other books with a high number of citations included the *Gu Jin Yi Tong Da Quan* 古今医统大全 (c. 1556) (*n* = 16), *Zhang Shi Yi Tong* 张氏医通 (c. 1695) (*n* = 16) and *Za Bing Yuan Liu Xi Zhu* 杂病源流犀烛 (c. 1773) (*n* = 16). Twenty books obtained five or more included citations of CHM treatment.

Frequency of Treatment Citations by Dynasty

The earliest citation with CHM intervention was identified in the *Huang Di Nei Jing Su Wen* 黄帝内经素问. This citation was obtained

Table 3.5.   Dynastic Distribution of Treatment Citations

Dynasty	No. of Treatment Citations
Before Tang Dynasty (to 618 CE)	1
Tang and 5 Dynasties (618–960)	5
Song and Jin Dynasties (961–1271)	26
Yuan Dynasty (1272–1368)	17
Ming Dynasty (1369–1644)	123
Qing Dynasty (1645–1911)	133
Ming Guo/Republic of China (1912–1949)	11
Total	316

by the search term *xiao ke* 消渴 (for a possible translation, see the above section "Definitions of the Condition and Aetiology").

The majority of the citations with CHM treatments were found from classical books published during the Ming (c. 1369–1644) and Qing dynasties (c. 1645–1911) (Table 3.5). Around 80% of the citations (*n* = 256) were identified during these two dynasties.

Treatment with Chinese Herbal Medicine

The 316 CHM citations describing treatment information were all considered possibly related to diabetes as they met the inclusion criteria. Of these, 26 citations were judged as being "most likely diabetes citations" by following the symptom grading criteria mentioned above. Data extracted from the "possible diabetes citations" data set and "most likely diabetes citations" sub-data set were analysed for frequently used formulae and herbs.

Most Frequent Formulae in Possible Diabetes Citations

A total of 316 formulae were identified from the possible diabetes citations data set. Of these, 51 (16.1%) citations did not specify any formula names. All formulae were described as oral administration.

The most frequently cited oral formulae names and their herb ingredients are presented in Table 3.6. Herbal ingredients were obtained from the earliest citation if variants were seen under the same formula name. Consistent with contemporary CHM management for diabetes, the four most frequently cited formulae — *Liu wei di huang wan* 六味地黄丸 (with variant formula names), *Shen qi wan* 肾气丸, *Tiao wei cheng qi tang* 调胃承气汤 and *Bai hu jia ren shen*

Table 3.6. **Most Frequent Oral Formulae in Possible Diabetes Citations**

Formula Name	Herb Ingredients	Number of Citations (n)
Liu wei di huang wan / Liu wei di huang wan jia jian/ Liu wei di huang tang jia sheng mai san 六味地黄丸/六味地黄丸加减/六味地黄汤加生脉散	Shan yao 山药, shan zhu yu 山茱萸, mu dan pi 牡丹皮, ze xie 泽泻, fu ling 茯苓, shu di huang 熟地黄 (*Dong Yuan Shi Xiao Fang* 东垣试效方, c. 1266)	32
Shen qi wan / Ba wei wan / Shen qi wan jia jian / Fu gui ba wei wan / Fu gui ba wei jia jian / Jia jian ba wei wan 肾气丸/八味丸/肾气丸加减/附桂八味丸/附桂八味加减/加减八味丸	Shu di huang 熟地黄, shan yao 山药, shan zhu yu 山茱萸, ze xie 泽泻, mu dan pi 牡丹皮, fu ling 茯苓, fu zi 附子, rou gui 肉桂 (*Su Wen Bing Ji Qi Yi Bao Ming Ji* 素问病机气宜保命集, c. 1186)	31
Tiao wei cheng qi tang / tiao wei cheng qi tang jia jian 调胃承气汤/调胃承气汤加减	Da huang 大黄, gan cao 甘草, mang xiao 芒硝 (*Dong Yuan Shi Xiao Fang* 东垣试效方, c. 1266)	23
Bai hu jia ren shen tang / Ren shen bai hu tang 白虎加人参汤/人参白虎汤	Ren shen 人参, shi gao 石膏, zhi mu 知母, gan cao 甘草, jing mi 粳米 (*Dong Yuan Shi Xiao Fang* 东垣试效方, c. 1266)	18
San huang wan / san huang tang 三黄丸/三黄汤	Da huang 大黄, huang qin 黄芩, huang lian 黄连 (*Dong Yuan Shi Xiao Fang* 东垣试效方, c. 1266)	14

Table 3.6. (*Continued*)

Formula Name	Herb Ingredients	Number of Citations (n)
Ren shen bai zhu tang 人参白术汤	Ren shen 人参, bai zhu 白术, dang gui 当归, shao yao 芍药, da huang 大黄, zhi zi 栀子, jing jie sui 荆芥穗, bo he 薄荷, jie geng 桔梗, zhi mu 知母, ze xie 泽泻, fu ling 茯苓, lian qiao 连翘, gua lou 瓜蒌, ge gen 葛根, gan cao 甘草, huo xiang 藿香, qing mu xiang 青木香, rou gui 肉桂, shi gao 石膏, han shui shi 寒水石, hua shi 滑石 (*Ren Zhai Zhi Zhi Fang Lun* 仁斋直指方论, c. 1264)	7
Qing liang yin zi 清凉饮子	Sheng ma 升麻, fang feng 防风, gan cao 甘草, fang ji 防己, di huang 地黄, dang gui 当归, chai hu 柴胡, qiang huo 羌活, gan cao 甘草, huang qi 黄芪, zhi mu 知母, huang qin 黄芩, long dan cao 龙胆草, shi gao 石膏, huang bo 黄柏, hong hua 红花, tao ren 桃仁, xing ren 杏仁 (*Dong Yuan Shi Xiao Fang* 东垣试效方, c. 1266)	7
Bai hu tang 白虎汤	Shi gao 石膏, zhi mu 知母, gan cao 甘草, jing mi 粳米 (*Yi Men Fa Lv* 医门法律, c. 1658)	7
Lan xiang yin zi/ Gan lu gao 兰香饮子/甘露膏	Ban xia 半夏, gan cao 甘草, bai dou kou 白豆蔻, ren shen 人参, lan xiang ye 兰香叶, sheng ma 升麻, lian qiao 连翘, jie geng 桔梗, fang feng 防风, zhi mu 知母, shi gao 石膏 (*Gu Jin Yi Tong Da Quan* 古今医统大全, c. 1556)	7

(*Continued*)

Table 3.6. *(Continued)*

Formula Name	Herb Ingredients	Number of Citations (n)
Bai fu ling wan 白茯苓丸	Fu ling 茯苓, fu pen zi 覆盆子, huang lian 黄连, ren shen 人参, gua lou 瓜蒌, di huang 地黄, bi xie 萆薢, xuan shen 玄参, ji nei jin 鸡内金, shi hu 石斛, she chuang 蛇床 (*Ji Feng Pu Ji Fang* 鸡峰普济方, c. 1133)	4
Hu fen san 胡粉散	Hu fen 胡粉, qian dan 铅丹, ze xie 泽泻, shi gao 石膏, chi shi zhi 赤石脂, bai shi zhi 白石脂, gua lou 瓜蒌, gan cao 甘草 (*Mai Yin Zheng Zhi* 脉因证治, c. 1279–1368)	4
Ren shen san 人参散	Ren shen 人参, bai zhu 白术, ze xie 泽泻, gua lou 瓜蒌, jie geng 桔梗, zhi zi 栀子, lian qiao 连翘, ge gen 葛根, huang qin 黄芩, da huang 大黄, bo he 薄荷, fu ling 茯苓, gan cao 甘草, shi gao 石膏, hua shi 滑石, han shui shi 寒水石, sha ren 砂仁 (*Huang Di Su Wen Xuan Ming Lun Fang* 黄帝素问宣明论方, c. 1172)	3
Shi bu wan 十补丸	Fu zi 附子, rou gui 肉桂, ba ji tian 巴戟天, bu gu zhi 补骨脂, gan jiang 干姜, yuan zhi 远志, tu si zi 菟丝子, chi shi zhi 赤石脂, hou po 厚朴, chuan jiao 川椒 (*Tai Ping Hui Min He Ji Ju Fang* 太平惠民和剂局方, c. 1078)	3
Yu nv jian 玉女煎	Di huang 地黄, shi gao 石膏, zhi mu 知母, yuan shen 元参, niu xi 牛膝, huang lian 黄连, tian men dong 天门冬, mai dong 麦冬, fu ling 茯苓, gan cao 甘草, pi pa 枇杷 (*Lin Zheng Zhi Nan Yi An* 临证指南医案, c. 1746)	3

Table 3.6. (*Continued*)

Formula Name	Herb Ingredients	Number of Citations (n)
Ge gen wan 葛根丸	Ge gen 葛根, gua lou 瓜蔞, qian dan 铅丹, fu zi 附子 (*Mai Yin Zheng Zhi* 脉因证治, c. 1279–1368)	3
Huang qi wan 黄芪丸	Huang qi 黄芪, mu li 牡蛎, gua lou 瓜蔞, gan cao 甘草, mai dong 麦冬, di gu pi 地骨皮, bai shi zhi 白石脂, ze xie 泽泻, zhi mu 知母, huang lian 黄连, shu yu 薯蓣, shu di huang 熟地黄 (*Pu Ji Fang* 普济方, c. 1309)	3
Huang qi tang 黄芪汤	Huang qi 黄芪, fu shen 茯神, gua lou 瓜蔞, gan cao 甘草, mai dong 麦冬, di huang 地黄 (*Wai Tai Mi Yao* 外台秘要, c. 752)	3

Note:

1. Formula ingredients are based on the earliest book within the group of included citations.
2. Formulae with the same name can vary in their ingredients and the same combination of ingredients may have different names. In this data, formulae with the same name that have variations in a few ingredients are grouped together while those with large variations in ingredients are separated. Also, formulae with the same ingredients but different names have been grouped together.
3. The use of some herbs/ingredients may be restricted in some countries; for example, herbs such as *fu zi* 附子, *qian dan* 铅丹 and *hu fen* 胡粉 can be toxic. Readers are advised to comply with the relevant regulations.

tang 白虎加人参汤 — were also recommended in contemporary CM guidelines and textbooks.[8,14] These formulae proposed to treat different CM syndromes of diabetes, including *yin* 阴 deficiency of the Kidney, deficiencies of both *yin* 阴 and *yang* 阳, excessive heat in the Stomach, and *yin* 阴 deficiency, with excessive heat, respectively.

Most Frequent Herbs in Possible Diabetes Citations

A total of 207 herbal ingredients were identified from the 316 possible diabetes citations. Same ingredients with different Chinese names or preparation methods, but similar clinical functions, were merged for frequency analysis. The most frequently reported herb was *gan cao* 甘草, which was obtained from 147 formulae (see Table 3.7). It was not surprising that *gan cao* 甘草 had the largest number as it had been widely used in CHM formulation for harmonising other herbs. The benefits of *gan cao* 甘草 include tonifying *qi* 气 and nourishing the Spleen for treating CM syndromes relating to *qi* 气 deficiency of diabetes.

Table 3.7. Most Frequent Oral Herbs in Possible Diabetes Citations

Herb Name	Scientific Name	No. of Citations (n)
Gan cao 甘草	*Glycyrrhizae* spp.	147
Fu ling 茯苓	*Poria cocos* (Schw.) Wolf.	117
Ze xie 泽泻	*Alisma orientalis* (Sam.) Juzep.	98
Shu di huang 熟地黄	*Rehmannia glutinosa* Libosch.	88
Zhi mu 知母	*Anemarrhena asphodeloides* Bge.	85
Shan yao 山药	*Dioscorea opposita* Thunb.	81
Ren shen 人参	*Panax ginseng* C. A. Mey.	79
Shan zhu yu 山茱萸	*Cornus officinalis* Sieb. et Zucc.	77
Shi gao 石膏	Hydrated calcium sulfate	77
Mu dan pi 牡丹皮	*Paeonia suffruticosa* Andr.	72
Gua lou 瓜蒌	1. *Trichosanthes kirilowii* Maxim. 2. *Trichosanthes rosthronii* Harms	65
Mai dong 麦冬	*Ophiopogon japonicus* (L.f) Ker-Gawl.	58
Huang lian 黄连	1. *Coptis chinensis* Franch. 2. *Coptis deltoidea* C. Y. Cheng et Hsiao 3. *Coptis teeta* Wall.	56
Da huang 大黄	1. *Rheum palmatum* L. 2. *Rheum tanguticum* Maxim. ex Balf. 3. *Rheum officinale* Baill.	55
Rou gui 肉桂	*Cinnamomum cassia* Presl	55
Di huang 地黄	*Rehmannia glutinosa* Libosch.	48
Huang qin 黄芩	*Scutellaria baicalensis* Georgi	45

Table 3.7. (*Continued*)

Herb Name	Scientific Name	No. of Citations (n)
Fu zi 附子	*Aconitum carmichaelii* Debx.	44
Huang qi 黄芪	1. *Astragalus membranaceus* (Fisch.) Bge. var. *mongholicus* (Bge.) Hsiao 2. *Astragalus membranaceus* (Fisch.) Bge.	34
Ge gen 葛根	*Pueraria lobata* (Willd.) Ohwi	31

Note: The use of some herbs/ingredients may be restricted in some countries; for example, herbs such as *fu zi* 附子 can be toxic. Readers are advised to comply with relevant regulations.

Functions of other most frequently cited herbal ingredients include expelling dampness (e.g., *fu ling* 茯苓, *shan yao* 山药 and *ze xie* 泽泻), nourishing *yin* 阴 (e.g., *shu di huang* 熟地黄, *mu dan pi* 牡丹皮 and *mai dong* 麦冬), dispersing heat (e.g., *zhi mu* 知母, *shi gao* 石膏 and *huang lian* 黄连), tonifying *qi* 气 and nourishing the Spleen (e.g., *ren shen* 人参), and nourishing *yang* 阳 (e.g., *rou gui* 肉桂 and *fu zi* 附子). These functions are also consistent with contemporary CM practice guidelines in managing different syndromes of diabetes according to its complex aetiology.

Most Frequent Formulae in Most Likely Diabetes Citations

Twenty-six citations describing the characteristic symptom "sweet urine" (*Niao tian* 尿甜) were further considered as "most likely diabetes citations". Twenty-one formulae with distance names were identified from these citations while five formulae were unnamed. Three formulae were identified as single herb formulae; these are *zhu sha* 朱砂, *gua lou* 瓜蒌 and *huang qi* 黄芪. All the cited formulae were for oral use.

The most frequently reported formulae in "most likely diabetes citations" were consistent with the ones from the "possible diabetes citations" pool with the largest number cited. Three formulae were found cited in more than two citations (see Table 3.8). *Shen qi wan*

Table 3.8. Most Frequent Oral Formulae in Most Likely Diabetes Citations

Formula Name	Herb Ingredients	No. of Citations (n)
Shen qi wan / Ba wei wan / Shen qi wan jia jian 肾气丸/八味丸/肾气丸加减	Shu di huang 熟地黄, shan yao 山药, shan zhu yu 山茱萸, ze xie 泽泻, mu dan pi 牡丹皮, fu ling 茯苓, fu zi 附子, rou gui 肉桂, wu wei zi 五味子, lu rong 鹿茸, yi zhi ren 益智仁 (*Ken Tang Yi Lun* 肯堂医论, c. 1602)	4
Liu wei di huang wan 六味地黄丸	Shan yao 山药, shan zhu yu 山茱萸, mu dan pi 牡丹皮, ze xie 泽泻, fu ling 茯苓, shu di huang 熟地黄 (*Dan Xi Xin Fa* 丹溪心法, c. 1347)	3
Qi wei bai zhu san 七味白术散	Ren shen 人参, bai zhu 白术, fu ling 茯苓, gan cao 甘草, mu xiang 木香, huo xiang 藿香, ge gen 葛根 (*Zhang Shi Yi Tong* 张氏医通, c. 1695)	2

Note:

1. Formula ingredients are based on the earliest book within the group of included citations.

2. Formulae with the same name can vary in their ingredients and the same combination of ingredients may have different names. In these data, formulae with the same name that have variations in a few ingredients are grouped together while those with large variations in ingredients are separated. Also, formulae with the same ingredients but different names have been grouped together.

3. The use of some herbs/ingredients may be restricted in some countries; for example, herbs such as *fu zi* 附子 can be toxic. Some herbs may be restricted under the Convention on International Trade in Endangered Species of Wild Fauna and Flora (CITES; e.g., *lu rong* 鹿茸). Readers are advised to comply with relevant regulations.

肾气丸 (*n* = 4, with variant formula names) and *Liu wei di huang wan* 六味地黄丸 (*n* = 3) also appeared to be two of the most frequently cited formulae in the "possible diabetes citations" formula list. Ingredients from the formula *Qi wei bai zhu san* 七味白术散 (*n* = 2) could also be identified in one of the most cited formulae *Ren shen bai zhu tang* 人参白术汤 in the "possible diabetes citations" pool. In CM practice, *Qi wei bai zhu san* 七味白术散 is prescribed for tonifying *qi* 气 and promoting body fluids (*jin* 津), which may be beneficial for treating diabetes patients with *qi* 气 and *yin* 阴 deficiency.

Most Frequent Herbs in Most Likely Diabetes Citations

The formulae obtained from the "most likely diabetes citations" were further analysed for herb ingredients. A total of 72 herb ingredients were identified from the included formulae. The most frequently cited herb ingredient list was similar to the list from "possible diabetes citations" (see Table 3.9). *Fu ling* 茯苓, obtained from 16 citations, was the most frequently reported herb in this pool. In CHM practice, *fu ling* 茯苓 is widely used to treat Spleen deficiency and damp reten-

Table 3.9.   Most Frequent Oral Herbs in Most Likely Diabetes Citations

Herb Name	Scientific Name	No. of Citations (n)
Fu ling 茯苓	*Poria cocos* (Schw.) Wolf.	16
Gan cao 甘草	*Glycyrrhizae* spp.	11
Shan zhu yu 山茱萸	*Cornus officinalis* Sieb. et Zucc.	10
Ren shen 人参	*Panax ginseng* C. A. Mey.	9
Shan yao 山药	*Dioscorea opposita* Thunb.	9
Ze xie 泽泻	*Alisma orientalis* (Sam.) Juzep.	9
Shu di huang 熟地黄	*Rehmannia glutinosa* Libosch.	9
Mu dan pi 牡丹皮	*Paeonia suffruticosa* Andr.	8
Rou gui 肉桂	*Cinnamomum cassia* Presl	7
Fu zi 附子	*Aconitum carmichaelii* Debx.	7
Mu xiang 木香	*Aucklandia lappa* Decne.	4
Bai zhu 白术	*Atractylodes macrocephala* Koidz.	4
Yuan zhi 远志	1. *Polygala tenuifolia* Willd. 2. *Polygala sibirica* L.	4
Lu rong 鹿茸	1. *Cervus nippon* Temminck 2. *Cervus elaphus* Linnaeus	4
Huang lian 黄连	1. *Coptis chinensis* Franch. 2. *Coptis deltoidea* C. Y. Cheng et Hsiao 3. *Coptis teeta* Wall.	4

Note: The use of some herbs/ingredients may be restricted in some countries; for example, herbs such as *fu zi* 附子 can be toxic. Some other herbs may be restricted under the Convention on International Trade in Endangered Species of Wild Fauna and Flora (CITES; e.g., *lu rong* 鹿茸). Readers are advised to comply with relevant regulations.

tion, as it carries the therapeutic function of nourishing the Spleen and expelling dampness, which could be beneficial for patients with diabetes syndromes related to Spleen deficiency and damp retention. Some classical literature also noted that *fu ling* 茯苓 could also have the function of generating body fluids (*jin* 津),[18,19] which could be helpful in solving the polydipsia symptom caused by *yin* 阴 deficiency or internal Heat. *Fu ling* 茯苓 also plays different roles according to the formulation principles, which could be beneficial for strengthening the formula efficacy with other herbs. For example, in *Shen qi wan* 肾气丸, the function that *fu ling* 茯苓 carries, which eliminates dampness and diuresis, could assist the herb *gui zhi* 桂枝 to promote *yang* 阳 and *qi* 气 to resolve dampness and phlegm. In the formula *Liu wei di huang wan* 六味地黄丸, *fu ling*'s 茯苓, expelling dampness in the Spleen function could assist the herb *shan yao* 山药 in nourishing the Spleen, while in *Qi wei bai zhu san* 七味白术散, *fu ling* 茯苓 also plays a similar role in resolving dampness and the Spleen with other herbs.

Discussion of Chinese Herbal Medicine for Diabetes

Findings from the ZHYD showed that most of the included citations describing CHM management for diabetes were from the Ming and Qing dynasties. It is not surprising that since more books were published, more knowledge about diabetes existed during this period. While many named or unnamed formulae have been identified from classical literature, the most frequently reported formulae were also recommended in contemporary CM guidelines and textbooks.[3,4] The formula and herb function vary among the most frequently cited CHM therapies; these include tonifying Kidney *yin* 阴 and *yang* 阳, clearing heat, nourishing the Spleen and *qi* 气, and promoting body fluids. These functions were consistent with the complex aetiology of diabetes according to contemporary guidelines.

The most frequently reported formulae in the "most likely diabetes citations" and "possible diabetes citations" were consistent, including *Shen qi wan* 肾气丸, *Liu wei di huang wan* 六味地黄丸 and *Qi wei bai zhu san* 七味白术散. These formulae have a focus on tonifying the Kidney, *yin* and Spleen, as well as generating body fluids.

It should also be noted that several toxic ingredients such as *hu fen* 胡粉, *qian dan* 铅丹 and *fu zi* 附子 were identified in the most frequently reported formulae in the possible diabetes citations pool. *Hu fen* 胡粉 (lead carbonate) and *qian dan* 铅丹 (lead oxide) were traditionally used for treating skin lesions and clearing toxins in CHM practice. They may also have been used for managing diabetes with the excessive heat toxin syndrome. However, these two ingredients are either restricted or forbidden for use in CM practice due to safety concerns in some countries.

Fu zi 附子 carries the function of warming the meridian and clearing heat and dampness. It could be beneficial for managing diabetes patients who have a deficiency of both *yin* 阴 and *yang* 阳, *yang* 阳 deficiency of the Spleen and Kidney, and cold syndromes. *Fu zi* 附子 is also one of the recommended herbs listed in contemporary guidelines and CM textbooks.[3,4] However, the aconitine contained in the herb may cause acute cardiovascular disease when inappropriately prescribed. To reduce its toxicity, some preparation methods have been invented (such as water wash and steam). In China, *zhi fu zi* 制附子 or *shu fu zi* 熟附子 is usually prescribed rather than the raw herb *sheng fu zi* 生附子. CM practitioners should be cautious when prescribing this herb in managing diabetes.

Acupuncture and Related Therapies

A total of 10 citations describing acupuncture and related therapies met the inclusion criteria and were included for analysis. These citations were obtained from seven classical books. The *Pu Ji Fang* 普济方 (c. 1406) (*n* = 3) and *Ren Zhai Zhi Zhi Fang Lun* 仁斋直指方论 (c. 1264) (*n* = 2) were two of the books that had more than one citation.

Frequency of Treatment Citations by Dynasty

Half of the identified citations (*n* = 5, 50%) were published during the Ming dynasty (c. 1369–1644) (Table 3.10). One citation was

Table 3.10.   Dynastic Distribution of Treatment Citations

Dynasty	No. of Treatment Citations
Song and Jin dynasties (961–1271)	3
Ming Dynasty (1369–1644)	5
Qing Dynasty (1645–1911)	1
Japan (Qing Dynasty)	1
Total	10

found in a Japanese book *Zhen Jiu Xue Gang Yao* 针灸学纲要 (c. 1766), published during the Qing dynasty. The earliest acupuncture citations were identified from the *Ren Zhai Zhi Zhi Fang Lun* 仁斋直指方论 (c. 1264). These citations introduced several acupuncture points for treating different symptoms possibly related to diabetes: BL20 *Pishu* 脾俞 and CV12 *Zhongwan* 中脘 were used to treat people with polydipsia. ST36 *Zusanli* 足三里 was used to treat people with polyphagia (针灸法: 脾俞二穴, 中脘一穴, 治饮不止渴. 三里二穴, 治食不充饥.). The earliest citation describing moxibustion therapy was from the *Bian Que Xin Shu* 扁鹊心书 (c.1146): applying moxibustion to the CV4 *Guanyuan* 关元 point (正法先灸关元二百壮, 服金液丹一斤而愈).

Treatment with Acupuncture and Related Therapies

Of the 10 acupuncture and related therapies citations, seven citations listed acupuncture as a therapy. The remaining three citations mentioned moxibustion, alone or in combination with acupuncture therapy (Table 3.11). Acupuncture points and meridians were obtained from these citations for further analysis.

Most Frequent Acupuncture Points in Acupuncture Citations

A total of 10 acupuncture points was found in the included citations. Acupuncture point KI3 *Taixi* 太溪 was obtained from seven citations with the highest frequency (see Table 3.12). KI3 *Taixi* 太溪 is the *yuan*

Table 3.11. Acupuncture Treatments in Diabetes Citations

Acupuncture Treatment	No. of Citations (n)
Acupuncture	7
Acupuncture and moxibustion	2
Moxibustion	1

Table 3.12. Most Frequent Acupuncture Points in Possible Diabetes Citations

Acupuncture Point	No. of Citations (n)
KI3 *Taixi*太溪	7
CV12 *Zhongwan* 中脘	3
ST36 *Zusanli* 足三里	3
BL20 *Pishu* 脾俞	2

xue of the Kidney meridian. In acupuncture practice, KI3 *Taixi* 太溪, when stimulated, carries the function of tonifying Kidney *yin* 阴 and *yang* 阳, and dispersing Heat and resolving polyuria. It could be used to treat diabetes relating to Kidney *yin* 阴 and/or *yang* 阳 deficiency syndromes. Other acupuncture points with more than one citation include CV12 *Zhongwan* 中脘 (*n* = 3), ST36 *Zusanli* 足三里 (*n* = 3) and BL20 *Pishu* 脾俞 (*n* = 2). Although they are located in different meridians, their therapeutic functions are similar. These include nourishing the Spleen and tonifying *qi* 气, and expelling dampness, which may be beneficial for resolving Spleen *qi* deficiency and the damp retention syndrome of diabetes.

Discussion of Acupuncture for Diabetes

There are a limited number of citations describing acupuncture and other related therapies for classical literature evidence evaluation. In most contemporary CM guidelines and textbooks, acupuncture and other related therapies are not in any recommendation list for the management of diabetes. One possible reason is that these invasive treatments may induce further skin infection due to the small vascular disease of diabetes. When comparing the evidence of acupuncture for diabetes from classical literature with the listings of acupuncture therapies in contemporary textbooks (see Chapter 2), the most frequently cited acupuncture points are all recommended in modern literature. The overall points carry the functions of tonifying Kidney *yin* 阴 and *yang* 阳 and Spleen *qi* 气.

Classical Literature in Perspective

After thousands of years of exploration, ancient CM practitioners formed a comprehensive understanding of diabetes and established fundamental knowledge of it. CM classical literature recorded its aetiology and pathogenesis, syndrome differentiations and treatments in detail. It continues to guide contemporary clinical practice. In classical literature, diabetes was diagnosed by its characteristic symptoms of sweet urine, emaciation, polydipsia, polyphagia and polyuria. The first disease term, *xiao ke* 消渴, that described diabetes symptoms was identified as early as the Warring States (474–221 BCE) period. Various terms were then developed to describe diabetes, according to its complex aetiology and pathogenesis and typical symptoms. Most of the identified citations were found in books published during the Ming (c. 1369–1644) and Qing dynasties (c. 1645–1911).

The aetiology and pathogenesis of diabetes were discussed comprehensively in classical literature. Many citations pointed out that overconsumption of food and wine and an indulgence in sexual activities were the two main factors of diabetes, as they cause body fluid exhaustion and deficient Heat in the *zang* 脏 and *fu* 腑. The knowledge of diabetes in classical literature is generally consistent with that of contemporary CM knowledge.

There are many Chinese herbal formulae and herbs identified in the "possible" diabetes citations. By comparison, the number is small in the "most likely" diabetes pool. The most frequently reported formulae *Shen qi wan* 肾气丸, *Liu wei di huang wan* 六味地黄丸, *Qi wei bai zhu san* 七味白术散 and *Tiao wei cheng qi tang* 调胃承气汤

in both pools are also recommended in current CM textbooks and guidelines. Herbs commonly mentioned for managing diabetes symptoms were aligned with the complex aetiology and pathogenesis of diabetes. The general functions that these herbs carried are: tonifying *qi* 气 and nourishing the Spleen, tonifying Kidney *yin* 阴 and *yang* 阳, clearing Heat, and promoting body fluids.

Evidence of acupuncture and other related therapies for diabetes is limited in classical literature. Manual acupuncture and moxibustion were the two main therapies found for diabetes, with KI3 *Taixi* 太溪 being the most frequently mentioned acupuncture point. In contemporary CM practice, acupuncture and other related therapies are seldom recommended for diabetes patients. Secondary skin infection might be a concern regarding these invasive therapies.

The systematic review of classical CM literature showed that the aetiology, pathogenesis and treatment methods of diabetes had been explored in depth for thousands of years. The precious CM knowledge documented in classical literature continues to inform and guide the management of diabetes in contemporary CM clinical practice.

References

1. Needham J, Lu G, Sivin N. (2000) *Science and Civilisation in China*. Cambridge University Press, Cambridge.
2. 仝小林. (2014) 糖尿病中医防治标准 (草案). 科学出版社, 北京.
3. 仝小林. (2016) 糖尿病中医药临床循证实践指南. 科学出版社, 北京.
4. 周仲英. (2003) 中医内科学. 中国中医药出版社, 北京.
5. Hu R. (2014) *Zhong Hua Yi Dian "Encyclopaedia of Traditional Chinese Medicine"*. Hunan Electronic and Audio-Visual Publishing House, Changsha.
6. May BH, Lu C, Xue CC. (2012) Collections of traditional Chinese medical literature as resources for systematic searches. *J Altern Complement Med* **18**(12): 1101–1107.
7. May BH, Lu Y, Lu C, et al. (2013) Systematic assessment of the representativeness of published collections of the traditional literature on Chinese medicine. *J Altern Complement Med* **19**(5): 403–409.

8. 张伯礼, 吴勉华. (2017) 中医内科学. 中国中医药出版社, 北京.

9. 王永炎. (1997) 中医内科学. 上海科学技术出版社, 上海.

10. 吴勉华, 王新月. (2012) 中医内科学. 中国中医药出版社, 北京.

11. 张伯臾, 董建华, 周仲瑛. (1985) 中医内科学. 上海科学技术出版社, 上海.

12. 国家中医药管理局. (1994) 中医病证诊断疗效标准. 南京大学出版社, 南京.

13. 中华中医药学会. (2008) 中医内科常见病诊疗指南 *(*中医疾病部分*)*. 中国中医药出版社, 北京.

14. 中华中医药学会. (2011) 糖尿病中医药防治指南. 中国中医药现代远程教育 **9**(4): 148–151.

15. 范冠杰, 邓兆智. (2013) 专科专病中医临床诊治丛书—内分泌科专病与风湿病中医临床诊治. 人民卫生出版社, 北京.

16. 王永炎, 严世芸. (2009) 实用中医内科学. 上海科学技术出版社, 上海.

17. World Health Organization. (2007) WHO international standard terminologies on traditional medicine in the western pacific region. WHO Regional Office for the Western Pacific, Manila, Philippines.

18. 李时珍. (1596) 本草纲目. 南京.

19. 张介宾. (1624) 本草正.

4

Methods for Evaluating Clinical Evidence

OVERVIEW

This chapter describes the methods used to identify and evaluate a range of Chinese medicine (CM) interventions for Type 2 diabetes mellitus in clinical studies. Studies identified through a comprehensive search were assessed against eligibility criteria. A review of the methodological quality of the studies was undertaken using standardised methods. Results from included studies were evaluated to provide an estimate of the effects of a range of CM therapies.

Introduction

The use of Chinese medicine (CM) for Type 2 diabetes mellitus (T2DM) has been well described in contemporary literature and classical CM. Several systematic reviews have been conducted to evaluate the efficacy and safety of CM treatment for T2DM. Systematic reviews have been summarised in the relevant chapters.

This chapter describes the methods used to examine the use of CM interventions for T2DM in clinical studies following the *Cochrane Handbook for Systematic Reviews.*[1] Interventions have been categorised as follows:

- Chinese herbal medicine (CHM) (Chapter 5)
- Acupuncture and related therapies (Chapter 7)
- Other CM therapies (Chapter 8)
- Combination CM therapies (Chapter 9)

References to clinical trials were obtained and assessed by an expert group. Randomised controlled trials (RCTs), non-randomised controlled clinical trials (CCTs) and non-controlled studies were evaluated in detail. CCTs were evaluated using the same approach as RCTs and have been described separately. Evidence from non-controlled clinical studies is more difficult to evaluate, therefore the approach was taken to describe the characteristics of the study, details of the intervention and any adverse events. References to the following studies comprise a letter followed by a number: CHM (e.g., H1), acupuncture and related therapies (e.g., A1), other CM therapies (e.g., O1), and combinations of CM therapies (e.g., C1) (Table 4.1).

Search Strategy

English and Chinese databases were searched for evidence and the methods followed the *Cochrane Handbook of Systematic Reviews.*[1] English databases included PubMed, Excerpta Medica Database (Embase), Cumulative Index of Nursing and Allied Health Literature (CINAHL), and the Cochrane Central Register of Controlled Trials (CENTRAL), including the Cochrane Library, and Allied and Complementary Medicine Database (AMED), while Chinese databases included China BioMedical Literature (CBM), China National Knowledge Infrastructure (CNKI), Chongqing VIP (CQVIP) and Wanfang. Databases were searched until 5 April 2018. No restrictions were applied. Search terms were mapped to controlled vocabulary (where applicable) in addition to being searched for as keywords.

To conduct a comprehensive search of the literature, searches were run according to the study design (reviews, controlled trials, non-controlled studies). This was done for each of the three intervention types (CHM, acupuncture and related therapies, and other CM therapies), resulting in the following nine searches in each of the nine databases:

1. CHM reviews.
2. CHM-controlled trials (randomised and non-randomised).

3. CHM non-controlled studies.
4. Acupuncture and related therapies reviews.
5. Acupuncture and related therapies controlled trials (randomised and non-randomised).
6. Acupuncture and related therapies non-controlled studies.
7. Other CM therapies reviews.
8. Other CM therapies controlled trials (randomised and non-randomised).
9. Other CM therapies non-controlled studies.

Studies of combination CM therapies were identified through the above searches. In addition to electronic databases, reference lists of systematic reviews and included studies were searched for in additional publications. Clinical trials registries were searched to identify ongoing or completed clinical trials and, where required, trial investigators were contacted to obtain data. The searched trial registries included the Australian New Zealand Clinical Trial Registry (ANZCTR), the Chinese Clinical Trial Registry (ChiCTR), the European Union Clinical Trials Register (EU-CTR), and the US National Institutes of Health register (ClinicalTrials.gov).

If required, trial investigators were contacted to obtain further information. Trial investigators were contacted via email or telephone and were subjected to follow-ups after two weeks if no reply was received. Where no response was received after one month, any unknown information was marked "not available".

Inclusion Criteria

- Participants: Adults diagnosed with T2DM using the guidelines from the following organisations: WHO (1999),[2] Chinese Diabetes Society,[3,4] and American Diabetes Association,[5] or a description of diagnostic criteria including:
  - o FPG ≥ 126 mg/dL (7.0 mmol/L). Fasting is defined as no caloric intake for at least 8 h.[1]*

---

[1] In the absence of unequivocal hyperglycaemia, results should be confirmed by repeat testing.

- o Or a 2-h PG ≥ 200 mg/dL (11.1 mmol/L) during an oral glucose tolerance test. The test should be performed as described by the WHO, using a glucose load containing the equivalent of 75 g anhydrous glucose dissolved in water.*
- o Or A1C ≥ 6.5% (48 mmol/mol). The test should be performed in a laboratory using a method that is certified by the National Glycohemoglobin Standardization Program and standardised to the Diabetes Control and Complications Trial assay.*
- o Or in a patient with classic symptoms of hyperglycaemia or hyperglycaemic crisis, a random plasma glucose ≥ 200 mg/dL (11.1 mmol/L).

- • Interventions: CHM, acupuncture and related therapies, or other CM therapies (Table 4.1). Integrative medicine such as CHM plus pharmacotherapy was also investigated.
- • Comparators: Placebos, conventional therapies recommended in guidelines, including pharmacotherapy, diet therapy, and lifestyle interventions.
- • Outcome measures: Studies reported at least one of the pre-specified outcome measures (Table 4.2).

Table 4.1. Chinese Medicine Interventions Included in Clinical Evidence Evaluation

Category	Intervention
Chinese herbal medicines (CHM)	Oral CHM
Acupuncture and related therapies	Acupuncture, electro-acupuncture, ear-acupressure, moxibustion
Other CM therapies	*Tuina* 推拿 (Chinese massage), *qigong* therapy 气功, *taichi* therapy太極, *Ba duan jin* (*Qigong*) therapy八段錦
Combination CM	Combination therapies are defined as two or more CM interventions from different categories administered together, for example, CHM plus acupuncture, or CHM plus *qigong* 气功.

Exclusion Criteria

- Study type: Epidemiological studies, studies that compared one type of CM therapy to other CM therapies, and duplicated studies reporting the same results.
- Participants:
  o Pre-diabetic state.
  o Type 1 diabetes.
  o Gestational diabetes.
  o Other specific types of diabetes included in the ADA and CDS:
    ▪ Genetic defects of beta-cells,
    ▪ Genetic defects in insulin action,
    ▪ Diseases of the exocrine pancreas,
    ▪ Endocrinopathies,
    ▪ Drug or chemical induced,
    ▪ Infections,
    ▪ Uncommon forms of immune-mediated diabetes, and
    ▪ Other genetic syndromes sometimes associated with diabetes.
  o Diabetic complications and comorbidities.
- Intervention: CM interventions not commonly practised world-wide and CM intravenous interventions.
- Comparators: Control not routinely recommended for chronic cough in international clinical practice guidelines or no treatment control. Control therapies that included any type of CM therapies. Integrative Medicine studies that used different therapies in the intervention groups compared to the control group.

Outcomes

Pre-specified outcomes include blood glucose tests, body mass index, quality of life, β-cell function assessment, plasma lipid profile and adverse events (Table 4.2).

Table 4.2   Pre-specified Outcomes

Outcome Categories	Outcome Measures	Scoring
Blood glucose tests	1. Fasting blood glucose (FPG)	1. Pre-diabetes: 100–125 mg/dL (5.6–6.9 mmol/L) 2. Diabetes: FPG ≥126 mg/dL (7.0 mmol/L)
	2. Postprandial blood glucose (PBG)	1. Diabetes: PBG ≥200 mg/dL (11.1 mmol/L)
	3. Glycated haemoglobin (A1C)	1. Diabetes: A1C ≥6.5% (48 mmol/mol)
Body Mass Index	1. Body Mass Index	Obesity: BMI ≥30.0, lower is better
Quality of life	1. Diabetes-Specific Quality of Life (DSQL) scale	1. Score range 27–135, lower is better
	2. Adjusted Diabetes Quality of Life (A-DQoL) measure	2. Score range 46–230, lower is better
	3. Quality of Life Scale for patients with Type 2 Diabetes Mellitus (DMQLS)	3. Score range 87–435, lower is better
β-cell function	1. Fasting insulin (FINS)	1. Normal range 4–12 mU/mL, lower is better
	2. Homeostasis Model Assessment-Insulin Resistance (HOMA-IR)	2. HOMA1-IR = (Fasting plasma insulin mU/l × Fasting plasma glucose mmol/L)/22.5, lower is better.
	3. Homeostasis Model Assessment-Insulin Sensitivity (HOMA-IS)	3. HOMA-IS = 1/(FPG*FINS), higher is better.
	4. C-peptide (CP)	4. Normal range 0.9–3.9 ng/ml, lower is better
Plasma lipids[24]	1. Triglycerides (TG)	Normal range <1.7 mmol/L (150 mg/dl), lower is better
	2. Total cholesterol (TC)	Normal range <5.18 mmol/L (200 mg/dl), lower is better

Table 4.2   (*Continued*)

Outcome Categories	Outcome Measures	Scoring
	3. High-density lipids (HDL)	Normal range >1.04 mmol/L (40 mg/dl), higher is better
	4. Low-density lipids (LDL)	Normal range <3.37 mmol/L (130 mg/dl), lower is better
Adverse events	Adverse events reported by included studies.	

Abbreviations: A-DQOL, Adjusted Diabetes Quality of Life Measure; Cp, C-peptide; Fins, Fasting insulin; FPG, Fasting blood glucose; DMQLS, Quality of Life Scale for Patients with T2DM; DSQL, Diabetes-Specific Quality of Life Scale; FPG, Fasting blood glucose; Hb1AC, Haemoglobin A1C; HDL, High-density lipids; HOMA-IR, Homeostasis Model Assessment-Insulin Resistance; HOMA-IS, Homeostasis Model Assessment-Insulin Sensitivity; LDL, Low-density lipids; PBG, Postprandial blood glucose; Tc, Total cholesterol; Tg, Triglycerides.

Fasting Plasma Glucose

Fasting plasma glucose (FPG) is a diagnostic test for diabetes mellitus. Fasting is defined as having no caloric intake for at least eight hours, after which a blood sample will be taken. An FPG level from 100 to 125 mg/dL (5.6 to 6.9 mmol/L) is considered pre-diabetes, and an FPG level higher or equal to 126 mg/dL (7.0 mmol/L) on two separate tests confirms a diabetes diagnosis.[5]

Postprandial Blood Glucose

Postprandial blood glucose test measures blood glucose two hours after an oral glucose tolerance test. The oral glucose tolerance test uses a glucose load containing the equivalent of 75 g of anhydrous glucose dissolved in water. PBG ≥ 200 mg/dL (11.1 mmol/L) during an oral glucose tolerance test indicates diabetes.[5]

Glycated Haemoglobin

The American Diabetes Association Clinical Practice Recommendations recommends using glycated haemoglobin (A1C) to diagnose diabetes using a National Glycohemoglobin Standardisation Program certified and standardised to the Diabetes Control and Complications Trial. HbA1c ≥ 6.5% (48 mmol/mol) indicates diabetes.[5]

Body Mass Index

The body mass index (BMI) is a measurement of body fat that is commonly used to classify adults as being underweight, overweight or obese.[6] It is defined as the weight in kilograms divided by the square of the height in meters (kg/m^2) and is an important reflection and measurement for diabetes and weight management.[6,7] Obesity is classified as a BMI ≥ 30;[6] however in China, a BMI ≥ 28 is classified as obese.[3] A reduction in the BMI in T2DM patients reflects reduced body fat and reduced risk for complications of T2DM.

Diabetes-Specific Quality of Life Scale

There are many quality of life scales used in clinical practice and research; in this monograph, the diabetes-specific quality of life scales was included. The included scales are introduced briefly here. In the included scales, a higher score indicates a reduced quality of life.

Diabetes-Specific Quality of Life Scale (DSQL) is a 27-item scale that measures the quality of life of diabetic patients by using questions from four domains: the effect of diabetes on one's physiological function, mental health, social relationships, and treatment. Each question has a score of 1 to 5.[8] The Adjusted Diabetes Quality of Life (A-DQoL) measure is based on the Diabetes Quality of Life (DQoL) instrument. The DQoL was published in 1988 by the Diabetes Control and Complications Trial Research Group.[9] The DQoL contains 46 items and is used to measure health-related quality of life among diabetes patients based on three main domains: "satisfaction", "impact" and "worry". The A-DQoL also has 46 questions but includes four domains: "satisfaction", "impact", "worry related to society, family or employment" and "worry related to disease".[10]

A diabetes-specific quality of life scale specifically for Chinese patients was also developed — the Quality of Life Scale for Chinese patients with T2DM (DMQLS).[11] This instrument contains 87 items and includes four domains, including "disease", "physiological", "social", "psychological" and "satisfaction".

Fasting Insulin

Fasting insulin (FINS) levels are used to assess insulin sensitivity. Impaired insulin sensitivity precedes glucose intolerance in the development of T2DM. Elevated fasting insulin is a compensatory mechanism to prevent glucose intolerance and diabetes.[12] The normal range is 4–12 μU/ml. After treatment, the lower the range is, the better.[13]

Homeostasis Model Assessment-Insulin Resistance

Insulin resistance (IR) is defined as reduced responsiveness to normal levels of insulin by target tissues (mainly liver and skeletal muscle) to insulin action.[14] The ability to measure IR is important in order to understand the aetiopathology of T2DM, to examine the epidemiology and to assess the effects of the intervention.[15] The Homeostasis Assessment Model (HOMA) is a mathematical model of the glucose insulin feedback system in the homeostatic (overnight-fasted) state. The HOMA model measures values for insulin sensitivity and β-cell function, from simultaneous fasting plasma glucose and fasting insulin to C-peptide concentrations.[16] A high HOMA-IR indicates high levels of IR.

The equation for IR calculated using the fasting plasma insulin concentration (mU/l) and fasting plasma glucose (mmol/l) is:

HOMA1-IR = (Fasting plasma insulin × Fasting plasma glucose)/22.5.[17]

Homeostasis Model Assessment-Insulin Sensitivity

Insulin sensitivity (IS) is the ability of insulin to stimulate glucose uptake, promote peripheral glucose disposal and suppress hepatic glucose production.[18] IS can be determined using the updated HOMA computer model, which determines IS (%S) and the β-cell function (%B) from paired fasting plasma glucose and radioimmunoassay insulin or specific insulin, or C-peptide concentrations across a range of 1–2,200 pmol/l for insulin and 1–25 mmol/l for glucose.[19] The updated HOMA model accounts for variations in hepatic and peripheral glucose resistance (i.e., the reduction in the suppression of hepatic glucose output [by hyperglycaemia] and the reduction of peripheral glucose-stimulated glucose uptake). These modifications provide a more accurate representation of the physiological state. As IS decreases, insulin levels will become elevated; if continued, patients may develop glucose intolerance and then T2DM.[18] The equation for IS is calculated using fasting insulin concentrations (mU/l) and fasting plasma glucose (mmol/l): HOMA-IS = 1/(Fins × FPG).

Fasting Oh C-peptide

C-peptide is produced in equal amounts to insulin and can be used to assess endogenous insulin secretion by the pancreatic β-cells.[20] C-peptide can be measured in blood and urine. The normal range for a c-peptide test is 0.9–3.9 nanograms per millilitre (ng/mL).[21] High levels of c-peptide with a low level of blood glucose could be an indication of insulin resistance.

Plasma Lipids (Triglycerides, Cholesterol, Low-Density Lipoprotein, High-Density Lipoprotein)

Plasma lipid is the cholesterol content in the blood. Plasma lipid profile includes total cholesterol (TC), triglycerides (TG), high-density lipoproteins (HDL), intermediate-density lipoproteins (IDL), low-density lipoproteins (LDL), and very low-density lipoproteins (VLDL).[22] In this monograph, we focus on TC, TG, LDL and HDL. Elevated levels of triglycerides are often the result of: being overweight, physically inactive, smoking, excessive consumption of alcohol, and diets that are high in fat and carbohydrates.[23] Elevated LDL cholesterol levels and lower levels of HDL are associated with an increased risk for incident cardiovascular disease.[22]

Adverse Events

The number and type of adverse events reported by included studies.

Risk of Bias Assessment

The risk of bias was assessed for randomised controlled trials using the Cochrane Collaboration's tool.[1] In clinical trials, bias can be categorised as selection bias, performance bias, detection bias, attrition bias and reporting bias. Each domain is assessed to determine whether the bias is at a low, high or unclear risk. A low risk of bias indicates that bias is unlikely; high risk indicates plausible bias that seriously weakens confidence in the results, and unclear bias indicates a lack of information or uncertainty over potential bias and raises some doubt about the results. A risk of bias assessment is verified by two people and any disagreement that may arise is resolved by discussion or consultation with a third person.

The risk of bias is categorised using the following six domains:

- **Sequence generation**: The method used to generate the allocation sequence is given in sufficient detail to allow an assessment of whether it should produce comparable groups. Low risk of bias refers to a random number table or computer random generator. High risk of bias includes studies that describe a non-random sequence generation such as an odd or even date of birth or admission.
- **Allocation concealment**: The method used to conceal the allocation sequence is given in enough detail to determine whether intervention allocations could have been foreseen before or during enrolment. Low risk of bias includes central randomisation or sealed envelopes and a high risk of bias includes an open random sequence, etc.

- **Blinding of participants and personnel**: Measures used to describe if the study participants and personnel are blind to the intervention received. In addition, information relating to whether the blinding was effective is also assessed. Studies that ensure the blinding of participants and personnel are at low risk of bias. If the study is not blind or incompletely blind, it is at a high risk of bias.
- **Blinding of outcome assessors**: Measures used to describe if the outcome assessors are blind to knowing which intervention a participant received. In addition, information relating to whether the blinding was effective is also assessed. Studies that ensure that outcome assessors are blinded are at low risk of bias. If the study is not blind or incompletely blind, it is at a high risk of bias.
- **Incomplete outcome data**: Completeness of outcome data for each main outcome, including dropouts, exclusions from the analysis with numbers missing in each group, and reasons for drop-outs or exclusions. Studies with a low risk of bias would include all outcome data. However, if there is missing data, it is unlikely to relate to the true outcome or is balanced between groups. Studies at a high risk of bias would have unexplained missing data.
- **Selective reporting**: The study protocol is available, and the pre-specified outcomes are included in the report. Studies with a published protocol that includes all pre-specified outcomes in their reports would be at low risk of bias. Studies at a high risk of bias would not include all pre-specified outcomes or the outcome data may be reported incompletely.

Statistical Analyses

The frequency of CM syndromes, CHM formulae, herbs and acupuncture points reported in the included studies are presented using descriptive statistics. CM syndromes reported in two or more studies were presented, and the 10 most frequently reported CHM formulae and 20 most frequently reported herbs presented were used in at least two studies, though this was not always possible for CHM formulae. The top 10 acupuncture points used in two or more studies are presented or as available. Where data was limited, reports of single CM syndromes or acupuncture points were provided as a guide for the reader.

Definitions of statistical tests and results are described in the glossary. Dichotomous data is reported as a risk ratio (RR) with 95% confidence intervals (CI), and continuous data are reported as mean difference (MD) or standardised mean difference (SMD) with 95% CI. For dichotomous data, when the RR is greater than one and the upper and lower values of the 95% CI are both greater than one, this indicates we can be 95% certain that there is a difference between the groups and that the true effect lies within these CIs. The same is true for values less than one. In such cases, we say there is "significant difference" between the groups. For continuous data, when the MD is greater than zero and both the upper and lower values of the 95% CI are greater than zero, we say there is "significant difference" between the groups. The same is true on the negative side of the scale.[1] For all analyses, the RR or MD and 95% CI were reported, together with a formal test for heterogeneity using the I^2 statistic. An I^2 score greater than 50% was considered to indicate substantial heterogeneity.[1]

Sensitivity analyses were undertaken to explore potential sources of heterogeneity based on a low risk of bias for one of the risks of bias domains — sequence generation. Where possible and appropriate, planned subgroup analyses included the comparator type, fasting blood glucose level at baseline, treatment duration, and CM syndrome differentiation. Available case analysis with a random effects model was used in all analyses. The random effects model was used to take into account the clinical heterogeneity likely to be encountered within and between included studies and the variation in treatment effects between included studies.

Assessment Using Grading of Recommendations, Assessment, Development and Evaluation

The Grading of Recommendations, Assessment, Development and Evaluation (GRADE) approach was used.[25,26] The GRADE approach summarises and rates the strength and certainty of evidence in systematic reviews using a structured process for presenting evidence summaries. The results are presented in the summary of the findings tables. The results provide an important overview for T2DM outcomes.

A panel of experts was established to evaluate the certainty of evidence. The panel included the systematic review team, CM practitioners, integrative medicine experts, research methodologists and conventional medicine physicians. The experts were asked to rate the clinical importance of key interventions from CHM, acupuncture therapies, and other CM therapies, as well as comparators and outcomes. Results were collated, and based on the rating scores and subsequent discussion, a consensus on the content for the summary of findings tables was achieved.

The certainty of the evidence for each outcome was rated according to five factors outlined in the GRADE approach. The certainty of evidence may be rated based on:

- Limitations in study design (risk of bias),
- Inconsistency of results (unexplained heterogeneity),
- Indirectness of evidence (interventions, populations and outcomes that are important to the patients with the condition),
- Imprecision (uncertainty about the results), and
- Publication bias (selective publication of studies).

These five factors are additive, and a reduction in one or more factors will reduce the certainty of the evidence for that outcome. The GRADE approach also includes methods for assessing observational studies. GRADE summaries in this monograph only include RCTs.

Treatment recommendations can also be assessed using the GRADE approach, but due to the diverse nature of CM practice, treatment recommendations were not included with the summary of findings. Therefore, the reader should interpret the evidence with reference to the local practice environment. It should also be noted that the GRADE approach requires judgements about the strength and certainty of evidence and some subjective assessment. However, the experience of the panel members suggests that the judgements are reliable and transparent representations of the certainty of evidence.

The GRADE levels of evidence are grouped into four categories:

1) High certainty: Very confident that the true effect lies close to that of the estimate of the effect,
2) Moderate certainty: Moderately confident in the effect estimate: The true effect is likely to be close to the estimate of the effect, but there is a possibility that it is substantially different,
3) Low certainty: Confidence in the effect estimate is limited: The true effect may be substantially different from the estimate of the effect, and
4) Very low certainty: Very little confidence in the effect estimate: The true effect is likely to be substantially different from the estimate of effect.

References

1. Higgins JPT, Green S, eds. (2011, updated) *Cochrane Handbook for Systematic Reviews of Interventions Version 5.1.0*. The Cochrane Collaboration, 2011. Available from: www.cochrane-handbook. org2011.
2. World Health Organization. (1999) Definition, diagnosis and classification of diabetes mellitus and its complications: Report of a WHO consultation. Part 1, Diagnosis and classification of diabetes mellitus. Geneva, Switzerland.
3. 中华医学会糖尿病学分会. (2011) 中国2型糖尿病防治指南 (2010年版). 中国北京, 北京大学出版社.
4. 中华医学会糖尿病学分会. (2014) 中国2型糖尿病防治指南 (2013年版). 中华糖尿病杂志 **6**(7): 447–498.
5. American Diabetes Association. (2019) 2. Classification and diagnosis of diabetes: Standards of medical care in diabetes — 2019. *Diabetes Care* **42**(Supplement 1): S13.
6. World Health Organization. (2000) Obesity: Preventing and managing the global epidemic. WHO Technical Report Series 894. Geneva, Switzerland.

7. WHO Expert Consultation. (2004) Appropriate body-mass index for Asian populations and its implications for policy and intervention strategies. *Lancet* **363**(9403): 157–163.

8. 周凤琼. (1997) 世界卫生组织生存质量量表—糖尿病特异模块的研制及应用. 中山大学, 中国广州.

9. Jacobsen A, Barofsky I, Cleary P, Rand L. (1988) Reliability and validity of a diabetes quality-of-life measure for the diabetes control and complications trial (DCCT). The DCCT Research Group. *Diabetes Care* **11**(9): 725–732.

10. 丁元林, 孙丹莉, 倪宗瓚, 邓浩华. (2004) 糖尿病特异性生存质量量表的文化调适与修订. 中国行为医学科学 **13**(1): 102–103.

11. 王乐三, 孙振球, 蔡太生, 周智广. (2005) 2型糖尿病患者生活质量量表的研制与考评. 中南大学学报(医学版) **30**(1): 21–27.

12. Carrillo A, Gomez-Meade C. (2013) Fasting insulin. In: *Encyclopedia of Behavioral Medicine*. Gellman MD, Turner JR, eds. Springer, New York, p. 785.

13. Chinese Diabetes Society. (2017) Guidelines for the prevention and treatment of Type 2 diabetes mellitus in China. *Chin J Diabetes Mellitus* **10**(1): 4–67.

14. Moller DE, Kaufman KD. (2005) Metabolic syndrome: A clinical and molecular perspective. *Annu Rev Med* **56**: 45–62.

15. Wallace TM, Matthews DR. (2002) *The Assessment of Insulin Resistance in Man*. Oxford, UK, pp. 527–534.

16. Matthews D, Hosker J, Rudenski A, *et al.* (1985) Homeostasis model assessment: Insulin resistance and β-cell function from fasting plasma glucose and insulin concentrations in man. *Clinical and Experimental Diabetes and Metabolism* **28**(7): 412–419.

17. Wallace TM, Levy JC, Matthews DR. (2004) Use and abuse of HOMA modeling. *Diabetes Care* **27**(6): 1487–1495.

18. Sanchez J. (2013) Insulin sensitivity. In: *Encyclopedia of Behavioral Medicine*. Gellman MD, Turner JR, eds. Springer, New York, p. 1085.

19. Levy J, Matthews D, Hermans M. (1998) Correct homeostasis model assessment (HOMA) evaluation uses the computer program. *Diabetes Care* **21**(12): 2191–2192.

20. Jones AG, Hattersley AT. (2013) The clinical utility of C-peptide measurement in the care of patients with diabetes. *Diabetic Med* **30**(7): 803–817.

21. 中华医学会糖尿病学分会. (2018) 中国 2 型糖尿病防治指南 (2017 年版). 中华糖尿病杂志 **10**(1): 4–67.

22. Harlapur M, Shimbo D. (2013) Lipid, plasma. In: *Encyclopedia of Behavioral Medicine*. Gellman MD, Turner JR, eds. Springer, New York.

23. Barrett C. (2013) Triglyceride. In: *Encyclopedia of Behavioral Medicine*. Gellman MD, Turner JR, eds. Springer, New York, pp. 2008–2009.

24. 王鸿利. (2010) 实验诊断学. 2nd edition. 中国北京, 人民卫生出版社.

25. Schunemann H, Brozek J, Guyatt G, *et al.* (2013) *GRADE Handbook for Grading Quality of Evidence and Strength of Recommendations*. Group TGW, ed. The GRADE Working Group. Available from: www.guidelinedevelopment.org/handbook

26. Schünemann H, Higgins J, Vist G, *et al.* (2019, updated) Chapter 14: Completing "summary of findings" tables and grading the certainty of the evidence. In: *Cochrane Handbook for Systematic Reviews of Interventions version 6.0*. Higgins JPT, Thomas J, Chandler J, *et al.*, eds. Cochrane. Available from: www.training.cochrane.org/handbook

5

Clinical Evidence for Chinese Herbal Medicine

OVERVIEW

Clinical studies of Chinese herbal medicine (CHM) have tested the efficacy and safety for the treatment of type 2 diabetes mellitus (T2DM). This chapter evaluates 236 clinical studies on CHM for T2DM and includes 149 formulae and 202 herbs. The meta-analyses of randomised controlled trials and results from controlled clinical trials indicate that CHM showed benefits in improving biochemical indexes for people with T2DM. In addition, CHM was well tolerated by people with T2DM.

Introduction

Chinese herbal medicine (CHM) is an important Chinese medicine (CM) therapy for type 2 diabetes mellitus (T2DM). Contemporary clinical guidelines of CM for T2DM describe the use of formula according to syndrome differentiation (Chapter 2). Classical Chinese medicine text analysis indicates that CHM was the main CM therapy used to manage T2DM symptoms (Chapter 3). Many clinical studies have evaluated the potential role of CHM for people with T2CM. This chapter reviews the clinical evidence from randomised controlled trials (RCTs), controlled clinical trials (CCTs) and non-controlled studies. CHM oral preparations for T2DM include decoctions, granules, solutions, tablets and capsules. Many different herb combinations and formulae have been used to treat T2DM, and the most commonly evaluated in clinical trials are presented in this chapter.

Previous Systematic Reviews

The efficacy of CHM for T2DM has been evaluated in systematic reviews and meta-analyses. Several reviews evaluated the efficacy of CHM alone or in combination with conventional medicine for T2DM. In 2016, a review was conducted on the systematic reviews on traditional CM treatment of T2DM.[1] Eighteen systematic reviews and meta-analyses were considered, of which 15 analysed the efficacy of CHMs. The re-evaluation of the efficacy and safety of Chinese patent medicine and herbal extracts treatment for T2DM suggested some clinical efficacy of Chinese patent medicine when compared with conventional medicine or a placebo treatment. However, the Grading of Recommendations, Assessment, Development and Evaluation (GRADE) classification ranged from low to medium quality, and the authors advised clinicians to interpret the results with caution.

A Cochrane systematic review originally published in 2002 (and updated in 2009) assessed the effects of CHM in patients with T2DM and included 66 RCTs (8,302 participants).[2] Sixty-nine different herbal medicines were tested in the included trials, which compared herbal medicines with placebos, hypoglycaemic agents, or herbal medicines plus hypoglycaemic agents. Results showed that compared with the placebo, Holy basil leaves, *Xian zhen* tablets 仙真片, *Qi dan tong mai* tablets 芩丹通脉片, traditional Chinese formulae, *Huo xue jiang tang ping zhi* 活血降糖平脂, and Inolter improved blood glucose control. When CHM was compared with hypoglycaemic agents — including glibenclamide, tolbutamide or gliclazide — seven herbal medicines demonstrated significantly better metabolic control, including *Bu shen jiang tang tang* 补肾降糖汤, composite *Trichosanthis*, *Jiang tang kang* 降糖汤, *Ke tang ling* 克糖灵, *Shen qi jiang tang yin* 参芪降糖饮, *Xiao ke tang* 消渴汤 and *Yi shen huo xue tiao gan* 益肾活血调肝. In 29 trials that evaluated herbal medicines combined with hypoglycaemic agents, 15 different herbal preparations showed additional hypoglycaemic effects apart from hypoglycaemic agent monotherapy. Furthermore, two studies on herbal therapies, when combined with diet and behaviour change, showed better hypoglycaemic effects than just diet and behaviour change alone. In this review, no serious adverse effects from the herbal medicines were reported. However, these findings should be carefully interpreted due to the low methodological quality, small sample size, and a limited number of trials.

In 2007, Yang and colleagues reported on the effects of CHM plus conventional medicine compared to conventional medicine alone in the treatment for T2DM.[3] In this review, 20 studies were included (2,732 participants). The results showed that the therapeutic effect of CHM plus conventional medicine on T2DM was better than conventional medicine alone, where fasting plasma glucose (FPG), total triglyceride (TG), and total cholesterol (TC) levels were reduced. The methodological quality of the included RCTs was low, and therefore, no firm conclusion could be drawn.

In 2010, Zhang and colleagues reported on a systematic review of randomised controlled trials of CM treatment for T2DM.[4] The results showed that CM treatment of T2DM may be effective in reducing the FPG, postprandial blood glucose (PBG), and glycated haemoglobin (A1C) levels and improving insulin sensitivity, and that there is potential to improve diabetes symptoms.

A Ph.D. thesis (2012) reviewed 232 studies, and meta-analysis was performed on 170 RCTs.[5] Compared to a placebo, *semen Trigonellae* saponins capsules and Extracts of Touchi had beneficial effects on A1C and PBG level control, and the Korean red *Radix ginseng* and *semen Trigonella* saponins capsule had an effect on reducing the FPG level. CHM, when combined with hypoglycaemic agents, was better than hypoglycaemic agents alone to reduce the A1C, FPG, PBG, symptom score, and QOL score level. The authors found that 27.65% (47/170) of the included studies reported adverse effects.

A review published in 2018 included 58 RCTs involving 6,637 participants with T2DM, with trial periods averaging 12 weeks.[6] A total of 132 different CHMs were examined. This included studies comparing CHM with other interventions, and it evaluated primary outcomes of trials in accordance with the *Cochrane Handbook for Systematic Reviews of Intervention*. This review reported that for people with T2DM, CHMs were effective at controlling blood sugar and insulin resistance, and traditional CM clinical symptoms scores were reduced in 19 studies. However, evidence is limited because of the quality of the studies.

Identification of Clinical Studies

A search of nine databases identified 66,570 potentially relevant citations. After removing duplicates and excluding ineligible studies by reviewing the titles and abstracts (41,729 studies), the full-text articles of 3,229 citations were retrieved (Figure 5.1). After reading the full-text articles, 2,993 were not relevant and excluded from review in this chapter. Of the 236 studies, 210 were RCTs (H1–H210), 10 were CCTs (H211–H220), and 16 were non-controlled studies (H221–H236). Studies are denoted by the letter "H", and then followed by a number. Corresponding references can be found at the end of the chapter.

All studies were conducted in China. Effects of CHM generated from RCTs and CCTs were synthesised using meta-analysis.

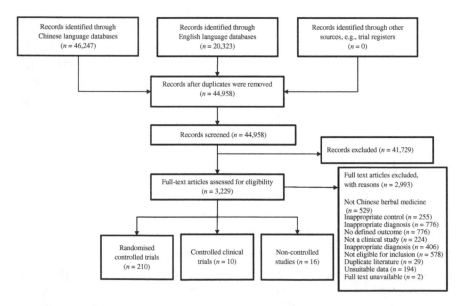

Figure 5.1. Flow chart of the study selection process: Chinese herbal medicine.

Non-controlled studies are summarised and described, but their results are not included in the meta-analysis.

The participants ranged from 39 to 87 years of age while an average course of T2DM ranged from two days to 30 years. All studies assessed T2DM only. Type 1 diabetes mellitus, gestational diabetes mellitus, specific types of diabetes, diabetic complications, and diabetes mellitus with other diseases (such as diabetes mellitus with hypertension and diabetes mellitus with cardiovascular disease) were not included. CM syndromes were reported at baseline in 146 studies and the most common syndrome was *qi* and *yin* deficiency 气阴两虚. Other common syndromes included *yin* deficiency and excessive heat 阴虚热盛, damp heat obstructing the Spleen 湿热困脾, phlegm-dampness and Blood stasis 痰湿血瘀, Spleen deficiency, and Liver *qi* stagnation.

Chinese Herbal Medicine Treatments

CHM alone was assessed in 60 studies (H1–H40, H200–H214, H222, H225, H232, H233, H236), and 176 studies combined CHM with conventional treatment recommended in guidelines (H41–H199, H215–H221, H223, H224, H226–H231, H234, H235). All CHM treatments were orally administrated. Oral preparation types included decoction, oral solution, capsules, granules, pills and tablets.

A total of 149 distinct formulae and 202 different herbs were investigated in the included clinical studies. The most common formulae were *Liu wei di huang wan* 六味地黄丸 (five studies), *Shen qi jiang tang ke li* 参芪降糖颗粒 (five studies), *Jin li da ke li* 津力达颗粒 (four studies), and *Huang lian su* 黄连素 (four studies). The most frequent herbs were *huang qi* 黄芪 (131), *sheng di huang* 生地黄 (115), *ge gen* 葛根 (95), *dan shen* 丹参 (86), *mai men dong* 麦门冬 (84), *shan yao* 山药 (83), *huang lian* 黄连 (83), *fu ling* 茯苓 (81), *tian hua fen* 天花粉 (77) and *zhi mu* 知母 (59). Controls included placebo, pharmacotherapies and lifestyle management, including diabetes self-management education, medical nutrition therapy, physical activity, and psychosocial care.

Randomised Controlled Trials of Oral Chinese Herbal Medicine

Oral CHM was tested in 210 RCTs (H1–H210) involving 19,805 people with T2DM. Fifty-one studies used CHM alone (H1–H40, H205–H210, H200–H204), while 159 studies assessed a combination of CHM with conventional medication (Integrative Medicine) (H41–H199). Most studies were two-arm design, five RCTs (H3, H9, H24, H28, H31) were three arms, and three RCTs (H19, H56, H207) were of four arms. CHM or integrative medicine was compared to pharmacologic therapy, placebo or lifestyle intervention with no pharmacologic therapy. Various types of hypoglycaemic agents were used, including biguanides, sulfonylureas, thiazolidinediones, α-Glucosidase inhibitors, meglitinides, DPP-4 inhibitors, GLP-1 receptor agonists, and insulins. Lifestyle management of T2DM includes diabetes self-management education and support (DSMES), medical nutrition therapy (MNT), physical activity, and psychosocial care.

All studies were in accordance with the 1999 World Health Organization (WHO) diagnostic criteria for T2DM. Included participants' age ranged from 20 to 87 years. Their duration of T2DM ranged from two days to 28 years, and the treatment duration ranged from two to 24 weeks. Only four studies (H2, H49, H85, H112) implemented follow-ups after treatment, and the longest follow-up duration was one year.

CM syndrome differentiation was described in 145 studies. The most common syndromes included *qi* and *yin* deficiency 气阴两虚, *yin* deficiency and excessive heat 阴虚热盛, damp heat obstructing the Spleen 湿热困脾, phlegm-dampness and Blood stasis 痰湿血瘀.

A total of 128 distinct formulae were assessed in the studies and the most common formula was *Liu wei di huang wan* 六味地黄丸, which was used in five studies (Table 5.1). A diverse range of herbs was used across in the formulae; in total, 183 distinct herbs were used and the most frequently used herb was *huang qi* 黄芪 (Table 5.2).

Table 5.1.   Frequently Reported Oral Formulae in Randomised Controlled Trials

Most Common Formulae	No. of Studies	Ingredients (Studies)
Liu wei di huang wan 六味地黄丸	5	*Shu di huang* 熟地黄, *shan zhu yu* 山茱萸, *mu dan pi* 牡丹皮, *shan yao* 山药, *fu ling* 茯苓, *ze xie* 泽泻 (H70, H85, H92, H116, H129)
Shen qi jiang tang granule 参芪降糖颗粒	4	*Ren shen* 人参, *wu wei zi* 五味子, *huang qi* 黄芪, *shan yao* 山药, *sheng di huang* 生地黄, *fu pen zi* 覆盆子, *mai men dong* 麦门冬, *fu ling* 茯苓, *tian hua fen* 天花粉, *ze xie* 泽泻, *gou qi zi* 枸杞子 (H29, H61, H119, H183)
Jin li da granule 津力达颗粒	4	*Ren shen* 人参, *huang jing* 黄精, *cang zhu* 苍术, *ku shen* 苦参, *mai dong* 麦冬, *sheng di huang* 生地黄, *he shou wu* 何首乌, *shan zhu yu* 山茱萸, *fu ling* 茯苓, *pei lan* 佩兰, *huang lian* 黄连, *zhi mu* 知母, *yin yang huo* 淫羊藿, *dan shen* 丹参, *ge gen* 葛根, *li zhi he* 荔枝核, *di gu pi* 地骨皮 (H19, H102, H117, H133)
Huang lian su tablets 黄连素片	4	Berberine tablets 盐酸小檗碱 (H90, H201, H203, H209)
Xiao ke fang 消渴方	3	*Huang lian* 黄连, *tian hua fen* 天花粉, *ren ru zhi/niu ru zhi* 人乳汁 (或牛乳), *ou* 藕, *sheng di huang* 生地黄, *sheng jiang* 生姜, *feng mi* 蜂蜜 (H63, H79, H85)
Yu quan wan 玉泉丸	3	*Ge gen* 葛根, *tian hua fen* 天花粉, *sheng di huang* 生地黄, *mai men dong* 麦门冬, *wu wei zi* 五味子, *gan cao* 甘草 (H57, H77, H178)
Shen di shen jin capsule 参地生津胶囊	2	*Ren shen* 人参, *shen di huang* 生地黄, *mai men dong* 麦门冬, *dan shen* 丹参, *san qi* 三七, *huang qi* 黄芪, *ge gen* 葛根, *shan yao* 山药 (H34, H159)
Tian mai xiao ke tablets 天麦消渴片	2	*Tian hua fen* 天花粉, *mai men dong* 麦门冬, *wu wei zi* 五味子 (H31, H186)
Da huang huang lian xie xin tang 大黄黄连泻心汤	2	*Da huang* 大黄, *huang lian* 黄连, *huang qin* 黄芩 (H30, H199)

(Continued)

105

Table 5.1.   (*Continued*)

Most Common Formulae	No. of Studies	Ingredients (Studies)
Yu nü jian 玉女煎	2	*Shi gao* 石膏, *shu di huang* 熟地黄, *zhi mu* 知母, *mai men dong* 麦冬, *niu xi* 牛膝 (H149, H85)
Ren shen bai hu tang 人参白虎汤	2	*Shi gao* 石膏, *zhi mu* 知母, *xi yang shen* 西洋参, *ge gen* 葛根, *yu zhu* 玉竹, *shu di hang* 熟地黄, *shan yao* 山药, *shan zhu yu* 山 茱萸, *ren shen* 人参, *gan cao* 甘草 (H17, H49)
Zhi bai di huang tang 知柏地黄汤	2	*Sheng di huang* 生地黄, *zhi mu* 知母, *shan yao* 山药, *tian hua fen* 天花粉, *mu dan pi* 牡丹皮, *ze xie* 泽泻, *tao ren* 桃仁, *fu ling* 茯苓 (H83, H127)
Ku gua capsule 苦瓜 胶囊	2	*Ku gua* 苦瓜 (H41, H42)

Ingredients are referenced to their original studies where possible. If herb ingredients varied across studies, the herb ingredients were sourced from the *Zhong Yi Fang Ji Da Ci Dian* 中医方剂大辞典.

Note: The use of some herbs may be restricted in some countries. Readers are advised to comply with relevant regulations.

Table 5.2.   Frequently Reported Orally Used Herbs in Randomised Controlled Trials

Most Common Herbs	Scientific Name	Frequency of Use
Huang qi 黄芪	*Astragalus membranaceus* (Fisch.) Bge.	118
Sheng di huang 生地黄	*Rehmannia glutinosa* (Gaertn.) Libosch.	102
Ge gen 葛根	*Pueraria lobata* (Willd.) Ohwi	86
Huang lian 黄连	*Coptis* spp.	78
Dan shen 丹参	*Salvia miltiorrhiza* Bge.	78
Mai men dong 麦门冬	*Ophiopogon japonicus* Ker-Gawler (Liliaceae)	75
Shan yao 山药	*Dioscorea opposita* Thunb.	74
Fu ling 茯苓	*Poria cocos* (Schw.) Wolf	70
Tian hua fen 天花粉	*Trichosanthes kirilowii* Maxim.	70
Zhi mu 知母	*Anemarrhena asphodeloides* Bge	51

Table 5.2. *(Continued)*

Most Common Herbs	Scientific Name	Frequency of Use
Bai zhu 白术	*Atractylodes macrocephala* Koidz.	47
Shan zhu yu 山茱萸	*Cornus officinalis* Sieb. et Zucc.	44
Ren shen 人参	*Panax ginseng* C. A. Meyer.	39
Wu wei zi 五味子	*Schisandra chinensis* (Turcz.) Baill.	37
Cang zhu 苍术	*Atractylodes lancea*	36
Ze xie 泽泻	*Alisma orientalis* (Sam.) Juzep.	36
Huang jing 黄精	*Polygonatum kingianum* Coll. et Hemsl.	35
Xuan shen 玄参	*Scrophularia ningpoensis* Hemsl.	32
Huang qin 黄芩	*Scutellaria baicalensis* Georgi	30
Mu dan pi 牡丹皮	*Paeonia suffruticosa* Andr.	28

Risk of Bias

All RCTs were described as "randomised". However, only 64 (30.5%) described an appropriate method of random sequence generation. Eleven studies (5.2%) described the method of allocation concealment, while 199 (94.8%) were judged to be of unclear risk of bias because they did not describe the details of allocation concealment. Blinding of participants and personnel was reported in six studies (2.9%), which were judged to be at low risk of bias, and 201 studies (95.7%) were judged as high risk. The method of blinding of outcome assessors was judged as a low risk of bias in seven studies (3.3%). All outcome data were available for 201 studies (95.7%), and they were assessed to be of low risk of bias for this domain. Selective outcome reporting was reported in 160 studies (76.2%) that were judged to be of unclear risk of bias, and 48 studies (22.8%) were judged as high risk because their reported outcomes did not match those that are pre-specified. A summary of the assessment of bias is presented in Table 5.3.

Outcomes

In the following sections, meta-analysis results are presented according to the outcome measure. For each outcome, studies are grouped

Table 5.3. Risk of Bias of Randomised Controlled Trials: Oral Chinese Herbal Medicines

Risk of Bias Domain	Low Risk n(%)	Unclear Risk n(%)	High Risk n(%)
Sequence generation	64(30.5)	123(58.6)	23(10.9)
Allocation concealment	11(5.2)	199(94.8)	0(0.0)
Blinding of participants	6(2.9)	3(1.4)	201(95.7)
Blinding of personnel	6(2.9)	3(1.4)	201(95.7)
Blinding of outcome assessors	7(3.3)	3(1.4)	200(95.3)
Incomplete outcome data	201(95.7)	9(4.3)	0(0.0)
Selective outcome reporting	2(1.0)	160(76.2)	48(22.8)

by the type of comparison: CHM versus placebo, CHM versus hypo-glycaemic agents, CHM plus hypoglycaemic agents integrative medicine (IM) versus hypoglycaemic agents, CHM versus lifestyle intervention only with no pharmacologic therapy, and CHM plus hypoglycaemic agents versus only lifestyle intervention with no pharmacologic therapy.

Sensitivity analyses were undertaken to explore potential sources of heterogeneity, based on a low risk of bias for sequence generation. Where possible, subgroup analysis included comparator drug class, FPG level at baseline (6–8 mmol/L, 8–10 mmol/L, ≥10 mmol/L), treatment duration (≤3 months, 3–6 months and ≥6 months), and CM syndrome differentiation.

Fasting Plasma Glucose

Two hundred of the 210 studies, including 18,428 participants, assessed FPG levels in patients with T2DM. A lower FPG value indicates greater improvement. Overall, meta-analysis for FPG was performed at the end of treatment based on different comparators.

Chinese Herbal Medicine vs. Placebo

Six RCTs (H205–H210) with 1,052 participants compared CHM with a placebo. The treatment duration ranged from 12 to 24 weeks.

The result showed that CHM was superior to the placebo in reducing FPG levels (MD −1.07 [−1.67, −0.48]; I^2 = 92.3%); however, heterogeneity was high.

Chinese Herbal Medicine vs. Lifestyle Intervention

Seven RCTs (H9, H19, H200–H204) with 525 participants compared CHM with lifestyle intervention. The treatment duration ranged from two to 24 weeks. The result showed that CHM was superior to lifestyle intervention at reducing FPG levels at the end of treatment (MD −1.11 [−1.54, −0.68]; I^2 = 65.0%).

Chinese Herbal Medicine vs. Pharmacotherapy

Thirty-nine RCTs (n = 3,484; H1–H25, H27–H40) compared CHM with hypoglycaemic agents. Different classes of pharmacotherapy were used as comparators, including biguanides, sulfonylureas, thiazolidinediones, a-Glucosidase inhibitors, and aspirin. Specific hypoglycaemic agents include metformin, glimepiride, glipizide, glyburide, pioglitazone, rosiglitazone, and acarbose. The treatment duration ranged from four to 24 weeks.

The overall meta-analysis result showed no difference in the FPG levels between the CHM group and pharmacological therapies (MD −0.16 [−0.33, 0.02]; I^2 = 76.1%) (Table 5.4). A meta-analysis of studies assessed as low risk for sequence generation produced a result that was more homogeneous (12 studies, 1,287 participants, MD −0.10 [−0.34, 0.15]; I^2 = 61%), but still with no difference between CHM and pharmacotherapy.

A subgroup analysis showed the benefit in reducing FPG levels in people receiving CHM compared to α-Glucosidase inhibitors (MD −0.60 [−0.99, −0.22]; I^2 = 74.5%); however, when compared to other classes of hypoglycaemic drugs and aspirin, CHM did not show more benefits. In 10 RCTs (H4, H12, H16, H27, H29, H31, H32, H37–H39), including 862 participants with high levels of FPG at baseline (≥10 mmol/L), the results showed that CHM was superior at reducing FPG levels (MD −0.49 [−0.76, −0.22]; I^2 = 50.9%). When

Table 5.4. Chinese Herbal Medicine vs. Pharmacotherapy: Fasting Plasma Glucose

Group	No. of Studies (Participants)	MD [95% CI], I^2%	Included Studies
All studies	39 (3,484)	−0.16 [−0.33, 0.02]; 76.1%	H1–25, H27–40
Low risk of bias SG	12 (1,287)	−0.10 [−0.34, 0.15]; 61.0%	H2, H8–H10, H13, H18, H19, H22–H24, H30, H35
Agent class			
Biguanides	24 (2,133)	−0.11 [−0.32, 0.10]; 72.4%	H1, H4, H5, H8, H10, H12, H15–H21, H23–H25, H28–H30, H32, H33, H35, H37, H39
α-Glucosidase inhibitors	3 (296)	−0.60 [−0.99, −0.22]*; 74.5%	H9, H11, H38
TZDs	5 (388)	−0.34 [−0.75, 0.07]; 43.5%	H2, H7, H22, H36, H40
Sulfonylureas	5 (545)	0.25 [−0.57, 1.07]; 91.0%	H3, H14, H27, H31, H34
Hypoglycaemic agents (not specified)	1 (64)	−0.10 [−0.96, 0.76]	H6
Aspirin	1 (58)	−0.86 [−2.11, 0.39]	H13
FPG level at baseline			
6–8 mmol/L	2 (194)	−0.24 [−0.07, 0.55]; 0.0%	H7, H23
8–10 mmol/L	27 (2,428)	−0.09 [−0.30, 0.12]; 76.9%	H1–H3, H5, H6, H8–H10, H11, H13–H15, H17–H22, H24, H25, H28, H30, H33, H34–H36, H40
≥10 mmol/L	10 (862)	−0.491 [−0.76, −0.22]*; 50.9%	H4, H12, H16, H27, H29, H31, H32, H37–H39

Table 5.4. *(Continued)*

Group	No. of Studies (Participants)	MD [95% CI], I²%	Included Studies
Treatment duration			
≤3 months	38 (3,404)	−0.15 [−0.33, 0.03]; 76.7%	H1–H8, H10–H25, H27–H40
≥6 months	1 (80)	−0.36 [−0.71, −0.01]*	H9
CM syndrome differentiation			
Qi and *yin* deficiency	8 (688)	−0.10 [−0.69, 0.49]; 86.6%	H3, H14, H15, H25, H29, H34, H36, H40
Yin deficiency and excessive heat	7 (489)	0.01 [−0.21, 0.23]; 32.7%	H5, H8, H17, H21, H22, H24, H35
Damp heat retention	5 (486)	0.07 [−0.48, 0.63]; 81.7%	H2, H7, H23, H32, H33
Phlegm-dampness and Blood stasis	1 (60)	−0.97 [−1.49, −0.45]*	H20

*Statistically significant

Abbreviations: CI, confidence interval; CM, Chinese medicine; FPG, fasting plasma glucose; MD, mean difference; SG, sequence generation; TZDs, thiazolidinedione.

subgroup analysis was based on treatment duration, one study with longer treatment duration showed a benefit in CHM when compared to pharmacotherapy (MD −0.36 [−0.71, −0.01]). Treatment duration of less than three months did not show any difference between the groups. Additional subgroup analysis showed that the CHM group is superior when compared to pharmacotherapy in people with the CM syndrome phlegm-dampness and Blood stasis (1 study, *n* = 60) (H20) (MD −0.97 [−1.49, −0.45]).

Chinese Herbal Medicine Plus Pharmacotherapy vs. Pharmacotherapy

A total of 155 RCTs (H3, H19, H24, H28, H31, H41–H45, H47, H49, H50–H72, H74–H111, H113–H124, H126–H131, H133,

H134, H136–H165, H167–H180, H182–H199), including 13,582 participants, assessed the effects of CHM plus hypoglycaemic agents versus hypoglycaemic agents alone; these studies used the same hypoglycaemic agents in both groups. The treatment duration ranged from two to 24 weeks. Different classes of hypoglycaemic agents were used across studies, including biguanides, sulfonylureas, thiazolidinediones, α-Glucosidase inhibitors, meglitinides, DPP-4 inhibitors, GLP-1 receptor agonists and insulins. Specific hypoglycaemic agents include metformin, gliclazide, glipizide, glibenclamide, gliclazone, glimepiride, pioglitazone, repaglinide, nateglinide, acarbose, sitagliptin, liraglutide and insulin.

The integrative use of CHM plus hypoglycaemic agents was superior to hypoglycaemic agents alone at reducing FPG levels at the end of treatment (MD −0.84 [−0.93, −0.75]; I^2 = 85.4%), although heterogeneity was high. A meta-analysis of studies assessed as low risk for sequence generation produced a similar result to that of the overall results (44 RCTs, 3,680 participants, MD −0.70 [−0.84, −0.57]; I^2 = 83%).

A subgroup analysis based on a pharmacotherapy drug class showed that except for DPP-4 inhibitors, CHM together with other hypoglycaemic agents were superior at reducing FPG levels than hypoglycaemic agents alone (Table 5.5). Combinations of different drug classes also showed a significant difference between groups. Additional subgroup analyses based on baseline levels of FPG, treatment duration, and CM syndrome differentiation all showed significant differences between groups (Table 5.5).

Postprandial Blood Glucose

A total of 179 studies, including 16,567 participants, assessed the postprandial blood glucose (PBG) level in people with T2DM. A lower value on PBG indicates greater improvement. Overall meta-analysis for PBG was performed at the end of treatment based on different comparators.

Table 5.5.   Chinese Herbal Medicine Plus Pharmacotherapy vs. Pharmacotherapy: Fasting Plasma Glucose

Group	No. of Studies (Participants)	MD [95% CI], I^2%	Included Studies
All studies	155 (13,582)	−0.84 [−0.93, −0.75]*; 85.4%	H3, H19, H24, H28, H31, H41–H45, H47, H49, H50–H72, H74–H111, H113–124, H126–H131, H133–134, H136–165, H167–180, H182–199
Low risk of bias SG	44 (3,680)	−0.70 [−0.84, −0.57]*; 83.0%	H19, H51, H57, H60, H63–H66, H78–H80, H82, H84, H86, H87, H90, H91, H96, H97, H100, H102, H106, H110, H116, H119, H122, H124, H126, H24, H129, H134, H140, H144, H146, H163, H165, H168, H173–H176, H183, H193, H199
Drug class			
Biguanides	57 (5,170)	−1.00 [−1.14, −0.87]*; 81.1%	H19, H24, H28, H41, H42, H44, H45, H47, H60–H63, H65, H66, H68, H69, H72, H74, H75, H77, H78, H83, H88, H90, H95, H101, H108, H109, H115, H116, H118, H120, H126, H130, H134, H137, H143, H145, H147, H150–H154, H156, H164, H165, H167, H170, H172, H174, H178, H183, H184, H190, H191, H199
Sulfonylureas	20 (1,931)	−0.80 [−1.08, −0.53]*; 85.5%	H3, H31, H49, H56, H81, H85, H87, H103, H111, H123, H127, H142, H146, H159, H161, H168, H169, H171, H185, H187
Insulin	13 (1,289)	−0.61 [−0.91, −0.30]*; 88.1%	H50, H58, H59, H79, H89, H102, H122, H140, H141, H175–H177, H182
TZDs	4 (326)	−1.36 [−1.69, −1.02]*; 33.4%	H53, H100, H139, H162
α-Glucosidase inhibitors	5 (409)	−0.54 [−0.91, −0.17]*; 81.0%	H57, H99, H113, H149, H186

(Continued)

Table 5.5. *(Continued)*

Group	No. of Studies (Participants)	MD [95% CI], I²%	Included Studies
Meglitinides	3 (220)	−0.59 [−0.96, −0.21]*; 0.0%	H70, H82, H93
DPP-4 inhibitors	2 (170)	−0.55 [−2.00, 0.89]; 95.0%	H91, H117
Biguanides and Sulfonylureas	17 (1228)	−0.71 [−0.93, −0.41]*; 47.7%	H51, H54, H76, H84, H94, H96–H98, H105, H121, H131, H148, H157, H188, H193, H194, H197
Biguanides and α-Glucosidase inhibitors	9 (607)	−0.83 [−1.22, −0.44]*; 93.3%	H55, H67, H71, H80, H107, H129, H144, H160, H163
FPG level at baseline			
6–8 mmol/L	88 (7,577)	−0.82 [−0.93, −0.72]*; 82.3%	H3, H24, H19, H28, H41, H42, H44, H45, H47, H49, H50, H55, H57, H62, H64–H69, H71, H72, H74, H77, H79, H80, H82–H84, H87–H94, H99, H100, H103, H104, H106, H110, H111, H114–H117, H119, H121, H124, H126, H127, H133, H134, H139, H141, H142, H144–H146, H149–H151, H153–H155, H158, H159, H161–H165, H168, H169, H171, H175, H176, H180, H184, H187–H189, H191, H193, H194, H199
8–10 mmol/L	59 (5,339)	−0.94 [−1.12, −0.75]*; 87.5%	H31, H43, H51–H54, H56, H58, H59, H61, H63, H70, H75, H76, H78, H81, H85, H95, H98, H101, H102, H105, H107–H109, H113, H118, H120, H122, H123, H128–H131, H137, H138, H140, H143, H147, H148, H152, H156, H157, H160, H167, H172–H174, H177–H179, H182, H183, H185, H190, H192, H195–H197
≥10 mmol/L	8 (666)	−0.45 [−0.68, −0.23]*; 73.3%	H60, H86, H96, H97, H136, H170, H186, H198

Table 5.5. (*Continued*)

Group	No. of Studies (Participants)	MD [95% CI], I²%	Included Studies
Treatment duration			
≤3 months	147 (12,744)	−0.83 [−0.92, −0.74]*; 85.6%	H3, H19, H24, H28, H31, H43–H45, H47, H49–H69, H71, H72, H74–H111, H113–H116, H118–H124, H126–H131, H133, H134, H136–H165, H167–H172, H174–H176, H178, H180, H182–H198
3–6 months	2 (176)	−1.16 [−2.14, −0.18]*; 90.6%	H41, H42
≥6 months	4 (404)	−0.82 [−1.10, −0.54]*; 20.5%	H70, H173, H179, H199
CM syndrome differentiation			
Qi and *yin* deficiency	43 (3,569)	−0.85 [−1.02, −0.67]*; 85.3%	H3, H47, H50, H54, H60, H61, H66, H74, H78, H81, H84, H91, H93, H94, H99, H103, H104, H109, H114, H119, H123, H124, H133, H137, H143, H146, H147, H150–H152, H156, H161, H163, H165, H170, H171, H175, H177, H180, H185, H187–H189
Yin deficiency and excessive heat	15 (1,140)	−0.70 [−0.88, −0.52]*; 59.0%	H63, H75, H79, H83, H87, H89, H110, H116, H126, H127, H24, H129, H153, H162, H193
Phlegm-dampness and Blood stasis	8 (737)	−0.78 [−1.06, −0.50]*; 85.9%	H58, H59, H76, H82, H113, H139, H164, H198
Damp heat retention	7 (481)	−0.62 [−0.91, −0.34]*; 70.4%	H62, H64, H90, H122, H138, H145, H174
Spleen deficiency	4 (278)	−0.69 [−1.23, −0.15]*; 94.4%	H80, H100, H149, H160
Liver *qi* stagnation	1 (80)	−0.40 [−0.67, −0.13]*	H140

*Statistically significant
Abbreviations: CI, confidence interval; CM, Chinese medicine; FPG, fasting plasma glucose; MD, mean difference; SG, sequence generation.

Chinese Herbal Medicine vs. Placebo

Six RCTs (H205–H210) with 1,052 participants compared CHM with a placebo. The treatment duration ranged from 12 to 24 weeks. The results showed that CHM was superior to a placebo at reducing PBG levels at the end of treatment (MD −1.69 [−2.87, −0.52]; I^2 = 96.2%), indicating improved blood sugar metabolism.

Chinese Herbal Medicine vs. Lifestyle Intervention

Six RCTs (H9, H19, H200–H202, H204) with 465 participants compared CHM with lifestyle intervention. The treatment duration ranged from two to 24 weeks. The results showed that CHM was superior to no treatment (MD −1.98 [−2.68, −1.29]; I^2 = 69.7%).

Chinese Herbal Medicine vs. Pharmacotherapy

Thirty-five RCTs (n = 3,268; H1–H21, H23–H25, H27, H29–H35, H38–H40) compared CHM with pharmacotherapy. One RCT compared CHM to aspirin, while the remaining RCTs studied different classes of hypoglycaemic agents. Specific hypoglycaemic agent includes metformin, glimepiride, glipizide, glyburide, pioglitazone, rosiglitazone and acarbose. Treatment duration ranged from four to 24 weeks.

At the end of the treatment, a meta-analysis showed that CHM resulted in lower PBG levels than pharmacotherapy (MD −0.45 [−0.76, −0.13], I^2 = 81.6%). A meta-analysis of studies assessed as low risk for sequence generation produced a similar result to that of the overall results (11 RCTs, 1,227 participants, MD −0.47 [−1.03, 0.1]; I^2 = 78.4%); however, no significant difference between groups was seen.

A subgroup analysis by drug class showed that CHM is better at reducing PBG levels than biguanides and aspirin, but not α-glucosidase inhibitors, TZDs or sulfonylureas (Table 5.6). Biguanides/metformin formed the biggest pool of studies with 22 RCTs and 2,037 participants, though the effect on PBG is similar to that of the overall result. When grouped by FPG levels at baseline, studies with lower FPG levels at baseline did not show any difference in PBG levels after CHM or pharmacotherapy treatment. However, studies with medium to high levels of FPG levels at baseline showed a significant difference between the CHM and pharmacotherapy groups at the end of treatment. Studies with a duration of three months or less (34 RCTs, 3,188 participants) showed that CHM lowered PBG levels more than the pharmacotherapy group. The same effect was not seen in a study that had treatment duration of more than six months. In T2DM participants with phlegm-dampness and Blood stasis, PBG was reduced more in the CHM group than the pharmacotherapy group. No significant differences were seen in other syndrome differentiation subgroup analyses (Table 5.6). All meta-analyses showed statistical heterogeneity, and this lowers confidence in estimates of the treatment effect.

Table 5.6. **Chinese Herbal Medicine vs. Pharmacotherapy: Postprandial Blood Glucose**

Group	No. of Studies (Participants)	MD [95% CI], I^2%	Included Studies
All studies	35 (3,268)	−0.45 [−0.76, −0.13]*; 81.6%	H1–21, H23–25, H27, H29–35, H38–40
Agents class			
Low risk of bias SG	11 (1,227)	−0.47 [−1.03, 0.10]; 78.4%	H2, H8–H10, H13, H18, H19, H23, H24, H30, H35
Biguanides	22 (2,037)	−0.47 [−0.85, −0.09]*; 80.2%	H1, H4, H5, H8, H10, H12, H15–H21, H23–H25, H29, H30, H32, H33, H35, H39
α-Glucosidase inhibitors	3 (296)	−1.30 [−2.48, −0.13]*; 88.6%	H9, H11, H38
TZDs	3 (268)	−0.03 [−1.82, 1.77]; 85.6%	H2, H7, H40
Sulfonylureas	5 (545)	0.13 [−0.71, 0.97]; 83.6%	H3, H14, H27, H31, H34

(Continued)

Table 5.6. *(Continued)*

Group	No. of Studies (Participants)	MD [95% CI], I^2%	Included Studies
Hypoglycaemic agents (not detailed)	1 (64)	−0.54 [−1.87, 0.79]	H6
Aspirin	1 (58)	−1.31 [−2.47, −0.15]*	H13
FPG level at baseline			
6–8 mmol/L	2 (194)	0.71 [−1.03, 2.46]; 88.6%	H7, H23
8–10 mmol/L	24 (2,272)	−0.39 [−0.77, −0.02]*; 80.9%	H1–H3, H5, H6, H8–H11, H13–H15, H17–H21, H24, H25, H30, H33–H35, H40
≥10 mmol/L	9 (802)	−0.87 [−1.43, −0.31]*; 76.2%	H4, H12, H16, H27, H29, H31, H32, H38, H39
Treatment duration			
≤3 months	34 (3,188)	−0.46 [−0.78, −0.13]*; 82.1%	H1–H8, H10–H21, H23–H25, H27, H29–H35, H38–H40
≥6 months	1 (80)	−0.19 [−0.10, 0.62]	H9
CM syndrome differentiation			
Qi and *yin* deficiency	7 (628)	−0.39 [−1.17, 0.39]; 85.1%	H3, H14, H15, H25, H29, H34, H40
Yin deficiency and excessive heat	6 (429)	−0.10 [−0.46, 0.26]; 27.1%	H5, H8, H17, H21, H22, H24, H35
Damp heat retention	5 (486)	0.43 [−0.60, 1.46]; 83.3%	H2, H7, H23, H32, H33
Phlegm-dampness and Blood stasis	1 (60)	−0.99 [−1.79, −0.19]*	H20

*Statistically significant

Abbreviations: CI, confidence interval; CM, Chinese medicine; FPG, fasting plasma glucose; MD, mean difference; SG, sequence generation; TZDs, thiazolidinedione.

Chinese Herbal Medicine Plus Hypoglycaemic Agents vs. Hypoglycaemic Agents

A total of 138 RCTs (H3, H19, H24, H31, H41–H45, H47, H49–H57, H60–H72, H74–H87, H89–H103, H105, H107–H111, H114–H119, H121–H123, H126–H131, H133, H134, H136–H139, H141–H145, H147–H153, H155–H164, H167–H176, H178–H180, H182, H183, H185–H191, H193–H196, H198, H199), including 11,979 participants, assessed the effects of CHM plus hypoglycaemic agents compared to hypoglycaemic agents alone. All studies used the same hypoglycaemic agent in both groups. Hypoglycaemic agents included biguanides, sulfonylureas (second generation), thiazolidinediones, α-glucosidase inhibitors, meglitinides, DPP-4 inhibitors, SGLT2 inhibitors, GLP-1 receptor agonists and insulins. Specific agents include metformin, gliclazide, glipizide, glibenclamide, glimepiride, gliclazone, pioglitazone, acarbose, voglibose, repaglinide, sitagliptin, liraglutide and insulin. The treatment duration ranged from two to 24 weeks.

Meta-analysis results showed that as integrative medicine, CHM plus hypoglycaemic agents was superior to hypoglycaemic agents alone (MD -1.23 [-1.38, -1.08], $I^2 = 88.5\%$). The heterogeneity remained high after a sensitivity analysis with studies with low risk of bias for sequence generation (Table 5.7).

Biguanides/metformin formed the biggest pool of studies with 51 RCTs and 4,673 participants, where the effect on PBG is similar to that of the overall result. The combination of CHM to TZDs, insulin and a DPP-4 inhibitor did not produce a better result than these agents alone (Table 5.7). The combined use of CHM with different classes of hypoglycaemic agents also produced a significant difference between groups, where the results are like the overall analysis (Table 5.7). Combinations of different drug classes also showed a significant difference between groups. Additional subgroup analyses based on baseline levels of FPG, the treatment duration, and CM syndrome differentiation all showed significant differences between groups (Table 5.7). Subgrouping by FPG levels at baseline showed a greater effect in PBG levels in the medium and high-level studies, although all subgroups produced a significant result. When

Table 5.7.   Chinese Herbal Medicine Plus Hypoglycaemic Agents vs. Hypoglycaemic Agents: Postprandial Blood Glucose

Group	No. of Studies (Participants)	MD [95% CI], I²%	Included Studies
Hypoglycaemic agents			
All studies	138 (11,979)	−1.23 [−1.38, −1.08]*; 88.5%	H3, H19, H24, H31, H41–H45, H47, H49–H57, H60–H72, H74–H87, H89–H103, H105, H107–H111, H114–H119, H121–H123, H126–H131, H133, H134, H136–H139, H141–H145, H147–H153, H155–H164, H167–H176, H178–H180, H182, H183, H185–H191, H193–H196, H198, H199
Low risk of bias SG	39 (3,287)	−1.24 [−1.56, −0.93]*; 93.0%	H19, H24, H51, H57, H60, H63–H66, H78–H80, H82, H84, H86, H87, H90, H91, H96, H97, H100, H102, H110, H116, H119, H122, H126, H129, H134, H144, H163, H168, H173–H176, H183, H193, H199
Drug class			
Biguanides	51 (4,673)	−1.38 [−1.62, −1.14]*; 88.3%	H19, H24, H41, H42, H44, H45, H47, H60–H63, H65, H66, H68, H69, H72, H74, H75, H77, H78, H83, H90, H95, H101, H108, H109, H115, H116, H118, H126, H130, H134, H137, H143, H145, H147, H150–H153, H156, H164, H167, H170, H172, H174, H178, H183, H190, H191, H199
Sulfonylureas	19 (1,831)	−1.30 [−1.74, −0.86]*; 87.0%	H3, H31, H49, H56, H81, H85, H87, H103, H111, H123, H127, H142, H159, H161, H168, H169, H171, H185, H187
Insulin	9 (811)	−1.19 [−2.00, −0.38]; 93.5%	H50, H79, H89, H102, H122, H141, H175, H176, H182
TZDs	4 (326)	−0.90 [−1.50, −0.31]; 57.0%	H53, H100, H139, H162

Table 5.7. (*Continued*)

Group	No. of Studies (Participants)	MD [95% CI], I²%	Included Studies
α-Glucosidase inhibitors	4 (337)	−1.16 [−1.97, −0.35]*; 89.1%	H57, H99, H149, H186
Meglitinides	3 (220)	−0.66 [−1.02, −0.28]*; 0.0%	H70, H82, H93
DPP-4 inhibitors	2 (170)	−1.54 [−3.17, 0.10]; 90.8%	H91, H117
Biguanides and Sulfonylureas	16 (1,130)	−1.15 [−1.63, −0.66]*; 82.2%	H51, H54, H76, H84, H94, H96–H98, H105, H121, H131, H148, H157, H188, H193, H194
Biguanides and α-Glucosidase inhibitors	9 (607)	−1.29 [−1.81, −0.77]*; 91.8%	H55, H67, H71, H80, H107, H129, H144, H160, H163
FPG level at baseline			
6–8 mmol/L	8 (666)	−0.79 [−1.49, −0. 08]*; 96.4%	H60, H86, H96, H97, H136, H170, H186, H198
8–10 mmol/L	79 (6,778)	−1.18 [−1.35, −1.01]*; 84.6%	H3, H19, H24, H41, H42, H44, H45, H47, H49, H50, H55, H57, H62, H64–H69, H71, H72, H74, H77, H79, H80, H82–H84, H87, H89–H94, H99, H100, H103, H110, H111, H114–H117, H119, H121, H126, H127, H133, H134, H139, H141, H142, H144, H145, H149–H151, H153, H155, H158, H159, H161–H164, H168, H169, H171, H175–H189, H191, H193, H194, H199
≥10 mmol/L	51 (4,535)	−1.38 [−1.67, −1.09]*; 89.3%	H31, H43, H51–H54, H56, H61, H63, H70, H75, H76, H78, H81, H85, H95, H98, H101, H102, H105, H107–H109, H118, H122, H123, H128–H131, H137, H138, H143, H147, H148, H152, H156, H157, H160, H167, H172–H174, H178, H179, H182, H183, H185, H190, H195, H196

(*Continued*)

Table 5.7. *(Continued)*

Group	No. of Studies (Participants)	MD [95% CI], I^2%	Included Studies
Treatment duration			
≤3 months	131 (11,239)	−1.21 [−1.36, −1.06]*; 88.4%	H3, H19, H24, H31, H43–H45, H47, H49–H57, H60–H69, H71, H72, H74–H103, H105, H107–H111, H114–H116, H118, H119, H121–H123, H126–H131, H133, H134, H136–139, H141–145, H147–153, H155–164, H167–H172, H174–H176, H178, H180, H182, H183, H185–H191, H193–196, H198
3–6 months	2 (176)	−1.98 [−3.86, −0.10]*; 93.3%	H41, H42
≥6 months	4 (404)	−1.32 [−1.94, −0.71]*; 79.7%	H70, H173, H179, H199
CM syndrome differentiation			
Qi and *yin* deficiency	38 (3,036)	−1.14 [−1.44, −0.83]*; 88.1%	H3, H47, H50, H54, H60, H61, H66, H74, H78, H81, H84, H91, H93, H94, H99, H103, H109, H114, H119, H123, H133, H137, H143, H147, H150–H152, H156, H161, H163, H170, H171, H175, H180, H185, H187–H189
Yin deficiency and excessive heat	15 (1,140)	−0.91 [−1.19, −0.63]*; 57.9%	H24, H63, H75, H79, H83, H87, H89, H110, H116, H126, H127, H129, H153, H162, H193
Phlegm-dampness and Blood stasis	5 (365)	−1.10 [−1.66, −0.54]*; 91.5%	H76, H82, H139, H164, H198
Damp heat retention	7 (481)	−0.72 [−1.41, −0.02]*; 89.6%	H62, H64, H90, H122, H138, H145, H174
Spleen deficiency	4 (278)	−1.05 [−1.40, −0.69]*; 70.1%	H80, H100, H149, H160

* Statistically significant

Abbreviations: CI, confidence interval; CM, Chinese medicine; FPG, fasting plasma glucose; MD, mean difference; SG, sequence generation; TZDs, thiazolidinedione.

subgrouping by treatment duration, studies that showed the greatest effect are seen in those that provided treatment for three to six months, although the treatment duration of <3 months or >6 months also produced a significant difference between groups. The heterogeneity remained high in the subgroup analysis.

Glycated Haemoglobin

A total of 151 studies with 13,708 T2DM participants assessed levels of A1C. A lower value on the A1C indicates greater improvement. Overall meta-analysis for A1C was performed at the end of treatment based on different comparators.

Chinese Herbal Medicine vs. Placebo

Five RCTs (H205–H207, H209, H210) with 572 participants compared CHM with a placebo, with the treatment duration ranging from 12 to 24 weeks. The result showed that CHM was superior to the placebo (MD −0.93 [−1.51, −0.35]; I^2 = 96.3%).

Chinese Herbal Medicine vs. Lifestyle Intervention

Five RCTs (H9, H19, H201–H203) with 413 participants compared CHM with lifestyle intervention only. The treatment duration ranged from two to 24 weeks. The result showed that CHM was superior to lifestyle intervention only in T2DM patients (MD −1.13 [−1.64, −0.63], I^2 = 71.0%).

Chinese Herbal Medicine vs. Hypoglycaemic Agents

Twenty-eight RCTs (n = H1–H4, H8–H10, H15, H17–H25, H28–H32, H35–H40) compared CHM with hypoglycaemic agents. Four classes of anti-diabetic agents were used as comparators, including biguanides, sulfonylureas, thiazolidinediones and α-glucosidase inhibitors. Specific agents included metformin, glimepiride, glipizide, glyburide, pioglitazone, rosiglitazone and acarbose. The treatment duration ranged from 4 to 24 weeks.

The overall meta-analysis result showed that there was no significant difference between the CHM group and the hypoglycaemic agents (MD −0.11 [−0.26, 0.04], I^2 = 75.6%). Studies with a low risk of bias for sequence generation produced a slightly more modest reduction with CHM and appeared to be more homogeneous (11 RCTs, 1,229 participants, MD −0.09 [−0.26, 0.08]; I^2 = 66.6%).

α-Glucosidase inhibitors were used as a comparator in two (H9, H38) of the 28 RCTs, including 184 participants. The result indicated that the value of A1C was reduced in people receiving CHM compared to α-Glucosidase inhibitors (MD −0.81 [−1.52, −0.09], I^2 = 92.1%). There was no statistical difference between CHM and biguanides, TZDs or sulfonylureas (Table 5.7). Twenty-seven out of 28 studies had treatment duration of less than three months, and a subgroup analysis showed no statistical difference between groups (Table 5.8). One study (n = 80; H9) treated participants for more than six months, and the result indicated that the value of A1C reduced more in patients receiving CHM (MD −0.45 [−0.69, −0.21]). The *qi* and *yin* deficiency subgroup included six RCTs (n = 388; H3, H15, H25, H29, H36, H40), and the result indicated that the value of A1C reduced in patients receiving CHM alone and the results were more homogenous (MD −0.31 [−0.57, −0.05], I^2 = 15.1%). T2DM

Table 5.8. Chinese Herbal Medicine vs. Hypoglycaemic Agents: A1C

Group	No. of Studies (Participants)	MD [95% CI], I^2%	Included Studies
All studies	28 (2,441)	−0.11 [−0.26, 0.04]; 75.6%	H1–H4, H8–H10, H15, H17–H25, H28–H32, H35–H40
Low risk of bias SG	11 (1,229)	−0.09 [−0.26, 0.08]; 66.6%	H2, H8–H10, H18, H19, H22–H24, H30, H35
Agent class			
Biguanides	20 (1,871)	−0.03 [−0.18, 0.11]; 66.3%	H1, H4, H8, H10, H15, H17–H21, H23–H25, H28–H30, H32, H35, H37, H39

Table 5.8. (*Continued*)

Group	No. of Studies (Participants)	MD [95% CI], I²%	Included Studies
α-Glucosidase inhibitors	2 (184)	−0.81 [−1.52, −0.09]*; 92.1%	H9, H38
TZDs	4 (264)	−0.19 [−0.45, 0.08]; 0.0%	H2, H22, H36, H40
Sulfonylureas	2 (122)	0.27 [−0.22, 0.77]; 0.0%	H3, H31
FPG level at baseline			
6–8 mmol/L	1 (70)	−0.08 [−0.32, 0.16]	H23
8–10 mmol/L	20 (1,762)	−0.09 [−0.24, 0.07], 70.7%	H1–H3, H8–H10, H15, H17–H22, H24, H25, H28, H30, H35, H36, H40
≥10 mmol/L	7 (609)	−0.16 [−0.74, 0.43], 86.0%	H4, H29, H31, H32, H37–H39
Treatment duration			
≤3 months	27 (2,361)	−0.09 [−0.25, 0.07]; 74.9%	H1–H4, H8, H10, H15, H17–H25, H28–H32, H35–H40
≥6 months	1 (80)	−0.45 [−0.69, −0.21]*	H9
CM syndrome differentiation			
Qi and *yin* deficiency	6 (388)	−0.31 [−0.57, −0.05]*; 15.1%	H3, H15, H25, H29, H36, H40
Yin deficiency and excessive heat	6 (429)	0.11 [−0.03, 0.25]; 17.6%	H8, H17, H21, H22, H24, H35
Damp heat retention	3 (290)	−0.01 [−0.18, 0.16]; 0.0%	H2, H23, H32
Phlegm-dampness and Blood stasis	1 (60)	−0.28 [−0.52, −0.04]*	H20

*Statistically significant

Abbreviations: CI, confidence interval; CM, Chinese medicine; FPG, fasting plasma glucose; MD, mean difference; SG, sequence generation; TZDs, thiazolidinedione.

participants with the CM syndrome phlegm-dampness and Blood stasis also showed a reduction in A1C in the CHM group; however, the result is only from one small study (Table 5.8). Overall, the heterogeneity remained high in the subgroup analysis.

Chinese Herbal Medicine Plus Hypoglycaemic Agents vs. Hypoglycaemic Agents

A total of 120 RCTs (H3, H19, H24, H28, H31, H41, H42, H44–H47, H51–H55, H59–H62, H64–H68, H70–H75, H77–H80, H82–H90, H92–H95, H99, H100, H102, H104–H106, H108, H110, H111, H113, H115, H116, H118, H119, H121–H126, H128, H130, H131, H133, H134, H137, H139–H145, H149–H151, H153, H155, H156, H158, H160–H168, H171–H173, H175–H184, H186–H189, H191, H192, H195, H196, H198, H199), including 10,497 participants, assessed the effects of CHM plus hypoglycaemic agents versus hypoglycaemic agents alone. All studies used the same hypoglycaemic agents in both groups, including biguanides, sulfonylureas, thiazolidinediones, α-glucosidase inhibitors, meglitinides, DPP-4 inhibitors, GLP-1 receptor agonists and insulins. Specific agents include metformin, gliclazide, glimepizide, gliquidone, glibenclamide, pioglitazone, repaglinide, nateglinide, sitagliptin, voglibose, acarbose and insulin.

CHM plus hypoglycaemic agents was superior to hypoglycaemic agents alone (MD −0.75 [−0.86, −0.64], I^2 = 93.2%). The heterogeneity remained high in a subgroup analysis except in one subgroup where meglitinides were combined with CHM (Table 5.9). CHM plus meglitinides were used as a comparator in three RCTs (H70, H82, H93), including 220 participants. The result indicated that the value of A1C was reduced in people receiving CHM plus meglitinides compared to meglitinides alone (MD −0.93 [−1.25, −0.60], I^2 = 31.8%). Additionally, for T2DM with the CM syndrome of Spleen *qi* deficiency and Liver *qi* stagnation, there was no benefit in adding CHM to hypoglycaemic agents compared to hypoglycaemic agents alone (Table 5.9).

Table 5.9. Chinese Herbal Medicine Plus Hypoglycaemic Agents vs. Hypoglycaemic Agents: A1C

Group	No. of Studies (Participants)	MD [95% CI], I^2%	Included Studies
All studies	120 (10,497)	−0.75 [−0.86, −0.64]*; 93.2%	H3, H19, H24, H28, H31, H41, H42, H44–H47, H51–H55, H59–H62, H64–H68, H70–H75, H77–H80, H82–H90, H92–H95, H99, H100, H102, H104–H106, H108, H110, H111, H113, H115, H116, H118, H119, H121–H126, H128, H130, H131, H133, H134, H137, H139–H145, H149–H151, H153, H155, H156, H158, H160–H168, H171–H173, H175–H184, H186–H189, H191, H192, H195, H196, H198, H199
Low risk of bias SG	36 (3,212)	−0.61 [−0.79, −0.43]*; 92.6%	H51, H60, H64–H66, H78–H80, H82, H84, H86, H87, H90, H100, H102, H106, H110, H19, H116, H119, H122, H124, H126, H24, H134, H140, H144, H163, H165, H168, H173, H175, H176, H181, H183, H199
Drug class			
Biguanides	47 (4,289)	−0.89 [−1.04, −0.73]*; 90.4%	H19, H24, H28, H41, H42, H44–H47, H60–H62, H65, H66, H68, H72, H74, H75, H77, H78, H83, H88, H90, H95, H108, H115, H116, H118, H126, H130, H134, H137, H143, H145, H150, H151, H153, H156, H164, H165, H167, H172, H178, H183, H184, H191, H199
Sulfonylureas	13 (1,161)	−0.41 [−0.67, −0.16]*; 78.8%	H3, H31, H73, H85, H87, H111, H123, H142, H161, H168, H171, H181, H187
Insulin	11 (1,069)	−0.79 [−1.23, −0.34]*; 94.2%	H59, H79, H89, H102, H122, H140, H141, H175–H177, H182

(Continued)

Table 5.9. *(Continued)*

Group	No. of Studies (Participants)	MD [95% CI], I²%	Included Studies
TZDs	4 (326)	−0.90 [−1.55, −0.25]*; 89.1%	H53, H100, H139, H162
α-Glucosidase inhibitors	4 (319)	−0.53 [−0.83, −0.23]*; 74.4%	H99, H113, H149, H186
Meglitinides	3 (220)	−0.93 [−1.25, −0.60]*; 31.8%	H70, H82, H93
Biguanides and Sulfonylureas	9 (669)	−0.54 [−0.85, −0.24]*; 79.3%	H51, H54, H84, H94, H105, H121, H125, H131, H188
Biguanides and α-Glucosidase inhibitors	7 (449)	−0.69 [−1.12, −0.25]*; 95.8%	H55, H67, H71, H80, H144, H160, H163
Fasting plasma glucose level at baseline			
6–8 mmol/L	4 (323)	−0.40 [−0.66, −0.13]*; 82.3%	H60, H86, H186, H198
8–10 mmol/L	73 (6,235)	−0.72 [−0.86, −0.59]*; 93.7%	H28, H41, H42, H44, H45, H47, H55, H62, H64–H68, H71, H72, H74, H3, H77, H79, H80, H82–H84, H87–H90, H92–H94, H99, H100, H104, H106, H110, H111, H115, H19, H116, H119, H121, H124, H126, H24, H133, H134, H139, H141, H142, H144, H145, H149–H151, H153, H155, H158, H161–H165, H168, H171, H175, H176, H180, H184, H187–H189, H191, H199
≥10 mmol/L	38 (3,381)	−0.87 [−1.06, −0.68]*; 88.4%	H31, H51–H54, H59, H61, H70, H75, H78, H85, H95, H102, H105, H108, H113, H118, H122, H123, H128, H130, H131, H137, H140, H143, H156, H160, H167, H172, H173, H177–H179, H182, H183, H192, H195, H196
Treatment duration			
≤3 months	113 (9,819)	−0.74 [−0.85, −0.62]*; 93.2%	H3, H19, H24, H28, H31, H44–H47, H51–H55, H59–H62,

Table 5.9. (*Continued*)

Group	No. of Studies (Participants)	MD [95% CI], I²%	Included Studies
			H64–H68, H71–H75, H77–H80, H82–H90, H92–H95, H99, H100, H102, H104–H106, H108, H110, H111, H113, H115, H116, H118,H119, H121–H126, H128, H130, H131, H133, H134, H137, H139–H145, H149–H151, H153, H155, H156, H158, H160–H168, H171, H172, H175, H176, H178, H180–H184, H186–H189, H191, H192, H195, H196, H198
3–6 months	2 (176)	−1.50 [−2.47, −0.53]*; 95.9%	H41, H42
≥6 months	4 (404)	−0.55 [−0.95, −0.15]*; 83.8%	H70, H173, H179, H199
Chinese medicine syndrome differentiation			
Qi and *yin* deficiency	34 (2,636)	−0.77 [−0.94, −0.60]*; 81.2%	H3, H47, H54, H60, H61, H66, H73, H74, H78, H84, H93, H94, H99, H104, H119, H123, H124, H133, H137, H143, H150, H151, H156, H161, H163, H165, H166, H171, H175, H177, H180, H187–H189
Yin deficiency and excessive heat	12 (1,042)	−0.65 [−1.11, −0.19]*; 97.9%	H75, H79, H83, H87, H89, H110, H116, H126, H24, H153, H162, H181
Phlegm-dampness and blood stasis	6 (521)	−0.35 [−0.51, −0.20]*; 67.4%	H59, H82, H113, H139, H164, H198
Damp heat retention	5 (359)	−0.70 [−1.11, −0.29]*; 78.0%	H62, H64, H90, H122, H145
Spleen deficiency	4 (278)	−0.87 [−1.81, 0.08]; 96.2%	H80, H100, H149, H160
Liver *qi* stagnation	1 (80)	0.0 [−0.37, 0.37]	H140

*Statistically significant

Abbreviations: CI, confidence interval; CM, Chinese medicine; FPG, fasting plasma glucose; MD, mean difference; SG, sequence generation; TZDs, thiazolidinedione.

Quality of Life Scale for Patients with Type 2 Diabetes Mellitus

One RCT (H181) of 200 participants assessed the quality of life using the quality of life scale for patients with type 2 diabetes mellitus (DMQLS). Lower scores on the DMQLS indicate greater improvement. After eight weeks of treatment, CHM *Ping tang* 平糖 capsules plus hypoglycaemic agents reported a greater benefit than glipizide alone (MD −3.4 [−6.08, −0.72]).

Body Mass Index

Thirty of the 210 studies, including 3,020 participants, assessed weight changes in T2DM patients using the body mass index (BMI). A lower value of the BMI indicates greater improvement. Overall meta-analysis for BMI was performed at the end of treatment based on different comparators.

Chinese Herbal Medicine vs. Placebo

Three RCTs (H205, H209, H210) with 257 participants compared CHM with a placebo. All studies had treatment duration of 12 weeks. The result showed that CHM was not superior to the placebo at improving BMI in T2DM patients (MD −0.61 [−1.45, 0.24]; I^2 = 0.0%).

Chinese Herbal Medicine vs. Lifestyle Intervention

Two RCTs (H19, H202) with 212 participants compared CHM with lifestyle intervention. Participants were treated for eight or 12 weeks. The result showed that CHM was not superior to lifestyle intervention at improving BMI in T2DM patients (MD −1.06 [−2.52, 0.40]; I^2 = 73.8%).

Chinese Herbal Medicine vs. Hypoglycaemic Agents

Twelve RCTs (*n* = 1,407; H2, H7, H8, H10, H19, H23, H25, H26, H30–H32, H35) compared CHM with hypoglycaemic agents. Three classes of agents were used as comparators, including biguanides, sulfonylureas and thiazolidinediones. Specific agents included metformin, glimepiride, glipizide, glyburide, pioglitazone and rosiglitazone. The treatment duration ranged from four to 12 weeks.

The overall result indicated no significant difference between the CHM group and hypoglycaemic group (MD −0.30 [−0.72, 0.11]; I^2 = 70.4%). A subgroup analysis based on low risk of bias for sequence generation, comparator drug class, and FPG level at baseline did not produce different results. T2DM participants with the CM syndrome of *qi* and *yin* deficiency and damp heat retention showed significant differences in BMI between the two groups (Table 5.10).

Table 5.10. Chinese Herbal Medicine vs. Hypoglycaemic Agents: Body Mass Index

Groups	No. of Studies (Participants)	MD [95% CI], I^2%	Included Studies
All studies	12 (1,407)	−0.30 [−0.72, 0.11]; 70.4%	H2, H7, H8, H10, H19, H23, H25, H26, H30–H32, H35
Low risk of bias SG	11 (1,229)	−0.09 [−0.26, 0.08]; 66.6%	H2, H8–H10, H18, H19, H22, H23, H24, H30, H35
Agents class			
Biguanides	8 (1,081)	−0.26 [−0.85, 0.34]; 76.0%	H8, H10, H19, H23, H25, H30, H32, H35
TZDs	3 (264)	−0.47 [−1.21, 0.28]; 72.1%	H2, H7, H26
Sulfonylureas	1 (62)	0.40 [−1.38, 2.18]	H31

(*Continued*)

Table 5.10. *(Continued)*

Groups	No. of Studies (Participants)	MD [95% CI], I^2%	Included Studies
FPG level at baseline			
6–8 mmol/L	2 (194)	−0.70 [−1.87, 0.46]; 72.3%	H7, H23
8–10 mmol/L	7 (951)	−0.21 [−0.81, 0.40]; 74.2%	H2, H8, H10, H19, H25, H30, H35
≥10 mmol/L	2 (202)	−0.53 [−1.53, 0.47]; 41.6%	H31, H32
CM syndrome differentiation			
Qi and *yin* deficiency	1 (84)	−1.22 [−2.17, −0.27]*	H25
Yin deficiency and excessive heat	2 (178)	0.38 [−1.34, 2.09]; 84.1%	H8, H35
Damp heat retention	4 (414)	−0.65 [−1.04, −0.26]*; 53.5%	H2, H7, H23, H32

*Statistically significant

Abbreviations: CI, confidence interval; CM, Chinese medicine; FPG, fasting plasma glucose; MD, mean difference; SG, sequence generation; TZDs, thiazolidinedione.

Chinese Herbal Medicine Plus Hypoglycaemic Agents vs. Hypoglycaemic Agents

Fifteen RCTs (H19, H31, H41, H51, H55, H60, H71, H122, H130, H135, H145, H155, H165, H181, H186), including 1,165 participants, assessed the effects of CHM plus hypoglycaemic agents versus hypoglycaemic agents alone. Hypoglycaemic agents included biguanides, sulfonylureas, α-Glucosidase inhibitors and insulins. Specific agents include metformin, gliclazide, glibenclamide, glipizide, glimepiride, acarbose and insulin. The treatment duration ranged from four to 14 weeks.

Meta-analysis results showed that CHM plus hypoglycaemic agents were superior to hypoglycaemic agents alone at improving BMI (MD −0.95 [−1.60, −0.31], I^2 = 87.8%). A meta-analysis of studies assessed as low risk for sequence generation produced a result that was more homogeneous (seven studies, 627 participants MD −0.35 [−1.11, 0.41]; I^2 = 69.9%); however, no difference was found between groups.

A subgroup analysis by drug class showed that adding CHM to biguanides, sulfonylureas or combinations of different drug classes did not show any significant differences between the two groups. A subgroup analysis by FPG levels at baseline showed that in studies with low to medium levels, there was a benefit in adding CHM to hypoglycaemic agents, but not in studies that had a high level of FPG level at baseline (Table 5.11). A subgroup analysis by treatment duration (4–12 weeks) showed similar effects to the overall results. In studies that provided information on the CM syndrome, no syndrome showed benefit in the improvements of BMI using integrative medicine (Table 5.11).

Table 5.11. Chinese Herbal Medicine Plus Hypoglycaemic Agents vs. Hypoglycaemic Agents: Body Mass Index

Group	No. of Studies (Participants)	MD [95% CI], I^2%	Included Studies
All studies	15 (1,165)	−0.95 [−1.60, −0.31]*; 87.8%	H41, H51, H55, H60, H71, H19, H122, H130, H135, H145, H31, H155, H165, H181, H186
Low risk of bias SG	7 (627)	−0.35 [−1.11, 0.41]; 69.9%	H51, H60, H19, H122, H135, H165, H181
Drug class			
Biguanides	6 (417)	−1.27 [−2.70, 0.15]; 90.8%	H41, H60, H19, H130, H145, H165
Sulfonylureas	3 (331)	0.57 [0.21, 0.94]; 0.0%	H31, H168, H181
Insulin	2 (138)	−1.91 [−3.23, −0.58]*; I2 = 0.0%	H122, H135

(Continued)

Table 5.11. (*Continued*)

Group	No. of Studies (Participants)	MD [95% CI], I²%	Included Studies
α-Glucosidase inhibitors	1 (80)	−0.50 [−0.90, −0.10]*	H186
Biguanides and Sulfonylureas	1 (60)	−0.07 [−1.42, 1.28]	H51
Biguanides and α-Glucosidase inhibitors	2 (129)	−0.43 [−0.96, 0.10]; 0.0%	H55, H71
FPG level at baseline			
6–8 mmol/L	2 (154)	−0.42 [−0.77, −0.08]*; 0.0%	H60, H186
8–10 mmol/L	7 (514)	−1.48 [−2.72, −0.24]*; 89.6%	H41, H55, H71, H19, H145, H155, H165
≥10 mmol/L	4 (257)	−0.64 [−1.40, 0.12]; 17.1%	H51, H122, H130, H31
Treatment duration			
≤3 months	14 (1,075)	−0.62 [−1.11, −0.14]*; 75.2%	H51, H55, H60, H71, H19, H122, H130, H135, H145, H31, H155, H165, H181, H186
3–6 months	1 (90)	−4.91 [−6.05, −3.77]*	H41
CM syndrome differentiation			
Qi and *yin* deficiency	2 (169)	−0.04 [−0.73, 0.64]; 0.0%	H60, H165
Yin deficiency and excessive heat	1 (200)	0.61 [0.24, 0.98]	H181
Damp heat retention	2 (158)	−1.54 [−2.31, −0.78]; 0.0%	H122, H145
Spleen deficiency	1 (40)	−1.62 [−3.55, 0.31]	H135

*Statistically significant

Abbreviations: CI, confidence interval; CM, Chinese medicine; FPG, fasting plasma glucose; MD, mean difference; SG, sequence generation.

Triglyceride

A total of 112 studies, including 10,329 participants, assessed lipid metabolism in patients with T2DM by measuring triglyceride (TG). A lower value of TG indicates greater improvement. Overall meta-analysis for TG was performed at the end of treatment based on different comparators.

Chinese Herbal Medicine vs. Placebo

Five RCTs (H205–H207, H209, H210) with 572 participants compared CHM with a placebo, with treatment duration ranging from four to 12 weeks. The result showed that CHM was superior to the placebo at reducing TG levels in T2DM patients (MD −0.55 [−1.06, −0.03]; I^2 = 90.6%).

Chinese Herbal Medicine vs. Lifestyle Intervention

Four RCTs (H9, H201–H203) with 353 participants compared CHM with lifestyle intervention, with treatment duration ranging from eight to 12 weeks. The result showed that CHM was superior to lifestyle intervention (MD −0.40 [−0.52, −0.29]; I^2 = 40.6%).

Chinese Herbal Medicine vs. Pharmacotherapy

31 RCTs (n = 2,701; H1–H5, H7–H10, H12–H18, H20, H21, H23–H26, H28, H30–H33, H35, H37–H39) compared CHM with pharmacotherapy. The treatment duration ranged from four to 12 weeks. Different classes of hypoglycaemic agents were used as comparators, including biguanides, sulfonylureas, thiazolidinediones and α-glucosidase inhibitors. Specific agents included metformin, glipizide, glyburide, pioglitazone and acarbose. Aspirin was also used as a comparator.

The overall meta-analysis result showed a significant difference between the CHM group and pharmacotherapy group (MD −0.38 [−0.51, −0.26], I^2 = 86.3%). A meta-analysis of studies assessed as low risk for sequence generation produced a similar result to that of the overall results (11 RCTs, 1,227 participants, MD −0.29 [−0.50, −0.08]; I^2 = 72.7%).

A subgroup analysis by drug class showed that there was no difference between CHM and aspirin; however, results are based on one study with 58 participants (Table 5.12). Another study with 80 participants and treatment duration of more than six months did not show any significant difference between groups; interestingly, studies with treatment duration of less than three months presented with significant reduction in TG in the CHM group. However, heterogeneity was high (Table 5.12). In studies that provided information on the CM syndrome, T2DM participants with *qi* and *yin* deficiency and damp heat showed benefit in the improvements of BMI using integrative medicine (Table 5.12).

Table 5.12. Chinese Herbal Medicine vs. Pharmacotherapy: Triglyceride

Group	No. of Studies (Participants)	MD [95% CI], I^2%	Included Studies
All studies	31 (2,701)	−0.38 [−0.51, −0.26]*; 86.3%	H1–H5, H7–H10, H12–H18, H20, H21, H23–H26, H28, H30–H33, H35, H37–H39
Low risk of bias SG	11 (1,227)	−0.29 [−0.50, −0.08]*; 72.7%	H2, H8–H10, H13, H18, H23, H24, H26, H30, H35
Agents class			
Biguanides	22 (2,013)	−0.38 [−0.53, −0.22]*; 88.1%	H1, H4, H5, H8, H10, H12, H15–H18, H20, H21, H23–H25, H28, H30, H32, H33, H35, H37, H39
α-Glucosidase inhibitors	2 (184)	−0.49 [−0.91, −0.07]*; 78.5%	H9, H38
TZDs	3 (264)	−0.36 [−0.55, −0.18]*; 0.0%	H2, H7, H26

Table 5.12. (*Continued*)

Group	No. of Studies (Participants)	MD [95% CI], I^2%	Included Studies
Sulfonylureas	3 (182)	−0.53 [−0.81, −0.25]*; 55.9%	H3, H14, H31
Aspirin	1 (58)	0.11 [−0.28, 0.50]	H13
FPG level at baseline			
6–8 mmol/L	2 (194)	−0.29 [−0.67, 0.10]; 69.3%	H7, H23
8–10 mmol/L	20 (1,768)	−0.40 [−0.56, −0.24]*; 76.3%	H1, H2, H3, H5, H8–H10, H13–H15, H17, H18, H20, H21, H24, H25, H28, H30, H33, H35
≥10 mmol/L	8 (679)	−0.39 [−0.62, −0.16]*; 94.7%	H4, H12, H16, H31, H32, H37–H39
Treatment duration			
≤3 months	30 (2,621)	−0.39 [−0.51, −0.26]*; 86.7%	H1–H5, H7, H8, H10, H12–H18, H20, H21, H23–H26, H28, H30–H33, H35, H37–H39
≥6 months	1 (80)	−0.24 [−0.60, 0.12]	H9
CM syndrome differentiation			
Qi and *yin* deficiency	4 (264)	−0.63 [−0.99, −0.28]*; 73.3%	H3, H14, H15, H25
Yin deficiency and excessive heat	6 (429)	−0.33 [−0.68, 0.02]; 75.2%	H5, H8, H17, H21, H24, H35
Damp heat retention	5 (486)	−0.21 [−0.39, −0.03]*; 50.3%	H2, H7, H23, H32, H33
Phlegm-dampness and Blood stasis	1 (60)	−0.91 [−1.34, −0.48]*	H20

*Statistically significant

Abbreviations: CI, confidence interval; CM, Chinese medicine; FPG, fasting plasma glucose; MD, mean difference; SG, sequence generation; TZDs, thiazolidinedione.

CHM plus Hypoglycaemic Agents vs. Hypoglycaemic Agents

Seventy-seven RCTs (H3, H24, H31, H28, H41–H43, H46–H48, H51, H52, H55, H56, H60, H62, H64–H66, H71, H73–H76, H81, H86–H88, H92–H94, H96, H98, H100, H105, H107, H111, H113, H116, H121–H124, H126, H129, H130, H132–H133, H136–H139, H142, H145–H146, H149, H155, H157–H159, H161, H162, H164, H165, H167, H170, H172, H175, H176, H181, H183, H186, H188, H190, H192, H195, H196), including 6,858 participants, assessed the effects of CHM plus hypoglycaemic agents versus hypoglycaemic agents alone. All studies used the same hypoglycaemic agents in both groups. The specific agents include metformin, gliclazide, gliquidone, glibenclamide, glipizide, glimezide, acarbose, pioglitazone, repaglinide, sitagliptin, liraglutide and insulin. The treatment duration ranged from four to 12 weeks.

Meta-analysis showed that CHM in addition to hypoglycaemic agents was superior to hypoglycaemic agents alone at reducing TG levels in T2DM patients (MD −0.40 [−0.49, −0.32], I^2 = 94.4%). A meta-analysis of studies assessed as low risk for sequence generation produced a result that was more homogeneous (21 RCTs, 2,055 participants, MD −0.28 [−0.37, −0.19]; I^2 = 75.3%). Subgroup analyses by drug class and FPG level at baseline showed similar effects on TG. Two studies with longer treatment durations showed no significant difference between studies (Table 5.13). In studies that provided details on CM syndrome differentiation, adding CHM to hypoglycaemic agents showed more benefit in reducing TG levels in patients with *qi* and *yin* deficiency, *yin* deficiency with excessive heat, phlegm-dampness and Blood stasis, and Spleen deficiency, but not those with damp heat retention (Table 5.13).

Total Cholesterol

A total of 108 of the 210 studies, including 9,995 participants, assessed lipid metabolism in patients with T2DM using total cholesterol (TC) levels. A lower value of TC indicates greater improvement

Table 5.13. Chinese Herbal Medicine Plus Hypoglycaemic Agents vs. Hypoglycaemic Agents: Triglyceride

Group	No. of Studies (Participants)	MD [95% CI], I²%	Included Studies
All studies	77 (6,856)	−0.40 [−0.49, −0.32]*; 94.4%	H3, H28, H31, H41–H43, H46–H48, H51, H52, H55, H56, H60, H62, H64–H66, H71, H73–H76, H81, H86–H88, H92–H94, H96, H98, H100, H105, H107, H111, H113, H116, H121–H124, H126, H24, H129, H130, H132, H133, H136–H139, H142, H145, H146, H149, H155, H157–H159, H161, H162, H164, H165, H167, H170, H172, H175, H176, H181, H183, H186, H188, H190, H192, H195, H196
Low risk of bias SG	21 (2,055)	−0.28 [−0.37, −0.19]*; 75.3%	H24, H51, H60, H64–H66, H86, H87, H96, H100, H116, H122, H124, H126, H129, H146, H165, H175, H176, H181, H183
Drug class			
Biguanides	26 (2,549)	−0.44 [−0.64, −0.25]*; 95.5%	H24, H28, H41, H42, H46, H47, H60, H62, H65, H66, H74, H75, H88, H116, H126, H130, H132, H137, H145, H164, H165, H167, H170, H172, H183, H190
Sulfonylureas	13 (1,253)	−0.26 [−0.40, −0.11]*; 83.3%	H3, H31, H56, H73, H81, H87, H111, H123, H142, H146, H159, H161, H181
Insulin	3 (357)	−0.40 [−0.81, 0.02]; 81.8%	H122, H175, H176
TZDs	4 (272)	−0.58 [−0.87, −0.30]*; 81.6%	H48, H100, H139, H162
α-Glucosidase inhibitors	3 (244)	−0.25 [−0.45, −0.06]*; 85.3%	H113, H149, H186
Meglitinides	1 (60)	−0.45 [−0.58, −0.32]*	H93
Biguanides and Sulfonylureas	9 (639)	−0.29 [−0.43, −0.15]*; 58.9%	H51, H76, H94, H96, H98, H105, H121, H157, H188

(Continued)

Table 5.13. (*Continued*)

Group	No. of Studies (Participants)	MD [95% CI], I²%	Included Studies
Biguanides and α-Glucosidase inhibitors	2 (183)	−0.75 [−0.84, −0.66]*; 0.0%	H136, H155
FPG level at baseline			
6–8 mmol/L	6 (531)	−0.27 [−0.41, −0.13]*; 49.9%	H60, H86, H96, H136, H170, H186
8–10 mmol/L	40 (3,470)	−0.46 [−0.58, −0.34]*; 95.2%	H3, H24, H28, H41, H42, H47, H55, H62, H64, H65, H66, H71, H74, H87, H88, H92–H94, H100, H111, H116, H121, H124, H126, H133, H139, H142, H145, H146, H149, H155, H158, H159, H161, H162, H164, H165, H175, H176, H188
≥10 mmol/L	26 (2,175)	−0.34 [−0.43, −0.24]*; 82.8%	H31, H43, H51, H52, H56, H75, H76, H81, H98, H105, H107, H113, H122, H123, H129, H130, H137, H138, H157, H167, H172, H183, H190, H192, H195, H196
Treatment duration			
≤3 months	75 (6,682)	−0.41 [−0.50, −0.32]*; 94.5%	H3, H24, H28, H31, H43, H46–H48, H51, H52, H55, H56, H60, H62, H64–H66, H71, H73–H76, H81, H86–H88, H92–H94, H96, H98, H100, H105, H107, H111, H113, H116, H121–H124, H126, H129, H130, H132, H133, H136–H139, H142, H145, H146, H149, H155, H157–H159, H161, H162, H164, H165, H167, H170, H172, H175, H176, H181, H183, H186, H188, H190, H192, H195, H196
3–6 months	2 (176)	−0.20 [−0.74, 0.34]; 86.5%	H41, H42

Table 5.13. (*Continued*)

Group	No. of Studies (Participants)	MD [95% CI], I²%	Included Studies
CM syndrome differentiation			
Qi and *yin* deficiency	19 (1,595)	−0.38 [−0.56, −0.21]*; 96.2%	H3, H47, H60, H66, H73, H74, H81, H93, H94, H123, H124, H133, H137, H146, H161, H165, H170, H175, H188
Yin deficiency and excessive heat	8 (812)	−0.31 [−0.54, −0.09]*; 92.0%	H24, H75, H87, H116, H126, H129, H162, H181
Phlegm-dampness and Blood stasis	5 (368)	−0.71 [−1.41, −0.01]*; 98.8%	H48, H76, H113, H139, H164
Damp heat retention	5 (361)	−0.13 [−0.30, 0.05]; 74.2%	H62, H64, H122, H138, H145
Spleen deficiency	2 (158)	−0.40 [−0.57, −0.23]*; 0.0%	H100, H149

*Statistically significant

Abbreviations: CI, confidence interval; CM, Chinese medicine; FPG, fasting plasma glucose; MD, mean difference; SG, sequence generation; TZDs, thiazolidinedione.

in lipid metabolism. Overall meta-analysis for TC was performed at the end of treatment based on different comparators.

Chinese Herbal Medicine vs. Placebo

Five RCTs (H205–H207, H209, H210) with 572 participants compared CHM to placebo with treatment duration ranging from 12 to 24 weeks. The result showed CHM was superior to placebo (MD −0.89 [−1.28, −0.49]; I² = 88.5%) at reducing TC levels in T2DM patients.

Chinese Herbal Medicine vs. Lifestyle Intervention

Four RCTs (H9, H201–H203) with 353 participants compared CHM to lifestyle intervention. The treatment duration ranged from eight to 24 weeks. The result showed CHM was superior to lifestyle intervention (MD −0.57 [−0.77, −0.38]; I^2 = 0.0%) at reducing TC levels in T2DM patients.

Chinese Herbal Medicine vs. Pharmacotherapy

Thirty-one RCTs (*n* = 2,701; H1–H5, H7–H10, H12–H18, H20, H21, H23–H26, H28, H30–H33, H35, H37–H39) compared CHM with WM. Different classes of hypoglycaemic agents were used as comparators, including biguanides, sulfonylureas, thiazolidinediones and α-glucosidase inhibitors. Specific agents included metformin, glipizide, glyburide, pioglitazone and acarbose. Aspirin was also used as a comparator.

Meta-analysis result showed that the CHM group reduced TC levels more than the pharmacotherapy group (MD −0.42 [−0.57, −0.26], I^2 = 83.1%). A meta-analysis of studies assessed as low risk for sequence generation produced a result that was more homogeneous (11 RCTs, 1,127 participants, MD −0.30 [−0.51, −0.09]; I^2 = 69.4%).

Subgroup analyses by drug class showed that compared to thiazolidinediones, sulfonylureas and aspirin, CHM did not reduce TC levels more (Table 5.14). CHM was not better than pharmacotherapy at reducing TC levels in studies with lower levels of FPG at baseline (Table 5.14). A shorter or longer duration of treatment did not affect

Table 5.14. Chinese Medicine vs. Pharmacotherapy: Total Cholesterol

Group	No. of Studies (Participants)	MD [95% CI], I^2%	Included Studies
All studies	31 (2,701)	−0.42 [−0.57, −0.26]*; 83.1%	H1–H5, H7–H10, H12–H18, H20, H21, H23–H26, H28, H30–H33, H35, H37–H39
Low risk of bias SG	11 (1,227)	−0.30 [−0.51, −0.09]*; 69.4%	H2, H8–H10, H13, H18, H23, H24, H26, H30, H35

Table 5.14. (*Continued*)

Group	No. of Studies (Participants)	MD [95% CI], I²%	Included Studies
Agents class			
Biguanides	22 (2,013)	−0.41 [−0.58, −0.24]*; 82.5%	H1, H4, H5, H8, H10, H12, H15–H18, H20, H21, H23–H25, H28, H30, H32, H33, H35, H37, H39
α-Glucosidase inhibitors	2 (184)	−0.91 [−1.33, −0.48]*; 82.5%	H9, H38
TZDs	3 (264)	−0.08 [−0.64, 0.48]; 83.1%	H2, H7, H26
Sulfonylureas	3 (182)	−0.46 [−1.02, 0.10]; 72.7%	H3, H14, H31
Aspirin	1 (58)	−0.40 [−0.90, 0.10]	H13
FPG level at baseline			
6–8 mmol/L	2 (194)	0.28 [0.04, 0.52]; 0.0%	H7, H23
8–10 mmol/L	20 (1,768)	−0.44 [−0.60, −0.28]*; 71.4%	H1–H3, H5, H8–H10, H13–H15, H17, H18, H20, H21, H24, H25, H28, H30, H33, H35
≥10 mmol/L	8 (679)	−0.57 [−0.88, −0.26]*; 89.0%	H4, H12, H16, H31, H32, H37–H39
Treatment duration			
≤3 months	30 (2,621)	−0.41 [−0.56, −0.25]*; 83.5%	H1–H5, H7, H8, H10, H12–H18, H20, H21, H23–H26, H28, H30–H33, H35, H37–H39
≥6 months	1 (80)	−0.66 [−1.05, −0.27]*	H9
CM syndrome differentiation			
Qi and *yin* deficiency	4 (264)	−0.52 [−0.91, −0.13]*; 75.6%	H3, H14, H15, H25

(*Continued*)

Table 5.14. (*Continued*)

Group	No. of Studies (Participants)	MD [95% CI], I²%	Included Studies
Yin deficiency and excessive heat	6 (429)	−0.14 [−0.31, 0.04]; 6.7%	H5, H8, H17, H21, H24, H35
Damp heat retention	5 (486)	−0.04 [−0.36, 0.27]; 77.0%	H2, H7, H23, H32, H33
Phlegm-dampness and Blood stasis	1 (60)	−0.42 [−0.57, −0.26]*	H20

*Statistically significant

Abbreviations: CI, confidence interval; CM, Chinese medicine; FPG, fasting plasma glucose; MD, mean difference; SG, sequence generation; TZDs, thiazolidinedione.

the results. In studies that provided CM syndrome differentiation, CHM did not reduce TC more than pharmacotherapy in T2DM patients with *yin* deficiency and excess heat or damp heat retention (Table 5.14).

CHM plus Hypoglycaemic Agents vs. Hypoglycaemic Agents

Seventy-three RCTs (H3, H24, H28, H31, H41–H43, H46–H48, H51, H52, H56, H60, H62, H64–H66, H71, H73–H76, H81, H86–H88, H92–H94, H96, H98, H100, H105, H107, H111, H113, H116, H121–H124, H126, H129, H130, H132, H33, H136–H139, H142, H145, H149, H155, H157–H159, H161, H162, H164–165, H167, H172, H175, H176, H181, H183, H186, H188, H190, H192, H195), including 6,524 participants, assessed the effects of CHM plus hypoglycaemic agents versus hypoglycaemic agents alone. The term "hypoglycaemic agents" includes biguanides, sulfonylureas, thiazolidinediones, α-glucosidase inhibitors, meglitinides, DPP-4 inhibitors, GLP-1 receptor agonists and insulins. Specific agents included metformin, gliclazide, gliquidone, glibenclamide, glipizide, glimezide, acarbose, pioglitazone, repaglinide, sitagliptin, liraglutide and insulin. The treatment duration ranged from four to 14 weeks.

CHM plus hypoglycaemic agents were superior to hypoglycaemic agents alone at reducing TC levels (MD −0.49 [−0.64, −0.33], I^2 = 97.3%). A meta-analysis of studies assessed as low risk for sequence generation produced a similar result to that of the overall results, with high heterogeneity.

A subgroup analysis showed that the combination of CHM with insulin or α-Glucosidase inhibitors was not superior at reducing TC levels (Table 5.15). Studies with FPG levels of 8 mmol/L at baseline showed the biggest estimate of effect in TC levels; however, the heterogeneity was high (Table 5.15). Studies with treatment duration shorter than three months (71 RCTs, n = 6,348) showed a significant difference between the two groups, but not in the two studies with longer treatment durations (Table 5.15). Additional analysis on studies that provided CM syndrome information showed that integrative medicine was superior to hypoglycaemic agents alone in patients with *qi* and *yin* deficiency, *yin* deficiency with excessive heat,

Table 5.15. Chinese Herbal Medicine Plus Hypoglycaemic Agents vs. Hypoglycaemic Agents: Total Cholesterol

Group	No. of Studies (Participants)	MD [95% CI], I^2%	Included Studies
All studies	73 (6,524)	−0.49 [−0.64, −0.33]*; 97.3%	H3, H24, H28, H31, H41–H43, H46–H48, H51, H52, H56, H60, H62, H64–H66, H71, H73–H76, H81, H86–H88, H92–H94, H96, H98, H100, H105, H107, H111, H113, H116, H121–H124, H126, H129, H130, H132, H133, H136–H139, H142, H145, H149, H155, H157–H159, H161, H162, H164, H165, H167, H172, H175, H176, H181, H183, H186, H188, H190, H192, H195
Low risk of bias SG	20 (1,955)	−0.49 [−0.77, −0.20]*; 96.9%	H24, H51, H60, H64–H66, H86, H87, H96, H100, H116, H122, H124, H126, H129, H165, H175, H176, H181, H183

(Continued)

145

Table 5.15. (*Continued*)

Group	No. of Studies (Participants)	MD [95% CI], I²%	Included Studies
Drug class			
Biguanides	25 (2,429)	−0. 56 [−0.79, −0.33]*; 85.0%	H24, H41, H42, H46, H47, H60, H62, H65, H66, H74, H75, H88, H116, H126, H130, H132, H137, H28, H145, H164, H165, H167, H172, H183, H190
Sulfonylureas	12 (1,153)	−0. 3 3[−0.54, −0.12]*; 85.0%	H3, H31, H56, H73, H81, H87, H111, H123, H142, H159, H161, H181
Insulin	3 (357)	−0.31 [−1.10, 0.48]; 88.3%	H122, H175, H176
TZDs	4 (272)	−0.85 [−1.29, −0.41]*; 89.8%	H48, H100, H139, H162
α-Glucosidase inhibitors	3 (244)	−0.36 [−0.82, 0.10]; 84.7%	H113, H149, H186
Meglitinides	1 (60)	−0.29 [−0.46, −0.12]*	H93
Biguanides and Sulfonylureas	9 (639)	−0.05 [−0.81, −0.71]*; 95.0%	H51, H76, H94, H96, H98, H105, H121, H157, H188
Biguanides and α-Glucosidase inhibitors	3 (218)	−0.78 [−1.48, −0.08]*; 88.5%	H71, H107, H129
FPG level at baseline			
6–8 mmol/L	5 (411)	−0.14 [−0.26, −0.02]; 0.0%	H60, H86, H96, H136, H186
8–10 mmol/L	38 (3,301)	−0.61 [−0.87, −0.36]; 98.3%	H3, H24, H28, H41, H42, H47, H62, H64–H66, H71, H74, H87, H88, H92–H94, H100, H111, H116, H121, H124, H126, H133, H139, H142, H145, H149, H155, H158, H159, H161, H162, H164, H165, H175, H176, H188
≥10 mmol/L	25 (2,130)	−0.39 [−0.59, −0.18]; 90.9%	H31, H43, H51, H52, H56, H75, H76, H81, H98, H105, H107, H113, H122, H123, H129, H130, H137, H138, H157, H167, H172, H183, H190, H192, H195

Table 5.15. (*Continued*)

Group	No. of Studies (Participants)	MD [95% CI], I²%	Included Studies
Treatment duration			
≤3 months	71 (6,348)	−0.49 [−0.65, −0.33]*; 97.4%	H3, H24, H28, H31, H43, H46–H48, H51, H52, H56, H60, H62, H64–H66, H71, H73–H76, H81, H86–H88, H92–H94, H96, H98, H100, H105, H107, H111, H113, H116, H121–H124, H126, H129, H130, H132, H133, H136–H139, H142, H145, H149, H155, H157, H158, H159, H161, H162, H164, H165, H167, H172, H175, H176, H181, H183, H186, H188, H190, H192, H195
3–6 months	2 (176)	−0.37 [−1.05, 0.30]; 88.2%	H41, H42
CM syndrome differentiation			
Qi and *yin* deficiency	17 (1,375)	−0.54 [−0.74, −0.34]*; 93.2%	H3, H47, H60, H66, H73, H74, H81, H93, H94, H123, H124, H133, H137, H161, H165, H175, H188
Yin deficiency and excessive heat	8 (812)	−0.57 [−1.05, −0.09]*; 97.2%	H24, H75, H87, H116, H126, H129, H162, H181
Phlegm-dampness and Blood stasis	5 (368)	−0.69 [−1.17, −0.21]*; 88.7%	H48, H76, H113, H139, H164
Damp heat retention	5 (361)	−0.64 [−1.21, −0.07]*; 85.3%	H62, H64, H122, H138, H145
Spleen deficiency	2 (158)	−0.80 [−2.00, 0.39]; 95.5%	H100, H149

*Statistically significant

Abbreviations: CI, confidence interval; CM, Chinese medicine; FPG, fasting plasma glucose; MD, mean difference; SG, sequence generation; TZDs, thiazolidinedione.

phlegm-dampness and Blood stasis, or damp heat retention, but not those with Spleen deficiency (Table 5.15).

Low-Density Lipoprotein

Eighty-one studies, including 7,818 participants, conducted an assessment of lipid metabolism in patients with T2DM using the low-density lipoprotein (LDL). A lower value on the LDL indicates greater improvement. Overall, meta-analysis for LDL was performed at the end of treatment based on different comparators.

Chinese Herbal Medicine vs. Placebo

Four RCTs (H205, H207, H209, H210) with 497 participants compared CHM with a placebo. The treatment duration ranged from 12 to 24 weeks. The result showed that CHM was superior to the placebo (MD −0.57 [−0.78, −0.34], I^2 = 59.4%).

Chinese Herbal Medicine vs. Lifestyle Intervention

Three RCTs (H9, H201, H202) with 293 participants compared CHM with lifestyle intervention and no oral hypoglycaemics. The treatment duration ranged from eight to 24 weeks. The result showed that CHM was superior to lifestyle intervention (MD −0.36 [−0.57 −0.16]; I^2 = 0.0%).

Chinese Herbal Medicine vs. Pharmacotherapy

Twenty-four RCTs (n = 2,169; H1–H3, H7–H9, H12–H14, H16–H18, H21, H24–H26, H28, H30–H33, H35, H37, H38) compared CHM with pharmacotherapy. Pharmacotherapy included different classes of hypoglycaemic agents and aspirin. Specific hypoglycaemic agents include metformin, glipizide, glyburide, pioglitazone and acarbose. The treatment duration ranged from four to 24 weeks.

Meta-analysis results indicated that CHM could lower the LDL level more than the pharmacotherapy group (MD −0.34 [−0.47,

−0.21], I^2 = 82.8%). Nine studies assessed as low risk of bias for sequence generation showed similar results to the overall studies, with increased heterogeneity (Table 5.16). A subgroup analysis by drug class showed that compared to sulfonylureas and aspirin, CHM was not superior at reducing LDL levels (Table 5.16). In studies that provided details on CM syndrome differentiation, a subgroup analysis showed that CHM is better at reducing LDL levels in patients with *yin* deficiency and excessive heat, but not in those with *qi* and *yin* deficiency or damp heat retention (Table 5.16).

Table 5.16. Chinese Herbal Medicine vs. Pharmacotherapy: Low-Density Lipoprotein

Group	No. of Studies (Participants)	MD [95% CI], I^2%	Included Studies
All studies	24 (2,169)	−0.34 [−0.47, −0.21]; 82.8%	H1–H3, H7–H9, H12–H14, H16–H18, H21, H24–H26, H28, H30–H33, H35, H37, H38
Low risk of bias SG	9 (1,058)	−0.39 [−0.69, −0.10]*, 89.5%	H2, H8, H9, H13, H18, H24, H26, H30, H35
Agents class			
Biguanides	15 (1,481)	−0.31 [−0.48, −0.15]*; 85.4%	H1, H8, H12, H16–H18, H21, H24, H25, H28, H30, H32, H33, H35, H37
α-Glucosidase inhibitors	2 (184)	−0.56 [−0.85, −0.27]*; 85.4%	H9, H38
TZDs	3 (264)	−0.23 [−0.42, −0.03]*; 0.0%	H2, H7, H26
Sulfonylureas	3 (182)	−0.49 [−1.17, 0.19]; 86.5%	H3, H14, H31
Aspirin	1 (58)	−0.38 [−0.77, 0.01]	H13

(Continued)

Table 5.16. *(Continued)*

Group	No. of Studies (Participants)	MD [95% CI], I²%	Included Studies
FPG level at baseline			
6–8 mmol/L	1 (124)	−0.28 [−0.53, −0.03]*	H7
8–10 mmol/L	16 (1,489)	−0.32 [−0.51, −0.13]*; 85.2%	H1–H3, H8, H9, H13, H14, H17, H18, H21, H24, H25, H28, H30, H33, H35
≥10 mmol/L	6 (496)	−0.43 [−0.62, −0.24]*; 75.7%	H12, H16, H31, H32, H37, H38
Treatment duration			
≤3 months	23 (2,089)	−0.34 [−0.47, −0.20]*; 83.5%	H1–H3, H7, H8, H12–H14, H16–H18, H21, H24–H26, H28, H30–H33, H35, H37, H38
≥6 months	1 (80)	−0.3 8[−0.68, −0.08]*	H9
CM syndrome differentiation			
Qi and *yin* deficiency	3 (204)	−0.31 [−0.75, 0.14]; 81.8%	H3, H14, H25
Yin deficiency and excessive heat	5 (369)	−0.30 [−0.46, −0.13]*; 28.3%	H8, H17, H21, H24, H35
Damp heat retention	4 (416)	−0.17 [−0.40, 0.06]; 46.9%	H2, H7, H32, H33

*Statistically significant
Abbreviations: CI, confidence interval; CM, Chinese medicine; FPG, fasting plasma glucose; MD, mean difference; SG, sequence generation; TZDs, thiazolidinedione.

Chinese Herbal Medicine Plus Hypoglycaemic Agents vs. Hypoglycaemic Agents

Fifty-four RCTs (H3, H24, H28, H31, H41, H48, H51, H52, H56, H62, H64–H66, H71, H74, H76, H81, H86, H88, H92–H94, H98, H105, H107, H113, H116, H121, H122, H124, H126, H132, H137,

H139, H145, H155, H157–H159, H161, H162, H164, H165, H167, H172, H175, H176, H181, H183, H186, H188, H192, H195, H196), including 4,926 participants, assessed the effects of CHM plus hypoglycaemic agents versus hypoglycaemic agents alone. Different classes of hypoglycaemic agents were used, and the treatment duration ranged from four to 14 weeks.

When results for all 54 studies were combined for analysis, CHM plus hypoglycaemic agents was superior to hypoglycaemic agents alone (MD −0.39 [−0.50, −0.28]; I^2 = 96.5%). Fifteen studies assessed as low risk of bias for sequence generation showed similar results to the overall studies, with increased heterogeneity (Table 5.17). A subgroup analysis by drug class showed that compared to insulin, CHM added to insulin was not superior at reducing LDL levels (Table 5.17). In studies that provided details on CM syndrome differentiation, a subgroup analysis showed that CHM is better at reducing LDL levels in patients with *yin* deficiency and excessive heat, but not in those with *qi* and *yin* deficiency or damp heat retention (Table 5.17).

Table 5.17. Chinese Herbal Medicine plus Hypoglycaemic Agents vs. Hypoglycaemic Agents: Low-Density Liproprotein

Group	No. of Studies (Participants)	MD [95% CI], I2%	Included Studies
All studies	54 (4,926)	−0.39 [−0.50, −0.28]*; 96.5%	H3, H24, H28, H31, H41, H48, H51, H52, H56, H62, H64–H66, H71, H74, H76, H81, H86, H88, H92–H94, H98, H105, H107, H113, H116, H121, H122, H124, H126, H132, H137, H139, H145, H155, H157–H159, H161, H162, H164, H65, H167, H172, H175, H176, H181, H183, H186, H188, H192, H195, H196
Low risk of bias SG	15 (1,587)	−0.45 [−0.75, −0.15]*; 98.0%	H24, H51, H64–H66, H86, H116, H122, H124, H126, H165, H175, H176, H181, H183

(Continued)

Table 5.17. (*Continued*)

Group	No. of Studies (Participants)	MD [95% CI], I2%	Included Studies
Drug class			
Biguanides	18 (1,807)	−0.53 [−0.78, −0.27]*; 97.8%	H28, H41, H62, H65, H66, H74, H88, H116, H126, H24, H132, H137, H145, H164, H165, H167, H172, H183
Sulfonylureas	7 (853)	−0.15 [−0.28, −0.03]*; 63.5%	H3, H31, H56, H81, H159, H161, H181
Insulin	3 (357)	−0.57 [−1.20, 0.07]; 96.9%	H122, H175, H176
TZDs	3 (206)	−0.52 [−0.66, −0.37]*; 0.0%	H48, H139, H162
α-Glucosidase inhibitors	2 (152)	0.05 [−0.26, 0.36]; 89.7%	H113, H186
Meglitinides	1 (60)	−0.21 [−0.30, −0.12]*	H93
Biguanides and Sulfonylureas	8 (579)	−0.26 [−0.44, −0.08]*; 79.9%	H51, H76, H94, H98, H105, H121, H157, H188
Biguanides and α-Glucosidase inhibitors	2 (110)	−0.39 [−0.66, −0.12]*; 78.1%	H71, H107
FPG level at baseline			
6–8 mmol/L	2 (174)	−0.17 [−0.38, 0.05]; 47.4%	H86, H186
8–10 mmol/L	30 (2,581)	−0.50 [−0.66, −0.33]*; 96.8%	H3, H24, H28, H41, H62, H64, H65, H66, H71, H74, H88, H92, H93, H94, H116, H121, H124, H126, H139, H145, H155, H158, H159, H161, H162, H164, H165, H175, H176, H188
≥10 mmol/L	19 (1,637)	−0.21 [−0.30, −0.12]*; 78.1%	H31, H51, H52, H56, H76, H81, H98, H105, H107, H113, H122, H137, H157, H167, H172, H183, H192, H195, H196

Table 5.17. (*Continued*)

Group	No. of Studies (Participants)	MD [95% CI], I2%	Included Studies
Treatment duration			
≤3 months	53 (4,836)	−0.40 [−0.51, −0.28]*; 96.5%	H3, H24, H28, H31, H48, H51, H52, H56, H62, H64–H66, H71, H74, H76, H81, H86, H88, H92–H94, H98, H105, H107, H113, H116, H121, H122, H124, H126, H132, H137, H139, H145, H155, H157–H159, H161, H162, H164, H165, H167, H172, H175, H176, H181, H183, H186, H188, H192, H195, H196
3–6 months	1 (90)	−0.10 [−0.42, 0.22]	H41
CM syndrome differentiation			
Qi and *yin* deficiency	12 (885)	−0.23 [−0.33, −0.13]*; 60.7%	H3, H66, H74, H81, H93, H94, H124, H137, H161, H165, H175, H188
Yin deficiency and excessive heat	5 (544)	−0.55 [−1.19, 0.09]; 99.1%	H24, H116, H126, H162, H181
Phlegm-dampness and Blood stasis	5 (368)	−0.54 [−1.31, 0.22]; 98.2%	H48, H76, H113, H139, H164
Damp heat retention	4 (299)	−0.51 [−1.34, 0.30]; 97.8%	H62, H64, H122, H145

*Statistically significant
Abbreviations: CI, confidence interval; CM, Chinese medicine; FPG, fasting plasma glucose; MD, mean difference; SG, sequence generation; TZDs, thiazolidinedione.

Studies with higher FPG levels at baseline and shorter treatment durations showed a significant difference between group results. A subgroup analysis by CM syndrome differentiation showed in patients with *qi* and *yin* deficiency. Adding CHM to hypoglycaemic agents is better at reducing LDL than using hypoglycaemics alone (Table 5.17).

High-Density Lipoprotein

Eighty studies of 7,395 participants conducted an assessment of lipid metabolism in patients with T2DM using high-density lipoprotein (HDL). A higher value on HDL indicates greater improvement. Overall meta-analysis for HDL was performed at the end of treatment based on different comparators.

Chinese Herbal Medicine vs. Placebo

Five RCTs (H205–H207, H209, H210) with 572 participants compared CHM with a placebo. The treatment duration ranged from 12 to 24 weeks. The result showed that CHM is superior to placebo at increasing HDL levels in T2CM patients (MD 0.07 [−0.13, −0.26]; $I^2 = 94.1\%$); however, high heterogeneity was observed.

Chinese Herbal Medicine vs. Lifestyle Intervention

Three RCTs (H9, H201, H202) with 293 participants compared CHM with lifestyle intervention. The treatment duration ranged from eight to 24 weeks. The result showed there was no statistical difference between CHM and lifestyle intervention (MD 0.12 [−0.004, 0.25]; $I^2 = 30.1\%$).

CHM vs. Pharmacotherapy

Twenty-one RCTs ($n = 1,594$; H1–H2, H7–H10, H12–H14, H16–H18, H21, H24–H26, H28, H31–H33, H35) compared CHM with pharmacotherapy. Comparator drugs used includes different classes of hypoglycaemic agents and aspirin. The treatment duration ranged from four to 24 weeks.

When the results for all 21 studies were combined for analysis, there were significant differences between the CHM and pharmacotherapy group (MD 0.08 [0.03, 0.13], I^2 = 65.4%). A meta-analysis of studies assessed as low risk for sequence generation produced a slightly better estimate of effect with increased heterogeneity (nine RCTs, 707 participants, MD 0.15 [0.06, 0.24]; I^2 = 72%). A subgroup analysis by drug class showed there was no difference between CHM and sulfonylureas and aspirin (Table 5.18). Another subgroup analysis based on FPG level at baseline and treatment duration showed similar results to the overall result (Table 5.18). In five studies that reported CM syndrome *yin* deficiency and excessive heat, CHM is better at improving HDL levels with low heterogeneity (MD 0.07 [0.01, 0.12], I^2 = 8.1%).

Table 5.18. **Chinese Herbal Medicine vs. Pharmacotherapy: High-Density Lipoprotein**

Group	No. of Studies (Participants)	MD [95% CI], I^2%	Included Studies
All studies	21 (1,594)	0.08 [0.03, 0.13]*; 65.4%	H1, H2, H7–H10, H12–H14, H16–H18, H21, H24–H26, H28, H31–H33, H35
Low risk of bias SG	9 (707)	0.15 [0.06, 0.24]*; 72.0%	H2, H8–H10, H13, H18, H24, H26, H35
Agents class			
Biguanides	14 (1,070)	0.10 [0.03, 0.16]*; 64.1%	H1, H8, H10, H12, H16–H18, H21, H24, H25, H28, H32, H33, H35
α-Glucosidase inhibitors	1 (80)	0.14 [0.03, 0.26]*	H9
TZDs	3 (264)	0.03 [−0.31, 0.38]; 85.8%	H2, H7, H26
Sulfonylureas	2 (122)	−0.06 [−0.18, 0.06]; 0.0%	H14, H31
Aspirin	1 (58)	0.10 [0.03, 0.16]*	H13
FPG level at baseline			
6–8 mmol/L	1 (124)	−0.21 [−0.41, −0.01]*	H7

(Continued)

Table 5.18. *(Continued)*

Group	No. of Studies (Participants)	MD [95% CI], I²%	Included Studies
8–10 mmol/L	15 (1,078)	0.11 [0.05, 0.17]*; 64.1%	H1, H2, H8–H10, H13, H14, H17, H18, H21, H24, H25, H28, H33, H35
≥10 mmol/L	4 (332)	0.04 [−0.05, 0.12]*; 41.6%	H12, H16, H31, H32
Treatment duration			
≤3 months	20 (1,514)	0.07 [0.02, 0.13]*; 66.8%	H1, H2, H7, H8, H10, H12–H14, H16–H18, H21, H24–H26, H28, H31–H33, H35
≥6 months	1 (80)	0.14 [0.03, 0.26]*	H9
CM syndrome differentiation			
Qi and *yin* deficiency	2 (144)	0.01 [−0.11, 0.12]; 0.0%	H14, H25
Yin deficiency and excessive heat	5 (369)	0.07 [0.01, 0.12]*; 8.1%	H8, H17, H21, H24, H35
Damp heat retention	4 (416)	0.05 [−0.13, 0.23]; 81.3%	H2, H7, H32, H33

*Statistically significant

Abbreviations: CI, confidence interval; CM, Chinese medicine; FPG, fasting plasma glucose; MD, mean difference; SG, sequence generation; TZDs, thiazolidinedione.

CHM plus Hypoglycaemic Agents vs. Hypoglycaemic Agents

Fifty-five RCTs (H24, H28, H31, H41, H48, H51, H52, H56, H62, H64–H66, H71, H74, H76, H81, H86, H88, H92–H94, H98, H105, H107, H113, H116, H121, H122, H124, H126, H132, H136, H137, H139, H145, H149, H155, H157–H159, H161, H162, H164, H165, H167, H172, H175, H176, H181, H183, H186, H188, H192, H195, H196), including 5,061 participants, assessed the effects of

CHM plus hypoglycaemic agents versus hypoglycaemic agents alone. Different classes of hypoglycaemic agent were used, and the treatment duration ranged from four to 14 weeks.

Meta-analysis results of all 55 studies showed that CHM plus hypoglycaemic agents were superior to hypoglycaemic agents alone at improving HDL levels (MD 0.15 [0.11, 0.19]; I^2 = 93.3%). A meta-analysis of results from studies with a low risk of bias for sequence generation produced a similar result (Table 5.19). A subgroup analysis by drug class showed that CHM in combination with biguanides, sulfonylureas, TZDs and meglitinides can improve HDL levels better than using the agents alone (Table 5.19). Another subgroup analysis using FPG level at baseline and treatment duration showed significant differences between groups with high heterogeneity (Table 5.19). In T2DM patients with *qi* and *yin* deficiency, *yin* deficiency and excessive heat and Spleen deficiency, integrative medicine was better at improving HDL levels than hypoglycaemic agents alone (Table 5.19).

Table 5.19. Chinese Herbal Medicine Plus Hypoglycaemic Agents vs. Hypoglycaemic agents: High-Density Lipoprotein

Group	No. of Studies (Participants)	MD [95% CI], I^2%	Included Studies
All studies	55 (5,061)	0.15 [0.11, 0.19]*; 93.3%	H24, H28, H31, H41, H48, H51, H52, H56, H62, H64–H66, H71, H74, H76, H81, H86, H88, H92–H94, H98, H105, H107, H113, H116, H121, H122, H124, H126, H132, H136, H137, H139, H145, H149, H155, H157–H159, H161, H162, H164, H165, H167, H172, H175, H176, H181, H183, H186, H188, H192, H195, H196
Low risk of bias SG	15 (1,587)	0.11 [0.03, 0.18]*; 93.4%	H24, H51, H64, H65, H66, H86, H116, H122, H124, H126, H165, H175, H176, H181, H183

(Continued)

Table 5.19.   (*Continued*)

Group	No. of Studies (Participants)	MD [95% CI], I²%	Included Studies
Drug class			
Biguanides	18 (1,807)	0.24 [0.14, 0.34]*; 95.8%	H28, H41, H62, H65, H66, H74, H88, H116, H126, H24, H132, H137, H145, H164, H165, H167, H172, H183
Sulfonylureas	6 (793)	0.10 [0.0, 0.19]*; 80.9%	H31, H56, H81, H159, H161, H181
Insulin	3 (357)	0.09 [−0.14, 0.33]; 97.5%	H122, H175, H176
TZDs	3 (206)	0.22 [0.05, 0.39]*; 76.2%	H48, H139, H162
α-Glucosidase inhibitors	3 (224)	0.13 [−0.0, 0.26]; 72.1%	H113, H149, H186
Meglitinides	1 (60)	0.17 [0.09, 0.25]*	H93
Biguanides and Sulfonylureas	8 (579)	0.07 [−0.03, 0.16]; 84.0%	H51, H76, H94, H98, H105, H121, H157, H188
Biguanides and α-Glucosidase inhibitors	2 (110)	−0.04 [−0.12, 0.04]; 21.1%	H71, H107
FPG level at baseline			
6–8 mmol/L	3 (277)	0.16 [0.01, 0.30]*; 85.5%	H86, H136, H186
8–10 mmol/L	30 (2613)	0.17 [0.12, 0.23]*; 95.1%	H24, H28, H41, H62, H64–H66, H71, H74, H88, H92–H94, H116, H121, H124, H126, H139, H145, H149, H155, H158, H159, H161, H162, H164, H165, H175, H176, H188
≥10 mmol/L	19 (1637)	0.09 [0.04, 0.14]*; 81.6%	H31, H51, H52, H56, H76, H81, H98, H105, H107, H113, H122, H137, H157, H167, H172, H183, H192, H195, H196
Treatment duration			
≤3 months	54 (4,971)	0.14 [0.10, 0.18]*; 92.7%	H24, H28, H48, H51, H52, H56, H62–H66, H71, H74, H76, H81,

Table 5.19. (*Continued*)

Group	No. of Studies (Participants)	MD [95% CI], I²%	Included Studies
			H86, H88, H92–H94, H98, H105, H107, H113, H116, H121, H122, H124, H126, H132, H136, H137, H139, H145, H31, H149, H155, H157–H159, H161, H162, H164, H165, H167, H172, H175, H176, H181, H183, H186, H188, H192, H195, H196
3–6 months	1 (90)	0.59 [0.49, 0.69]*	H41
CM syndrome differentiation			
Qi and *yin* deficiency	11 (825)	0.14 [0.10, 0.19]*; 65.6%	H66, H74, H81, H93, H94, H124, H137, H161, H165, H175, H188
Yin deficiency and excessive heat	5 (544)	0.09 [0.03, 0.15]*; 56.5%	H116, H126, H24, H162, H181
Phlegm-dampness and Blood stasis	5 (368)	0.42 [0.13, 0.72]*; 95.0%	H48, H76, H113, H139, H164
Damp heat retention	4 (299)	0.10 [−0.05, 0.26]; 90.9%	H62, H64, H122, H145
Spleen deficiency	1 (92)	0.20 [0.02, 0.38]*	H149

*Statistically significant
Abbreviations: CI, confidence interval; CM, Chinese medicine; FPG, fasting plasma glucose; MD, mean difference; SG, sequence generation; TZDs, thiazolidinedione.

Fasting Insulin

Sixty-four studies, including 5,736 participants, assessed the β-cell function of T2DM using the fasting insulin (FINS). A lower value on the FINS indicates greater improvement. Studies that used the unit of FINS μU/ml or pmol/l (pmol/l = μU/ml × 6.965) are included. Overall meta-analysis for FINS was performed at the end of treatment based on different comparators.

Chinese Herbal Medicine vs. Placebo

Three RCTs (H205, H207, H209) with 399 participants compared CHM to a placebo. The treatment duration ranged from 12 to 24 weeks. The result showed that CHM was superior to placebo (MD 1.11 [0.55, 1.68], $I^2 = 30.9\%$).

Chinese Herbal Medicine vs. Lifestyle Intervention

One RCT (H202) with 152 participants compared CHM with only lifestyle intervention and no oral hypoglycaemic. The treatment duration was eight weeks. The results showed that CHM was superior to lifestyle intervention (MD −2.92 [−4.67, −1.17]).

Chinese Herbal Medicine vs. Hypoglycaemic Agents

Thirteen RCTs ($n = 1,009$; H3, H7–H8, H10, H11, H16, H24, H25, H28, H29, H35, H36, H40) compared CHM with hypoglycaemic agents (four classes of agents were used as comparators, including biguanides, sulfonylureas, thiazolidinediones and α-Glucosidase inhibitors). Specific agents included metformin, glipizide, glyburide, pioglitazone and acarbose. All studies had treatment duration of fewer than 12 weeks, ranging from four to 12 weeks.

The overall result indicated an improvement in the CHM group, though it was lower than in the anti-diabetic medication group (MD −1.00 [−1.84, −0.15], $I^2 = 75.3\%$). A meta-analysis of results from studies with a low risk of bias for sequence generation did not show benefit in improving FINS levels using CHM compared to hypoglycaemic agents (Table 5.20). Ten studies with the baseline FPG level of 8–10 mmol/L showed significant differences between groups (Table 5.20). Studies with lower or higher baseline FPG levels did not have the same results, but only one or two studies were included, so the results are not conclusive. In studies that provided CM syndrome differentiation, there were no significant differences in improving FINS levels between CHM and hypoglycaemic agents (Table 5.20).

Table 5.20. Chinese Herbal Medicine vs. Hypoglycaemic Agents: Fasting Insulin

Group	No. of Studies (Participants)	MD [95% CI], I^2%	Included Studies
All studies	13 (1,009)	−1.00 [−1.84, −0.15]*; 75.3%	H3, H7, H8, H10, H11, H16, H24, H25, H28, H29, H35, H36, H40
Low risk of bias SG	4 (349)	−0.86 [−3.56, 1.85]; 85.9%	H8, H10, H24, H35
Agents class			
Biguanides	8 (589)	−0.68 [−1.79, 0.43]; 82.4%	H8, H10, H16, H24, H25, H28, H29, H35
α-Glucosidase inhibitors	1 (112)	−1.51 [−2.35, 0.67]	H11
TZDs	3 (248)	−1.46 [−3.04, 0.12]; 0.0%	H7, H36, H40
Sulfonylureas	1 (60)	−4.29 [−8.20, −0.38]*	H3
FPG level at baseline			
6–8 mmol/L	1 (124)	−1.65 [−5.22, 1.92]	H7
8–10 mmol/L	10 (765)	−1.19 [−2.09, −0.28]*; 72.1%	H3, H8, H10, H11, H24, H25, H28, H35, H36, H40
≥10 mmol/L	2 (120)	−0.14 [−2.64, 2.36]; 83.0%	H16, H29
CM syndrome differentiation			
Qi and *yin* deficiency	5 (328)	−1.17 [−2.98, 0.63]; 81.4%	H3, H25, H29, H36, H40
Yin deficiency and excessive heat	3 (520)	−0.31 [−3.83, 3.21]; 73.7%	H8, H24, H35
Damp heat retention	1 (124)	−1.65 [−5.22, 1.92]	H7

*Statistically significant
Abbreviations: CI, confidence interval; CM, Chinese medicine; FPG, fasting plasma glucose; MD, mean difference; SG, sequence generation; TZDs, thiazolidinedione.

Chinese Herbal Medicine Plus Hypoglycaemic Agents vs. Hypoglycaemic Agents

Fifty-one RCTs (H3, H24, H28, H41, H45, H49, H51, H56, H59, H63, H71, H73, H78, H79, H82, H90, H91, H98, H100, H106, H109, H111, H112, H116, H119, H120, H126, H127, H131, H133, H141, H142, H144–H146, H154, H155, H157, H158, H165, H168, H170, H171, H179, H180, H182, H186, H192, H194, H197, H199), including 4,341 participants, assessed the effects of CHM plus hypoglycaemic agents versus hypoglycaemic agents alone. Different classes of hypoglycaemic agents were included and the treatment duration ranged from four to 24 weeks.

At the end of treatment, CHM plus hypoglycaemic agents were superior to hypoglycaemic agents alone at reducing FINS levels (MD −1.45 [−2.06, −0.84], I^2 = 98.3%). A meta-analysis of results from studies with a low risk of bias for sequence generation showed similar results from the overall result (Table 5.21). A subgroup analysis by hypoglycaemic agent class showed there were varied results for

Table 5.21. Chinese Herbal Medicine plus Hypoglycaemic Agents vs. Hypoglycaemic Agents: Fasting Insulin

Group	No. of Studies (Participants)	MD [95% CI], I^2%	Included Studies
All studies	51 (4,341)	−1.45 [−2.06, −0.84]*; 98.3%	H3, H24, H28, H41, H45, H49, H51, H56, H59, H63, H71, H73, H78, H79, H82, H90, H91, H98, H100, H106, H109, H111, H112, H116, H119, H120, H126, H127, H131, H133, H141, H142, H144–H146, H154, H155, H157, H158, H165, H168, H170, H171, H179, H180, H182, H186, H192, H194, H197, H199
Low risk of bias SG	19 (1,535)	−1.53 [−2.17, −0.90]*; 90.4%	H24, H51, H63, H78, H79, H82, H90, H91, H100, H106, H112, H116, H119, H126, H144, H146, H165, H168, H199

Table 5.21. *(Continued)*

Group	No. of Studies (Participants)	MD [95% CI], I²%	Included Studies
Drug class			
Biguanides	16 (1,355)	−0.75 [−1.58, 0.08]; 95.7%	H24, H28, H41, H45, H63, H78, H90, H109, H116, H120, H126, H145, H154, H165, H170, H199
Sulfonylureas	10 (738)	−2.32 [−3.28, −1.37]*; 82.7%	H3, H49, H56, H73, H111, H127, H142, H146, H168, H171
Insulin	4 (374)	−0.15 [−1.28, 0.99]; 96.2%	H59, H79, H141, H182
TZDs	1 (66)	−2.16 [−3.04, −1.28]*	H100
α-Glucosidase inhibitors	1 (80)	−1.10 [−1.97, −0.23]*	H186
Meglitinides	1 (60)	−4.51 [−5.66, −3.36]*	H82
DPP-4 inhibitors	1 (60)	2.32 [−0.70, 5.34]	H91
Biguanides and Sulfonylureas	6 (522)	−0.51 [−0.97, −0.05]*; 20.3%	H51, H98, H131, H157, H194, H197
Biguanides and α-Glucosidase inhibitors	2 (132)	−2.01 [−2.64, −1.38]*; 0.0%	H71, H144
FPG level at baseline			
6–8 mmol/L	2 (200)	−1.37 [−2.18, −0.56]*; 11.5%	H170, H186
8–10 mmol/L	33 (2,731)	−1.91 [−3.30, −0.52]*; 98.8%	H3, H24, H41, H45, H49, H71, H79, H82, H90, H91, H100, H106, H111, H116, H119, H126, H127, H133, H28, H141, H142, H144–H146, H154, H155, H158, H165, H168, H171, H180, H194, H199
≥10 mmol/L	14 (1,290)	−0.37 [−0.72, −0.02]*; 80.2%	H51, H56, H59, H63, H78, H98, H109, H120, H131, H157, H179, H182, H192, H197

(Continued)

Table 5.21. *(Continued)*

Group	No. of Studies (Participants)	MD [95% CI], I²%	Included Studies
Treatment duration			
≤3 months	48 (4,007)	−1.74 [−2.37, −1.10]*; 98.3%	H3, H24, H28, H45, H49, H51, H56, H59, H63, H71, H73, H78, H79, H82, H90, H91, H98, H100, H106, H109, H111, H112, H116, H119, H120, H126, H127, H131, H133, H141, H142, H144, H145, H146, H154, H155, H157, H158, H165, H168, H170, H171, H180, H182, H186, H192, H194, H197
3–6 months	1 (90)	7.00 [5.98, 8.02]	H41
≥6 months	2 (244)	0.95 [−2.51, 4.41]; 92.4%	H179, H199
CM syndrome differentiation			
Qi and *yin* deficiency	12 (1,103)	−2.51 [−4.84, −0.18]*; 99.5%	H3, H14, H73, H78, H91, H109, H119, H133, H165, H170, H171, H180,
Yin deficiency and excessive heat	6 (480)	−2.43 [−4.03, −0.84]*; 90.7%	H63, H79, H116, H126, H127, H24
Phlegm-dampness and Blood stasis	2 (204)	−2.40 [−6.45, 1.64]; 98.0%	H59, H82
Damp heat retention	2 (120)	−1.31 [−2.14, −0.48]*; 0.0%	H90, H145
Spleen deficiency	1 (66)	−2.16 [−3.04, −1.28]*	H100

*Statistically significant

Abbreviations: CI, confidence interval; CM, Chinese medicine; FPG, fasting plasma glucose; MD, mean difference; SG, sequence generation; TZDs, thiazolidinedione.

different classes of drugs, the largest group of studies used biguanides, and there were no benefits seen in the addition of CHM to biguanides (Table 5.21). Another subgroup analysis based on FPG level at baseline and treatment duration showed similar results to the overall result

(Table 5.21). Studies with shorter treatment duration of fewer than three months showed a benefit in adding CHM to hypoglycaemic agents, but not in studies with longer treatment (Table 5.21). In studies that provided details on CM syndrome differentiation, a benefit was seen in adding CHM to hypoglycaemic agents in patients with *qi* and *yin* deficiency, *yin* deficiency and excessive heat, damp heat retention, and Spleen deficiency, but not in those with the CM syndrome of phlegm-dampness and Blood stasis (Table 5.21).

Insulin Resistance Index

Thirty-two studies, including 2,728 participants, assessed the β-cell function of T2DM using the insulin resistance index (IR). A lower value on the IR indicates greater improvement. Overall meta-analysis for IR was performed at the end of the treatment based on different comparators. Two studies (H24, H28) have three arms; results from each comparison are analysed.

Chinese Herbal Medicine vs. Placebo

One RCT (H209) with 116 participants compared CHM with a placebo. The treatment duration was 12 weeks. The result showed that there were no statistical differences between the CHM group and placebo group (MD −0.85 [−1.74, 0.04]).

Chinese Herbal Medicine vs. Hypoglycaemic Agents

Six RCTs (*n* = 444; H8, H11, H24, H25, H28, H36) compared CHM with hypoglycaemic agents. biguanides, thiazolidinediones and α-Glucosidase inhibitors were used as comparators, while specific agents included metformin, pioglitazone and acarbose. The treatment duration ranged from eight to 12 weeks.

The overall result indicated an improvement in the CHM group, which was better than in the hypoglycaemic agents' group (MD −0.85 [−1.59, −0.10], I^2 = 86.9%). A meta-analysis of results from studies with a low risk of bias for sequence generation reduced the heterogeneity; however, results showed no significant differences

Table 5.22. Chinese Herbal Medicine vs. Hypoglycaemic Agents: Insulin Resistance Index

Group	No. of Studies (Participants)	MD [95% CI], I^2%	Included Studies
All studies	6 (444)	−0.85 [−1.59, −0.10]*; 86.9%	H8, H11, H24, H25, H28, H36
Low risk of bias SG	2 (152)	−0.78 [−1.63, 0.08]; 5.2%	H8, H24
Agents class			
Biguanides	4 (272)	−0.91 [−2.22, 0.39]; 91.7%	H8, H24, H25, H28
α-Glucosidase inhibitors	1 (112)	−0.64 [−1.03, −0.25]*	H11
TZDs	1 (60)	−0.77 [−2.73, 1.19]	H36
CM syndrome differentiation			
Qi and *yin* deficiency	2 (144)	−1.85 [−3.36, −0.33]*; 56.8%	H25, H36
Yin deficiency and excessive heat	2 (152)	−0.78 [−1.63, 0.08]; 5.2%	H8, H24

*Statistically significant
Abbreviations: CI, confidence interval; CM, Chinese medicine; FPG, fasting plasma glucose; MD, mean difference; SG, sequence generation; TZDs, thiazolidinedione.

between groups. A subgroup analysis by drug class showed significant differences between the two groups in one study that used α-Glucosidase inhibitor acarbose, but not in biguanides or pioglitazone (Table 5.22). A subgroup analysis by CM differentiation showed more improvement in the CHM group than the hypoglycaemic group of patients with *qi* and *yin* deficiency (Table 5.22).

CHM plus Hypoglycaemic Agents vs. Hypoglycaemic Agents

Twenty-seven RCTs (H24, H28, H45, H49, H51, H59, H71, H82, H90, H98, H106, H112, H116, H119, H126, H127, H133, H141, H144, H154, H155, H165, H168, H182, H186, H194, H199), including 2,222 participants, assessed the effects of CHM plus hypoglycaemic agents versus hypoglycaemic agents alone. Hypoglycaemic agents included biguanides, sulfonylureas, α-glucosidase inhibitors, meglitinides and insulins. The treatment duration ranged from four to 24 weeks.

CHM plus hypoglycaemic agents were superior to hypoglycaemic agents alone (MD −0.93 [−1.17, −0.69]; I^2 = 97.2%); however, the heterogeneity was high. A meta-analysis of results from studies with a low risk of bias for sequence generation showed similar results. A subgroup analysis by drug class did not show significant differences between the two groups in studies that used sulfonylureas and the combination of biguanides and sulfonylureas (Table 5.23). A subgroup analysis by CM differentiation showed that the benefit of adding CHM to the hypoglycaemic group was better than hypoglycaemic agents alone in patients with *yin* deficiency and excessive heat and damp heat retention (Table 5.23).

Table 5.23. Chinese Herbal Medicine Plus Hypoglycaemic Agents vs. Hypoglycaemic Agents: Insulin Resistance Index

Group	No. of Studies (Participants)	MD [95% CI], I^2%	Included Studies
All studies	27 (2,222)	−0.93 [−1.17, −0.69]*; 97.2%	H24, H28, H45, H49, H51, H59, H71, H82, H90, H98, H106, H112, H116, H119, H126, H127, H133, H141, H144, H154, H155, H165, H168, H182, H186, H194, H199
Low risk of bias SG	13 (1,049)	−0.63 [−0.86, −0.39]*; 90.7%	H24, H51, H82, H90, H106, H112, H116, H119, H126, H144, H165, H168, H199
Drug class			
Biguanides	9 (739)	−0.72 [−1.15, −0.30]*; 97.1%	H24, H28, H45, H90, H116, H126, H154, H165, H199

(Continued)

Table 5.23. (*Continued*)

Group	No. of Studies (Participants)	MD [95% CI], I²%	Included Studies
Sulfonylureas	3 (238)	−0.68 [−1.98, 0.62]; 91.7%	H49, H129, H168
Insulin	3 (284)	−1.19 [−2.00, −0.39]*; 97.5%	H59, H141, H182
α-Glucosidase inhibitors	1 (80)	−0.40 [−0.67, −0.13]*	H186
Meglitinides	1 (60)	−1.40 [−1.85, −0.95]*	H82
Biguanides and Sulfonylureas	3 (193)	−0.28 [−0.58, 0.02]; 7.3%	H51, H98, H194
Biguanides and α-Glucosidase inhibitors	2 (132)	−0.84 [−1.19, −0.48]*; 0.0%	H71, H144
FPG level at baseline			
6−8 mmol/L	1 (80)	−0.40 [−0.67, −0.13]*	H186
8−10 mmol/L	21 (1,765)	−0.88 [−1.16, −0.61]*; 97.6%	H45, H49, H71, H82, H90, H106, H116, H119, H126, H127, H24, H133, H28, H141, H144, H154, H155, H165, H168, H194, H199
≥10 mmol/L	4 (317)	−1.10 [−1.91, −0.28]*; 95.3%	H51, H59, H98, H182
Treatment duration			
≤3 months	26 (2,116)	−0.97 [−1.22, −0.72]*; 96.7%	H24, H28, H45, H49, H51, H59, H71, H82, H90, H98, H106, H112, H116, H119, H126, H127, H133, H141, H144, H154, H155, H165, H168, H182, H186, H194
≥6 months	1 (106)	−0.10 [−0.19, −0.01]*	H199

Table 5.23. (*Continued*)

Group	No. of Studies (Participants)	MD [95% CI], I²%	Included Studies
CM syndrome differentiation			
Qi and *yin* deficiency	3 (393)	−1.52 [−3.26, 0.22]; 99.5%	H119, H133, H165
Yin deficiency and excessive heat	4 (330)	−0.82 [−1.10, −0.54]*; 0.0%	H24, H116, H126, H127
Phlegm-dampness and Blood stasis	2 (204)	−1.55 [−1.77, −1.33]*; 0.0%	H59, H82
Damp heat retention	1 (60)	−0.18 [−1.03, 0.67]	H90

*Statistically significant
Abbreviations: CI, confidence interval; CM, Chinese medicine; FPG, fasting blood glucose; MD, mean difference; SG, sequence generation.

Insulin Sensitivity Index

Twenty-five of the 210 studies, including 2,061 participants, assessed the β-cell function of T2DM using the insulin sensitivity index (IS). A higher value on the IS indicates greater improvement. Overall meta-analysis for IS was performed at the end of the treatment based on different comparators. Two studies (H3, H28) have three arms, while one study (H56) has four arms. The results from different comparisons were extracted and analysed.

Chinese Herbal Medicine vs. Hypoglycaemic Agents

Six RCTs (*n* = 399; H3, H8, H10, H16, H28, H40) compared CHM with hypoglycaemic agents. Three classes of agents were used as comparators, including biguanides, thiazolidinediones and sulfonylureas. Specific agents included metformin, pioglitazone and glipizide. The treatment duration ranged from four to 12 weeks.

The overall result indicated there is no significant difference in IS between the two groups (MD 0.29 [−0.15, 0.72], I^2 = 97.3%). Meta-analysis of results from studies with a low risk of bias for sequence generation showed similar results. A subgroup analysis by comparator agent class, FPG level at baseline, showed no significant difference between CHM and hypoglycaemic agents (Table 5.24). In studies that reported on CM differentiation, there is a significant

Table 5.24. Chinese Herbal Medicine vs. Hypoglycaemic Agents: Insulin Sensitivity Index

Group	No. of Studies (Participants)	MD [95% CI], I^2%	Included Studies
All studies	6 (399)	0.29 [−0.15, 0.72]; 97.3%	H3, H8, H10, H16, H28, H40
Low risk of bias SG	2 (179)	0.55 [−0.51, 1.61]; 99.4%	H8, H10
Agents class			
Biguanides	4 (275)	0.30 [−0.24, 0.84]; 98.4%	H8, H10, H16, H28
TZDs	1 (64)	0.32 [−0.17, 0.81]	H40
Sulfonylureas	1 (60)	0.20 [−0.26, 0.66]	H3
FPG level at baseline			
8–10 mmol/L	5 (339)	0.31 [−0.23, 0.85]; 97.8%	H3, H8, H10, H28, H40
≥10 mmol/L	1 (60)	0.18 [−0.03, 0.39]	H16
CM syndrome differentiation			
Qi and *yin* deficiency	3 (200)	0.15 [−0.03, 0.33]; 0.0%	H3, H109, H180
Yin deficiency and excessive heat	2 (120)	0.21 [0.10, 0.32]*; 0.0%	H63, H127
Spleen deficiency	1 (66)	1.16 [1.04, 1.28]*	H100
Phlegm-dampness and Blood stasis	1 (144)	0.56 [0.47, 0.66]*	H59

*Statistically significant

Abbreviations: CI, confidence interval; CM, Chinese medicine; FPG, fasting blood glucose; MD, mean difference; SG, sequence generation; TZDs, thiazolidinedione.

difference between the two groups (Table 5.24) in T2DM patients with *yin* deficiency and excessive heat, phlegm-dampness with Blood stasis and Spleen deficiency.

Chinese Herbal Medicine Plus Hypoglycaemic Agents vs. Hypoglycaemic Agents

Twenty-one RCTs (H49, H56, H59, H63, H3, H98, H100, H109, H111, H120, H121, H127, H130, H131, H28, H142, H158, H172, H180, H182, H194), including 1,710 participants, assessed the effects of CHM plus hypoglycaemic agents versus hypoglycaemic agents alone. Various hypoglycaemic agents were used, including metformin, glipizide, gliclazide, glimepiride, pioglitazone, repaglinide and insulins. All studies had a treatment duration of less than or equal to 12 weeks. The shortest treatment duration was four weeks.

Meta-analysis showed that CHM plus hypoglycaemic agents were superior to hypoglycaemic agents alone (MD 0.40 [0.23, 0.57], I^2 = 95.1%). Meta-analysis of results from studies with a low risk of bias for sequence generation showed that there was no difference between groups. A subgroup analysis by drug class showed a benefit in adding CHM to sulfonylureas, TZDs and the combination of biguanides with sulfonylureas (reduced heterogeneity). No significant difference was observed when CHM was added to biguanides or insulin (Table 5.25). A subgroup analysis using baseline FPG levels

Table 5.25. Chinese Herbal Medicine Plus Hypoglycaemic Agents vs. Hypoglycaemic Agents: Insulin Sensitivity Index

Group	No. of Studies (Participants)	WMD [95% CI], I^2%	Included Studies
All studies	21 (1,710)	0.40 [0.23, 0.57]*; 95.1%	H3, H49, H56, H59, H63, H98, H100, H109, H111, H120, H121, H127, H130, H131, H28, H142, H158, H172, H180, H182, H194

(Continued)

Table 5.25. (*Continued*)

Group	No. of Studies (Participants)	WMD [95% CI], I²%	Included Studies
Low risk of bias SG	2 (126)	0.69 [−0.24, 1.62]; 98.8%	H63, H100
Drug class			
Biguanides	6 (482)	0.14 [−0.16, 0.44]; 94.1%	H63, H109, H120, H130, H28, H172
Sulfonylureas	6 (448)	0.38 [0.14, 0.61]*; 89.2%	H3, H49, H56, H111, H127, H142
Insulin	2 (184)	4.49 [−3.48, 12.46]; 96.6%	H59, H182
TZDs	1 (66)	1.16 [1.04, 1.28]*	H100
Biguanides and Sulfonylureas	4 (270)	0.43 [0.34, 0.52]*; 9.2%	H98, H121, H131, H194
FPG level at baseline			
8–10 mmol/L	11 (826)	0.51 [0.26, 0.76]*; 94.2%	H3, H49, H100, H111, H121, H127, H28, H142, H158, H180, H194
≥10 mmol/L	10 (834)	0.29 [0.09, 0.50]*; 94.3%	H56, H59, H63, H98, H109, H120, H130, H131, H172, H182
CM syndrome differentiation			
Qi and *yin* deficiency	3 (200)	0.15 [−0.03, 0.33]; 0.0%	H3, H109, H180
Yin deficiency and excessive heat	2 (120)	0.21 [0.10, 0.32]*; 0.0%	H63, H127
Phlegm-dampness and Blood stasis	1 (144)	0.56 [0.47, 0.66]*	H59
Spleen deficiency	1 (66)	1.16 [1.04, 1.28]*	H100

*Statistically significant
Abbreviations: CI, confidence interval; CM, Chinese medicine; FPG, fasting blood glucose; MD, mean difference; SG, sequence generation; TZDs, thiazolidinedione; WMD, Weighted mean difference.

produced similar results to the overall result with high heterogeneity. In studies that provided information on CM differentiation, meta-analyses showed a benefit in adding CHM to hypogelycemic agents in patients with *yin* deficiency and excessive heat, phlegm-dampness and Blood stasis or Spleen deficiency, but no difference was found in those with *qi* and *yin* deficiency (Table 5.25).

C-peptide

Nine studies, including 966 participants, assessed β–cell function of T2DM patients using the C-peptide. A lower value on the C-peptide indicates greater improvement. Overall, meta-analysis for CP was performed at the end of treatment based on different comparators. One study (H56) has four arms. Results from different comparisons were extracted and analysed.

CHM plus Hypoglycaemic Agents vs. Hypoglycaemic Agents

All nine RCTs (H42, H56, H92, H144, H145, H157, H163, H177, H191) assessed the effects of CHM plus hypoglycaemic agents versus hypoglycaemic agents alone. Hypoglycaemic agents included biguanides, sulfonylureas, α-Glucosidase inhibitors, GLP-1 and insulins. Specific agents included metformin, gliclazide, liraglutide, acarbose, voglibose and insulin. The treatment duration ranged from four to 14 weeks.

Meta-analysis results showed that CHM plus hypoglycaemic agents were not superior to hypoglycaemic agents alone (MD 0.18 [−0.09, 0.46]; $I^2 = 81.9\%$). Meta-analysis of results from studies with a low risk of bias for sequence generation showed similar results (2(140), MD −0.18 [−1.07, 0.71]; $I^2 = 70.5\%$; H144, H163). A subgroup analysis based on drug class, treatment duration, FPG level at baseline, and CM syndrome differentiation was performed, but there was no significant difference between the groups.

Assessment Using Grading of Recommendations, Assessment, Development and Evaluation

An assessment of the quality of the evidence from RCTs was made using the Grading of Recommendations, Assessment, Development and Evaluation (GRADE). Interventions, comparators and outcomes to be included were selected based on a consensus process described in Chapter 4. The comparisons of CHM versus pharmacotherapy and CHM plus hypoglycaemic agents were considered critically important. FPG, PGB, A1C, TG, TC, FINS and adverse events (AEs) were considered the most important outcomes to assess the effects of CHM on glucose metabolism.

Oral Chinese Herbal Medicine vs. Pharmacotherapy

Evidence for CHM versus pharmacotherapy for treating T2DM was of low to moderate quality (Table 5.26). The results showed that oral

Table 5.26. GRADE: Chinese Herbal Medicine vs. Pharmacotherapy for Treating Type 2 Diabetes Mellitus

Outcome Mean Treatment Duration	Estimated Absolute Effect		Relative Effect (95% CI) No. of Participants (Studies)	Certainty of the Evidence (GRADE)
	Oral Chinese Herbal Medicine	Pharmacotherapy		
FPG 9.1 weeks	**6.98** MD: 0.16 lower (95% CI: 0.33 lower to 0.22 lower)	**7.14**	**MD −0.16** (−0.33, −0.22) 3,484 (39 RCTs)	⊕⊕⊕⊖ MODERATE[a]
PBG 9 weeks	**9.51** MD: 0.45 lower (95% CI: 0.76 lower to 0.13 lower)	**9.96**	**MD −0.45** (−0.76, −0.13) 3,286 (35 RCTs)	⊕⊕⊖⊖ LOW[a,b]
A1C 10.1 weeks	**6.98** MD: 0.11 lower (95% CI: 0.26 lower to 0.04 lower)	**7.09**	**MD −0.11** (−0.26, −0.04) 2,441 (28 RCTs)	⊕⊕⊖⊖ LOW[a,b]
TG 9.3 weeks	**1.99** MD: 0.38 lower (95% CI: 0.51 lower to 0.26 lower)	**2.37**	**MD −0.38** (−0.51, −0.26) 2,701 (31 RCTs)	⊕⊕⊖⊖ LOW[a,b]

Table 5.26. (*Continued*)

Outcome Mean Treatment Duration	Estimated Absolute Effect		Relative Effect (95% CI) No. of Participants (Studies)	Certainty of the Evidence (GRADE)
	Oral Chinese Herbal Medicine	Pharmacotherapy		
TC 9.3 weeks	**4.96** MD: 0.42 lower (95% CI: 0.57 lower to 0.26 lower)	**5.38**	**MD −0.42** (−0.57, −0.26) 2,701 (31 RCTs)	⊕⊕⊕⚪ MODERATE[a]
FINS 9. 54 weeks	**12.5** MD: 1 lower (95% CI: 1.84 lower to 0.15 lower)	**13.5**	**MD −1.00** (−1.84, −0.15) 1,009 (13 RCTs)	⊕⊕⚪⚪ LOW[a,b]

*Statistically significant result.

Abbreviations: CI, confidence interval; FINS, fasting insulin; FPG, fasting plasma glucose; GRADE, Grading of Recommendations, Assessment, Development and Evaluation; A1C, glycosylated haemoglobin; LDL, low-density lipoprotein; MD, mean difference; PBG, postprandial blood glucose; RCTs, randomised controlled trials; TC, total cholesterol; TG, triglyceride.

Note:
[a] Unexplained high statistical heterogeneity. [b] Funnel plot not symmetrical.

References:
FPG: H1–H25, H27–H40
PBG: H1–H21, H23–H25, H27, H29–H35, H38–H40
A1C: H1–H4, H8–H10, H15–H25, H28–H32, H35–H40
TG: H1–H5, H7–H10, H12–H18, H20–H21, H23–H26, H28, H30–H33, H35, H37–H39
TC: H1–H5, H7–H10, H12–H18, H20, H21, H23–H26, H28, H30–H33, H35, H37–H39

CHM could improve the glycolipid metabolism and fasting insulin level.

Safety issues were reported in 10 RCTs (H8, H11, H16, H22, H23, H25, H30, H32, H34, H35). The CHM groups had a total of 30 AEs. The most common AEs in the CHM group were diarrhoea (nine cases) and abdominal distension (three cases). Other AEs include nausea and vomiting (one case), dizziness (one case), gastrointestinal discomfort (two cases), and transient slight alanine aminotransferase and aspartate aminotransferase elevation (one case). The pharmacotherapy group had a total of 101 AEs, including gastrointestinal discomfort (79 cases), hypoglycaemia (six cases) and liver dysfunction (seven cases). Other symptoms include abdominal distension and pain, diarrhoea, anorexia, nausea and vomiting.

Oral Chinese Herbal Medicine Plus Pharmacotherapy vs. Pharmacotherapy

Evidence for CHM plus Pharmacotherapy versus Pharmacotherapy alone were of low to moderate quality (Table 5.27). The results showed that Oral CHM could improve the glycolipid metabolism and fasting insulin level.

Table 5.27. GRADE: Chinese Herbal Medicine Plus Pharmacotherapy vs. Pharmacotherapy

Outcome Mean Treatment Duration	Estimated Absolute Effect		Relative Effect (95% CI) No. of Participants (Studies)	Certainty of the Evidence (GRADE)
	Oral Chinese Herbal Medicine	Pharmacotherapy		
FPG 8.93 weeks	6.6 MD: 0.84 lower (95% CI: 0.93 lower to 0.75 lower)	7.44	MD −0.84 (−0.93, −0.75) 13,582 (155 RCTs)	⊕⊕◯◯ LOW[a,b]
PBG 9.06 weeks	9.08 MD: 1.23 lower (95% CI: 1.38 lower to 1.08 lower)	10.31	MD −1.23 (−1.38, −1.08) 11,979 (138 RCTs)	⊕⊕◯◯ LOW[a,b]
A1C 9.65 weeks	6.61 MD: 0.76 lower (95% CI: 0.86 lower to 0.65 lower)	7.37	MD −0.76 (−0.86, −0.65) 10,497 (120 RCTs)	⊕⊕◯◯ LOW[a,b]
TG 8.8 weeks	1.81 MD: 0.40 lower (95% CI: 0.49 lower to 0.32 lower)	2.21	MD −0.40 (−0.49, −0.32) 6,858 (77 RCTs)	⊕⊕◯◯ LOW[a,b]
TC 8.89 weeks	4.82 MD: 0.42 lower (95% CI: 0.64 lower to 0.33 lower)	5.31	MD −0.49 (−0.64, −0.33) 6,524 (73 RCTs)	⊕⊕⊕◯ MODERATE[a]
FINS 9.38 weeks	11.25 MD: 1.45 lower (95% CI: 2.06 lower to 0.84 lower)	12.7	MD −1.45 (−2.06, −0.84) 5,431 (51 RCTs)	⊕⊕◯◯ LOW[a,b]

*Statistically significant result.

Abbreviations: CI, confidence interval; FINS, fasting insulin; FPG, fasting plasma glucose; GRADE, Grading of Recommendations, Assessment, Development and Evaluation; A1C, glycosylated haemoglobin; LDL, low-density lipoprotein; MD, mean difference; PBG, postprandial blood glucose; RCTs, randomised controlled trials; TC, total cholesterol; TG, triglyceride.

Note:
ᵃ Unexplained high statistical heterogeneity. ᵇ Funnel plot not symmetrical.

References:

FPG: H3, H19, H24, H28, H31, H41–H45, H47, H49 –72, H74–H111, H113–H124, H126–H131, H133–H134, H136–H165, H167–H180, H182–H199

PBG: H3, H19, H24, H31, H41–H45, H47, H49–H57, H60–H72, H74–H87, H89–H103, H105, H107–H111, H114–H119, H121–H132, H126–H131, H133–H134, H136–H139, H141–H145, H147–H153, H155–H164, H167–H176, H178–H180, H182, H183, H185–H191, H193–H196, H198, H199

A1C: H3, H19, H24, H28, H31, H41, H42, H44–H47, H51–H55, H59–H62, H64–H68, H70–H75, H77–H80, H82–H90, H92–H95, H99, H100, H102, H104–H106, H108, H110, H111, H113, H115, H116, H118, H119, H121–H126, H128, H130, H131, H133, H134, H137, H139, H140–H145, H149–H151, H153, H155, H156, H158, H160–H168, H171–H173, H175–H184, H186–H189, H191, H192, H195, H196, H198, H199

TG: H24, H28, H31, H41–H43, H46–H48, H51, H52, H55, H56, H60, H62, H64–H66, H71, H73, H74–H76, H3, H81, H86–H88, H92–H94, H96, H98, H100, H105, H107, H111, H113, H116, H121–H124, H126, H129, H130, H132, H133, H136–H139, H142, H145, H146, H149, H155, H157–H159, H161, H162, H164, H165, H167, H170, H172, H175, H176, H181, H183, H186, H188, H190, H192, H195, H196

TC: H3, H24, H28, H31, H41–H43, H46–H48, H51, H52, H56, H60, H62, H64–H66, H71, H73–H75, H76, H81, H86–H88, H92–H94, H96, H98, H100, H105, H107, H111, H113, H116, H121–H124, H126, H129, H130, H132, H133, H136–H139, H142, H145, H149, H155, H157–H159, H161, H162, H164, H165, H167, H172, H175, H176, H181, H183, H186, H188, H190, H192, H195

Safety issues were reported in 28 RCTs (H41, H51, H60, H64, H75, H78, H79, H84, H89, H92, H94, H101, H104, H116, H119, H124, H126, H133, H157, H159, H162, H164, H168, H176, H177, H192, H193, H196). The total number of AEs reported in the integrative medicine groups and pharmacotherapy group was 74 and 140, respectively. Gastrointestinal discomfort (45 cases) was the most common AE in the integrative medicine group. Other reported AEs include abdominal distention and pain, diarrhoea, anorexia, constipation, nausea and vomiting. In the hypoglycaemic group, hypoglycaemia was the most common AE (44 cases).

Randomised Controlled Trial Evidence for Individual Oral Formulae

Several studies tested the same individual formula for T2DM. Meta-analyses were able to be conducted for these formulas/products: *Liu wei di huang wan* 六味地黄丸, *Shen qi jiang tang ke li* 参芪降糖颗粒, *Jin li da ke li* 津力达颗粒, *Huang lian su* tablets 黄连素片, *Xiao ke fang* 消渴方, *Yu quan wan* 玉泉丸, *Shen di sheng jin jiao nang* 参地生津胶囊, *Tian mai xiao ke pian* 天麦消渴片, *Da huang huang lian xie xin tang* 大黄黄连泻心汤, *Yu nv jian* 玉女煎, *Ren shen bai hu tang* 人参白虎汤, *Zhi bo di huang tang* 知柏地黄汤 and *Ku gua jiao nang* 苦瓜胶囊. The evidence for the top 10 individual oral formulae used in two or more studies was separately analysed.

Liu wei di huang wan 六味地黄丸

Five studies (*n* = 730; H70, H85, H92, H116, H129) tested *Liu wei di huang wan* 六味地黄丸 as an adjunct to pharmacotherapy. When used as integrative medicine, *Liu wei di huang wan* 六味地黄丸 resulted in greater improvements in levels of:

- Reduced FPG (MD −0.82 [−1.02, −0.64], I^2 = 12.6%) (H70, H85, H92, H116, H129),
- Reduced PBG (MD −1.15 [−1.58, −0.72], I^2 = 63.0%) (H70, H85, H92, H116, H129),
- Reduced A1C (MD −1.07 [−1.27, −0.87], I^2 = 0.0%) (H70, H85, H92, H116),
- Reduced TG (MD −0.41 [−0.55, −0.27], I^2 = 61.4%) (H92, H116, H129),
- Reduced TC (MD −1.16 [−1.61, −0.71], I^2 = 86.4%) (H92, H116, H129), and
- Increased HDL (MD 0.30 [0.18, 0.42], I^2 = 0.0%) (H92, H116).

The addition of *Liu wei di huang wan* 六味地黄丸 to pharmacotherapy showed a trend to reduce LDL, but there were no significant differences between the groups (MD −0.92 [−1.90, 0.06], I^2 = 86.4%) (H92, H116).

Shen qi jiang tang ke li 参芪降糖颗粒

Shen qi jiang tang ke li 参芪降糖颗粒 was evaluated, and meta-analyses were possible for three studies (*n* = 348; H61, H119, H183).

These studies showed that the *Shen qi jiang tang* granule 参芪降糖颗粒, when added to pharmacotherapy, was superior to pharmacotherapy at the end of treatment measurements of FPG (MD -1.78 [-2.68, -0.89], I^2 = 87.6%), PBG (MD -3.28 [-5.16, -1.40], I^2 = 90.5%) and A1C (MD -1.51 [-1.82, -1.19], I^2 = 56.5%).

Jin li da ke li 津力达颗粒

Jin li da ke li 津力达颗粒 was evaluated in four studies (n = 430; H19, H102, H117, H133). Compared to pharmacotherapy alone, *Jin li da ke li* 津力达颗粒, when added to pharmacotherapy, resulted in a greater reduction in FPG (MD -1.31 [-1.57, -1.05], I^2 = 0) and PBG levels (MD -2.03 [-2.90, -1.17], I^2 = 78.2%) in all four studies. When used as integrative medicine, *Jin li da ke li* 津力达颗粒 showed a benefit in the reduction of A1C at the end of treatment for three studies (MD -1.12 [-1.61, -0.69], I^2 = 47.8%) (H19, H102, H133).

Xiao ke fang 消渴方

Xiao ke fang 消渴方 was evaluated in three studies (n = 450; H63, H79, H85). In the three studies, *Xiao ke fang* 消渴方, when added to pharmacotherapy, resulted in a greater reduction in FPG (MD -0.68 [-1.26, -0.11], I^2 = 81.7%) and PBG levels (MD -0.89 [-1.49, -0.28], I^2 = 74.0%). Compared to pharmacotherapy alone, the integrative use of *Xiao ke fang* 消渴方 was superior at reducing the A1C level (MD -0.66 [-1.24, -0.08], I^2 = 82.6%; H79, H85). FINS was also measured in two studies; however, no statistical difference was found between the integrative medicine group and pharmacotherapy group (MD -0.84 [-1.77, 0.08], I^2 = 50.8%) (H79, H63).

Yu quan wan 玉泉丸

Yu quan wan 玉泉丸 was evaluated in three studies (n = 284; H57, H77, H178). *Yu quan wan* 玉泉丸 plus pharmacotherapy is superior to pharmacotherapy alone in reducing the values of FPG (MD -0.39 [-0.71, -0.03], I^2 = 0.0%) and PBG (MD -1.29 [-1.76, -0.83], I^2 = 47.3%). A1C was measured in two studies that showed a better reduction in the integrative medicine group compared to pharmacotherapy alone (MD -0.67 [-1.31, -0.03], I^2 = 82.3%) (H77, H178).

Tian mai xiao ke pian 天麦消渴片

Tian mai xiao ke pian 天麦消渴片 was evaluated in two studies (*n* = 142; H31, H186). Compared to pharmacotherapy alone, when used as integrative medicine, *Tian mai xiao ke pian* 天麦消渴片 resulted in greater improvements in the BMI (MD −0.48 [−0.87, −0.20], I^2 = 0.0%), but not in FPG, PBG, A1C, TG, TC, LDL and HDL levels.

Zhi bo di huang tang 知柏地黄汤

Two studies evaluated *Zhi bo di huang tang* 知柏地黄汤 as an adjunct therapy to pharmacotherapy (*n* = 100; H83, H127). When used as integrative medicine, *Zhi bo di huang tang* 知柏地黄汤 resulted in greater improvements in FPG (MD −0.66 [−1.01, −0.30], I^2 = 0.0%) and PBG (MD −1.19 [−1.74, −0.67], I^2 = 0.0%) levels.

Ku gua jiao nang 苦瓜胶囊

Two studies (*n* = 176; H41, H42) evaluated *Ku gua jiao nang* 苦瓜胶囊. When compared to metformin alone, *Ku gua jiao nang* 苦瓜胶囊 resulted in greater improvements in levels of blood glucose measurements, although the heterogeneity was high:

- Reduced FPG (MD −1.16 [−2.14, −0.18], I^2 = 90.6%),
- Reduced PBG (MD −1.98 [−3.86, −0.10], I^2 = 93.3%), and
- Reduced A1C (MD −1.50 [−2.47, −0.53], I^2 = 95.9%).

No significant differences were observed between groups in TG (MD −0.20 [−0.74, 0.34], I^2 = 86.5%) or TC (MD −0.37 [−1.05, 0.30], I^2 = 88.2%) levels.

Frequently Reported Orally Used Herbs in Meta-analyses Showing Favourable Effect

The most frequent herbs used in studies from favorable meta-analyses were calculated (Table 5.28). Studies were pooled according to 13

Table 5.28. Frequently Reported Herbs in Meta-analyses Showing Favorable Effect

Outcome Category	No. of Meta-analyses (studies)	Herbs	Scientific Name	Frequency of Use
CHM vs. Pharmacotherapy				
Blood glucose (FPG, PBG, A1C)	1 (35)	Huang qi 黄芪	*Astragalus membranaceus* (Fisch.) Bge.	18
		Huang lian 黄连	*Coptis chinensis* Franch.	17
		Sheng di huang 生地黄	*Rehmannia glutinosa* Libosch.	15
		Dan shen 丹参	*Salvia miltiorrhiza* Bge.	13
		Ge gen 葛根	*Pueraria lobata* (Willd.) Ohwi	12
		Mai men dong 麦门冬	*Ophiopogon japonicus* (Thunb.) Ker-Gawl.	10
		Ren shen 人参	*Panax ginseng* C. A. Meyer.	9
		Shan yao 山药	*Dioscorea opposita* Thunb.	9
		Zhi mu 知母	*Anemarrhena asphodeloides* Bge.	9
		Fu ling 茯苓	*Poria cocos* (Schw.) Wolf	8
Blood lipid metabolism (TG, TC, LDL, HDL)	4 (20)	Huang lian 黄连	*Coptis chinensis* Franch.	11
		Sheng di huang 生地黄	*Rehmannia glutinosa* Libosch.	9
		Dan shen 丹参	*Salvia miltiorrhiza* Bge.	6
		Ge gen 葛根	*Pueraria lobata* (Willd.) Ohwi	6
		Zhi mu 知母	*Anemarrhena asphodeloides* Bge.	5
		Huang qi 黄芪	*Astragalus membranaceus* (Fisch.) Bge.	5
		Chai hu 柴胡	*Bupleurum chinense* DC	4
		Huang qin 黄芩	*Scutellaria baicalensis* Georgi	4
		Tian hua fen 天花粉	*Trichosanthes kirilowii* Maxim.	4
		Ren shen 人参	*Panax ginseng* C. A. Meyer.	4

(Continued)

Table 5.28. (*Continued*)

Outcome Category	No. of Meta-analyses (studies)	Herbs	Scientific Name	Frequency of Use
β–cell Function (FINS, IR)	2 (2)	Huang lian黄连	*Coptis chinensis* Franch.	2
CHM plus Hypoglycaemic agents vs. Hypoglycaemic agents				
Blood glucose (FPG, PBG, A1C)	3 (103)	Huang qi 黄芪	*Astragalus membranaceus* (Fisch.) Bge.	64
		Sheng di huang 生地黄	*Rehmannia glutinosa* Libosch.	44
		Ge gen 葛根	*Pueraria lobata* (Willd.) Ohwi	41
		Dan shen 丹参	*Salvia miltiorrhiza* Bge.	38
		Mai men dong 麦门冬	*Ophiopogon japonicus* (Thunb.) Ker-Gawl.	37
		Tian hua fen 天花粉	*Trichosanthes kirilowii* Maxim.	36
		Huang lian 黄连	*Coptis chinensis* Franch.	36
		Fu ling 茯苓	*Poria cocos* (Schw.) Wolf	35
		Shan yao 山药	*Dioscorea opposita* Thunb.	32
		Shan zhu yu 山茱萸	*Cornus officinalis* Sieb. & Zucc.	25
BMI	1 (15)	Ge gen 葛根	*Pueraria lobata* (Willd.) Ohwi	7
		Bai zhu 白术	*Atractylodes macrocephala* Koidz.	6
		Fu ling 茯苓	*Poria cocos* (Schw.) Wolf	6
		Cang zhu 苍术	*Atractylodes lancea* (Thunb.) DC	5
		Huang qi 黄芪	*Astragalus membranaceus* (Fisch.) Bge.	5
		Mai men dong 麦门冬	*Ophiopogon japonicus* (Thunb.) Ker-Gawl.	5
		Wu wei zi 五味子	*Schisandra chinensis* (Turcz.) Baill.	4
		Dang shen 党参	*Codonopsis pilosula* (Franch.) Nannf.	4

Table 5.28. *(Continued)*

Outcome Category	No. of Meta-analyses (studies)	Herbs	Scientific Name	Frequency of Use
		Shan yao 山药	*Dioscorea opposita* Thunb.	4
		Ze xie 泽泻	*Alisma orientalis* (Sam.) Juzep.	4
		Huang lian 黄连	*Coptis chinensis* Franch.	4
Blood lipid metabolism (TG, TC, LDL, HDL)	4 (52)	Huang qi 黄芪	*Astragalus membranaceus* (Fisch.) Bge.	34
		Sheng di huang 生地黄	*Rehmannia glutinosa* Libosch.	23
		Tian hua fen 天花粉	*Trichosanthes kirilowii* Maxim.	22
		Shan yao 山药	*Dioscorea opposita* Thunb.	21
		Dan shen 丹参	*Salvia miltiorrhiza* Bge.	19
		Huang lian 黄连	*Coptis chinensis* Franch.	19
		Mai men dong 麦门冬	*Ophiopogon japonicus* (Thunb.) Ker-Gawl.	17
		Ge gen 葛根	*Pueraria lobata* (Willd.) Ohwi	16
		Shan zhu yu 山茱萸	*Cornus officinalis* Sieb. & Zucc.	15
		Fu ling 茯苓	*Poria cocos* (Schw.) Wolf	15

Abbreviations: BMI, body mass index; FINS, fasting insulin; FPG, fasting plasma glucose; A1C, glycosylated haemoglobin A1C; HDL, high-density liproprotein; IR, insulin resistance; LDL, low-density liproprotein; PBG, plasma blood glucose; TC, total cholesterol; TG, triglyceride.

outcome measures. Analysis was conducted according to categories of outcomes, which included blood glucose metabolism, blood lipid metabolism, BMI and β-cell function. Only one study reported on the quality of life for people with T2DM, so herb frequency analysis was not conducted for this outcome.

Safety of Oral Chinese Herbal Medicine in Randomised Controlled Trials

Out of the 210 studies, 94 RCTs mentioned AEs. Of these, 43 studies provided specific details about the AEs (Table 5.29). AEs were analysed where the nature and number of events were reported.

Table 5.29.   Adverse Events

Comparisons	No. of Studies	Intervention Group AEs	Control Group AEs
Chinese herbal medicine vs. placebo	6	Total AEs = 56 moderate constipation (2), abdominal distenstion (1), mild AEs and no other information (24), ALT eleveation (2), AST elevation (2), mild to moderate constipation (5), drug-related adverse events (6), serious adverse events (1), adverse events leading to abscission (2), abnormal liver function (8), urinary tract infection, lumbar disc surgery, ankle swelling (1).	Total AEs = 25 moderate constipation (2), mild AEs and no other information (7), abdominal cramping and diarrhoea (1), mild to moderate constipation (1), drug-related adverse events (2), serious adverse events (2), mild liver dysfunction (3), urinary red blood cells (4), nausea and vomiting, insomnia (1)
Chinese herbal medicine vs. lifestyle intervention	1	Total AEs = 1 mild epigastric discomfort (1)	Total AEs = 1 mild pruritus (1)
CHM vs. pharmacotherapy	10	Total AEs = 30: abdominal distention (3), diarrhoea (9),	Total AEs = 101: Hypoglycaemia (6), liver dysfunction (7),

Table 5.29. *(Continued)*

Comparisons	No. of Studies	Intervention Group AEs	Control Group AEs
		nausea and vomiting (1), dizziness (1), gastrointestinal discomfort (2), transient slight ALT and AST elevation (1), non severe AEs and no other information (13)	gastrointestinal discomfort (10), abdominal distention & pain (58), diarrhoea (4), anorexia (2), nausea and vomiting (5), non-severe AEs and no other information (9)
CHM plus hypoglycaemic agents vs. hypoglycaemic agents	28	Total AEs = 74: digestive tract discomfort (specific unknown) (13), abdominal pain and diarrhoea (8), constipation (1), abdominal distension (6), nausea (16), loss of appetite (1), hypoglycaemia (18 cases), weakness (1), hypertension (2), insomnia (1), dizziness (2), one case of cardiovascular events caused by hypoglycaemia (1), increased the number of urine stools (3), drug-related adverse reactions (unknown) (1)	Total AEs = 140: digestive tract discomfort (24), abdominal pain and diarrhoea (6), constipation (1), hypoglycaemia (44), weakness (9), elevated transaminase (2), nausea and vomiting (11), dizziness and headache (4), abdominal distension (29), rash (1), cardiovascular events caused by hypoglycaemia (5), drug-related adverse reactions (unknown) (4)

Abbreviations: AE, adverse events; ALT, Alanine aminotransferase; AST, Aspartate aminostransferase; CHM, Chinese herbal medicine.

Chinese Herbal Medicine vs. Placebo

In six RCTs of CHM versus a placebo, two studies (H206, H207) reported no AEs. The total number of AEs reported in the CHM group placebo group was 56 and 25, respectively. The most common AE in the CHM group was abnormal liver enzyme levels (12 cases) followed by constipation (seven cases) (H205, H208–H210). The most common AEs in the placebo group was red blood cell in urine (four cases), followed by constipation (three cases) and mild liver dysfunction (three cases) (H205, H209, H210).

Chinese Herbal Medicine vs. Lifestyle Intervention

Four studies that compared CHM to lifestyle intervention reported on AEs. Three RCTs (H9, H19, H204) reported no AEs occurred during the study period in both groups. In the one study that reported AEs, one case of epigastric discomfort was reported in the CHM group, and one case of mild pruritus was reported in the lifestyle intervention group.

Chinese Herbal Medicine vs. Pharmacotherapy

Twelve studies (H1, H3–H5, H7, H9, H17, H19, H20, H27, H38, H39) reported no AEs during the treatment period. In the studies that had AEs (H8, H32, H35), the total number of AEs reported in the CHM group was 30, and 101 AEs were reported in the pharmacotherapy group. The most common AE in the CHM group was diarrhoea (nine cases) and abdominal distention (three cases). In the pharmacotherapy group, the most common AEs were gastrointestinal discomfort (79 cases), liver dysfunction (seven cases) and hypoglycaemia (six cases, H30, H16, H22). The AEs included abdominal distention and pain, diarrhoea, anorexia, nausea and vomiting (H8, H11, H16, H23, H25, H32, H35), non-severe AEs and no other information (nine cases) (H30).

Chinese Herbal Medicine Plus Hypoglycaemic Agents vs. Hypoglycaemic Agents

Sixty-six RCTs mentioned AEs in this group of studies (H3, H19, H41, H47, H49, H51, H52, H57, H58, H60, H62, H64, H66, H70–H72, H74, H75, H78–H80, H82, H84, H87, H89, H92–H94, H96, H98, H100, H101, H104, H105, H109, H111, H113, H116, H119, H122, H124, H126, H130, H133, H142, H145, H153, H155, H157–H162, H164, H168, H171, H176, H177, H179, H183, H192, H193, H195, H196, H199).

Thirty-eight RCTs (H3, H19, H47, H49, H52, H57, H58, H62, H66, H70–H72, H74, H80, H82, H87, H93, H96, H98, H100, H105, H109, H111, H113, H122, H130, H142, H145, H153, H155, H158, H160, H161, H171, H179, H183, H195, H199) reported no AEs in both groups.

Twenty-eight studies (H41, H51, H60, H64, H75, H78, H79, H84, H89, H92, H94, H101, H104, H116, H119, H124, H126, H133, H157, H159, H162, H164, H168, H176, H177, H192, H193, H196) provided information on the AEs.

The total number of AEs reported in the CHM plus hypoglycaemic agents group was 74, and the total was 140 in the hypoglycaemic agents group. The most common AE in the integrative medicine group was gastrointestinal discomfort such as abdominal distention and pain, diarrhoea, constipation, nausea and vomiting. Hypoglycaemia (44 cases) was the most common AE in the control group.

Controlled Clinical Trials of Oral Chinese Herbal Medicine

Ten controlled clinical trials (H211–H220) investigated the effect of CHM in 961 participants. Four studies (H211–H214) evaluated CHM versus hypoglycaemic agents alone, and six studies (H215–H220) evaluated CHM and hypoglycaemic agents versus hypoglycaemic agents alone.

Comparators included metformin, glyburide and insulin glargine. Treatment duration ranged from eight to 24 weeks. Six different Chinese herbal formulae (H213, H214, H216, H217, H219, H220), three Chinese herbal manufactured products (*Yi qi zi yin pian* 益气滋阴片, *Xiao tang ling jiao nang* 消糖灵胶囊 and *Yi tang jiao nang* 益糖胶囊 (H211, H212, H218), and one single herb (*Fan bai cao* 翻白草, *Potentilla discolor* Bge.) (H215) were used in the studies (Table 5.30). All formulae were orally administrated. Fifty-eight herbs were used in the formulae and the most common included *huang qi* 黄芪, *sheng di huang* 生地黄, *ge gen* 葛根, *mai dong* 麦冬, *shan yao* 山药, *cang zhu* 苍术, *dan shen* 丹参, *di gu pi* 地骨皮, *mu dan pi* 牡丹皮, *nv zhen zi* 女贞子 and *zhi mu* 知母. Metformin was used as a control in seven studies (H212–H216, H218, H219), insulins in

Table 5.30.   Frequently Reported Orally Used Herbs in Controlled Clinical Trials

Most Common Herbs	Scientific Name	Frequency of Use
Huang qi 黄芪	*Astragalus membranaceus* (Fisch.) Bge	7
Sheng di huang 生地黄	*Rehmannia glutinosa* Libosch.	7
Ge gen 葛根	*Pueraria lobata* (Willd.) Ohwi	5
Mai men dong 麦冬	*Ophiopogon japonicus* (Thunb.) Ker-Gawl.	5
Shan yao 山药	*Dioscorea opposita* Thunb.	5
Cang zhu 苍术	*Atractylodes lancea* (Thunb.) DC	4
Dan shen 丹参	*Salvia miltiorrhiza* Bge.	4
Di gu pi 地骨皮	*Lycium Chinense* Mill	4
Mu dan pi 牡丹皮	*Paeonia suffruticosa* Andr.	4
Nv zhen zi 女贞子	*Ligustrum lucidum* Ait.	4
Zhi mu 知母	*Anemarrhena asphodeloides* Bge.	4
Huang lian 黄连	*Coptis chinensis* Franch.	3
Tian hua fen 天花粉	*Trichosanthes kirilowii* Maxim.	3
Xuan shen 玄参	*Scrophularia ningpoensis* Hemsl.	3

Note: The use of some herbs may be restricted in some countries. Readers are advised to comply with relevant regulations.

two studies (H217, H220), and glyburide plus metformin in one study (H211).

Fasting Plasma Glucose

Chinese Herbal Medicine vs. Hypoglycaemic Agents

Four studies (n = 319; H211–H214) compared CHM with hypoglycaemic agents. The result indicated that although there was a trend of reducing FPG in the CHM group, no significant difference was seen between the groups (MD −0.57 [−1.16, 0.02]; I^2 = 69.9%).

Chinese Herbal Medicine Plus Hypoglycaemic Agents vs. Hypoglycaemic Agents

Six studies (H215–H220) of 642 participants assessed the effects of CHM plus hypoglycaemic agents to hypoglycaemic agents alone. The result indicated that the value of FPG was reduced in people receiving CHM plus hypoglycaemic agents, compared to control groups (MD −1.218 [−2.30, −0.14]; I^2 = 94.8%). The heterogeneity was high.

Postprandial Blood Glucose

Chinese Herbal Medicine vs. Hypoglycaemic Agents

Four studies (n = 319; H211–H214) compared CHM with hypoglycaemic agents alone. The result indicated an improvement in the CHM group, and the value of PBG was lower than in the conventional medicine group (MD −1.37 [−2.21, −0.52], I^2 = 64.9%).

CHM Plus Hypoglycaemic Agents vs. Hypoglycaemic Agents

Six studies (H215–H220) of 642 participants assessed the effects of CHM in addition to hypoglycaemic agents to hypoglycaemic agents alone. The result indicated that the PBG level was reduced in the integrative medicine group compared to hypoglycaemic agents (MD −2.14 [−3.10, −1.17], I^2 = 87.4%), although the heterogeneity was high.

Glycoslated Haemoglobin A1C

Chinese Herbal Medicine vs. Hypoglycaemic Agents

Three studies (*n* = 219; H212–H214) compared CHM to hypoglycaemic agents. The result indicated a greater improvement in the A1C level of the CHM group (MD −0.48 [−0.62, −0.33]; I^2 = 0.0%).

CHM plus Hypoglycaemic Agents vs. Hypoglycaemic Agents

Three studies (H216, H217, H219) of 272 participants compared CHM plus hypoglycaemic agents to hypoglycaemic agents alone. The result showed a greater reduction in the A1C level in people receiving CHM plus hypoglycaemic agents (MD −0.87 [−1.03, −0.71], I^2 = 35.8%).

Body Mass Index

One study (*n* = 66; H213) compared CHM with metformin. There was a trend in BMI reduction; however, there was no significant difference between the two groups (MD −0.21 [−1.23, 0.81]).

Triglycerides

Chinese Herbal Medicine vs. Hypoglycaemic Agents

Three studies (*n* = 253; H211, H212, H214) compared CHM with hypoglycaemic agents. No significant differences were found between these groups (MD −0.62 [−1.51, 0.27], I^2 = 96.2%).

Chinese Herbal Medicine Plus Hypoglycaemic Agents vs. Hypoglycaemic Agents

Two studies (H216, H218) of 300 participants assessed the effects of CHM plus hypoglycaemic agents versus hypoglycaemic agents alone. The result indicated that there was no significant difference between the integrative medicine group and hypoglycaemic agents, although the value of TG did reduce (MD −0.49 [−1.26, 0.28], I^2 = 92.7%).

Total Cholesterol

Chinese Herbal Medicine vs. Hypoglycaemic Agents

Four studies (n = 319; H211−H214) compared CHM with hypogly-caemic agents alone. The result indicated a greater improvement in the CHM group (MD −0.44 [−0.82, −0.05]; I^2 = 62.4%).

Chinese Herbal Medicine Plus Hypoglycaemic Agents vs. Hypoglycaemic Agents

Two studies (H216, H218) of 300 participants assessed the effects of CHM plus hypoglycaemic agents versus hypoglycaemic agents alone. The result indicated that adding CHM to hypoglycaemic agents was not superior to hypoglycaemic agents (MD −0.407 [−1.180, 0.366], I^2 = 91.4%).

Low-density Lipoprotein

Chinese Herbal Medicine vs. Hypoglycaemic Agents

Two studies (n = 153; H212, H214) compared CHM with hypogly-caemic agents alone. There were no significant differences between the CHM group and hypoglycaemic agents, although there is a trend in reduction of LDL (MD −0.11 [−0.78, 0.56], I^2 = 83.1%).

Chinese Herbal Medicine and Hypoglycaemic Agents vs. Hypoglycaemic Agents

One study (H216) of 100 participants assessed the effects of CHM plus hypoglycaemic agents versus hypoglycaemic agents alone. The result indicated that the integrative medicine group showed greater reduction in LDL levels compared to hypoglycaemic agents alone (MD −0.19 [−0.33, −0.05]).

High-density Lipoprotein

Two studies (n = 153; H212, H214) compared CHM with hypoglycaemic agents alone. The result indicated that there were no significant differences between the groups at improving HDL levels (MD 0.15 [−0.15, 0.46], I^2 = 87.2%).

Fasting Insulin

Three studies (n = 219; H212–H214) compared CHM with hypoglycaemic agents. The result indicated a greater reduction in FINS in the CHM group (MD −4.05 [−6.00, −2.09], I^2 = 84.1%), although considerable statistical heterogeneity was observed.

Insulin Resistance Index

One study (n = 67; H214) compared CHM with hypoglycaemic agents alone. The result indicated that there were no significant differences between the groups at improving IR (MD −3.91 [−9.36, 1.54]).

Safety of Oral Chinese Herbal Medicine in Controlled Clinical Trials

In four studies of CHM versus hypoglycaemic agents for treating T2DM, two studies (H212, H214) reported no AEs. The other two studies did not report on AEs.

Three studies (H216, H217, H220) mentioned AEs when CHM plus hypoglycaemic agents (IM) were compared with hypoglycaemic agents. Two studies (H216, H220) reported no AEs. One study (H217) reported six cases of AEs in the IM group, including skin rash (three cases), hypoglycaemia (one case) and diarrhoea (two cases). Five cases of AEs were reported in the hypoglycaemic group, including skin rash (two cases), hypoglycaemia (two cases) and edema (one case) (H217).

Non-controlled Studies of Oral Chinese Herbal Medicine

Sixteen non-controlled studies (H221–H236) evaluated CHM in 884 participants with T2DM. The treatment duration ranged from four to 24 weeks. Five case series (H222, H225, H232, H233, H236) assessed oral CHM alone, including four studies using extracted CHM capsules. One study (H225) selected a variety of Chinese patent medicines (*Tang niao kang pian* 糖尿康片, *Huang lian jiang tang pian* 黄连降糖片 and Liu xian yin六仙饮) according to the syndrome type. The other three studies (H232, H233, H236) used *Yi jin jiang tang ke li* 益津降糖胶囊, *Xiao ke ping jiao nang* 消渴平胶囊 and *Shen qi jiang tang ke li* 参芪降糖颗粒. Eleven studies (H221, H223, H224, H226–H231, H234, H235) assessed the effect of integrative CHM; these studies used a combination of CHM and hypoglycaemic agents recommended in guidelines, such as biguanides, sulfonylureas, thiazolidinediones and α-Glucosidase inhibitors. Some studies (H221–H224, H226–H231, H234, H235) did not indicate the specific type of hypoglycaemic agent used.

Eight formulae (H221–H224, H226, H227, H229, H235) with a distinctive name were studied. The most commonly used formula was *Chai hu shu gan san* 柴胡疏肝散. It was used in two studies (H221, H235). One study (H225) used individualised syndrome differentiation and treatment. A total of 105 herbs were used in the formulae and the most common herbs were *gan cao* 甘草, *fu ling* 茯苓, *huang qi* 黄芪, *mai dong* 麦冬, *zhi mu* 知母, *bai shao* 白芍,

chai hu 柴胡, *chen pi* 陈皮, *shan zhu yu* 山茱萸 and *sheng di huang* 生地黄.

Safety of Chinese Herbal Medicine in Non-controlled Studies

Four studies (H224, H229, H231, H234) reported no AEs. Two studies reported details of AEs: H225, H226 — after the taking of Chinese medicine of individualised syndrome differentiation, which included dry stools (two cases) (this was improved after adjusting the dosage), and H234, H235 — 19 cases of AEs were reported after taking *Tang wei jiao nang* 糖威胶囊; these included gastrointestinal upset (12 cases), dizziness and palpitation (seven cases).

Clinical Evidence for Commonly Used Chinese Herbal Medicine Treatments

Twenty-six studies (H17, H19, H29–H31, H49, H61, H63, H70, H79, H83, H85, H92, H102, H116, H117, H119, H127, H129, H133, H135, H149, H183, H186, H199, H210) evaluated 11 formulae recommended in the clinical practice guidelines and textbooks that were referred to in Chapter 2. These include *Liu wei di huang wan* 六味地黄丸, *Shen qi jiang tang ke li* 参芪降糖颗粒, *Jin li da ke li* 津力达颗粒, *Xiao ke fang* 消渴方, *Tian mai xiao ke pian* 天麦消渴片, *Yu nv jian* 玉女煎, *Da huang huang lian xie xin tang* 大黄黄连泻心汤, *Ren shen bai hu tang* 人参白虎汤, *Zhi bo di huang tang* 知柏地黄汤, *Ge gen qin lian tang* 葛根芩连汤 and *Shen ling bai zhu san* 参苓白术散. Evidence for *Liu wei di huang wan* (H70, H85, H92, H116, H129), *Shen qi jiang tang granule* (H29, H61, H119, H183), *Jin li da granule* (H19, H102, H117, H133), *Xiao ke fang* (H63, H79, H85), *Tian mai xiao ke tablets* (H31, H186), *Yu nv jian* (H149, H85), *Da huang huang lian xie xin tang* (H30, H199), *Ren shen bai hu tang* (H17, H49) and *Zhi bo di huang tang* (H83, H127) have been reported in the previous section of RCT evidence for individual oral formulae. *Ge gen qin lian tang* and *Shen ling bai zhu san* were evaluated in two studies (H135, H210) separately.

Ge gen qin lian tang 葛根芩连汤

One study (H210) including 98 participants compared *Ge gen qin lian tang* 葛根芩连汤 to a placebo. *Ge gen qin lian tang* 葛根芩连汤 was statistically different to the placebo at reducing FPG level study (MD −1.13 [−1.96, −0.30]). The same effect was not seen in PBG, A1C, BMI, TG, TC, LDL or HDL levels at the end of the treatment period. No significant differences were observed between groups.

Shen ling bai zhu san 参苓白术散

Shen ling bai zhu san 参苓白术散 plus insulin was compared to insulin alone in one study (*n* = 40). At the end of the treatment period, the BMI was assessed in one study. No significant difference was observed between the groups (MD −1.62 [−3.55, 0.31]; H135).

Summary of Chinese Herbal Medicine Clinical Evidence

In total, 236 clinical studies evaluated CHM for T2DM. RCTs were the most common study design (210 studies). CHM alone or combined with hypoglycaemic agents as intervention and hypoglycaemic agents as the control were the most common. All studies were in accordance with the 1999 World Health Organization (WHO) diagnostic criteria for T2DM. All participants had a T2DM diagnosis without other concurrent conditions. In studies that described CM syndromes, internal deficiency of *qi* and *yin* was the most frequent. Nearly all CHM interventions were orally administrated. The most common formulae were *Liu wei di huang wan* 六味地黄丸 (five studies), *Shen qi jiang tang* granule 参芪降糖颗粒 (four studies), *Jin li da* granule 津力达颗粒 (four studies), *Huang lian su* tablets 黄连素片 (four studies), *Xiao ke fang* 消渴方 (three studies) and *Yu quan wan* 玉泉丸 (three studies). The three most common herbs were *huang qi* 黄芪, *sheng di huang* 生地黄 and *ge gen* 葛根. The most common comparator in the studies was biguanides.

Chinese Herbal Medicine

CHM was superior to conventional medicine for treating T2DM in terms of reducing PBG, TG, TC and LDL, increasing HDL, and improving the FINS and IR. However, the results had moderate to high statistical heterogeneity.

In terms of FPG, although the overall efficacy of CHM is not as good as conventional medicine for treating T2DM, in subgroup analysis, including patients with a disease duration of five to 10 years and a baseline fasting blood glucose level >10 mmol/L, meta-analysis results show that CHM is superior to conventional medicine — although heterogeneity remained high in the subgroups.

CHM was superior to a placebo and is the only lifestyle intervention in terms of reducing FPG, PBG, A1C, TC and LDL, increasing HDL, and improving FINS. However, the number and size of the placebo and lifestyle intervention studies were small.

The pooled results showed moderate to high statistical heterogeneity that could not be explained by a subgroup analysis. The reasons for heterogeneity may include baseline fasting plasma glucose levels, course of disease and age of patients, different CHM interventions in terms of treatment duration, dosage, etc.

As for safety, the AE total in the CHM group was less than a third of the conventional medicine group. The most common AE in the CHM group was abdominal distention and diarrhoea. The GRADE assessment indicated that the evidence was of low to moderate quality. Despite the positive results, some caution should be taken when interpreting the findings because the studies had methodological shortfalls; almost all the included studies were at risk of bias in terms of randomisation and blinding, which may overestimate the effect. Overall, CHM shows promising effects as compared with conventional medicine for treating T2DM and appears to be safe.

Integrative Medicine

CHM combined with hypoglycaemic agents showed more benefits than hypoglycaemic agents alone in terms of reducing the value of blood glucose (including FPG, PBG, A1C), BMI, and improving blood lipids (including TG, TC, LDL, HDL) and β-cell function (including FINS, IR, IS). However, there were methodological short-falls, and the studies had unclear sequence generation and allocation concealment, plus a lack of blinding of participants and personnel. In addition, the pooled results had considerable heterogeneity, which may have been due to inconsistency across studies in terms of a patient's condition, compliance, CHM, study protocols, treatment duration, and outcome measurement. Also, a subgroup analysis does not reduce heterogeneity.

The total number of AEs in the integrative medicine group was about half of that of the hypoglycaemic agents group. The result should be interpreted cautiously as the number of studies was limited and the comparative effect size was very small. The evidence analysis using the GRADE approach showed that the studies were of low to moderate quality.

Overall, the effect of CHM combined with conventional medi-cine, including hypoglycaemic agents for T2DM, remains uncertain as the evidence is of low quality. However, CHM appears to be safe.

In summary, the best available evidence indicates that oral CHM can improve disease conditions and appears to be safe. A wide range of CHM interventions show promising benefits for people with T2DM. However, there is no outstanding herb or individual formula that outperforms the others. This is because the consistent studies assessing the same CM syndromes and formula over the same period of time are limited. Although the comparative effectiveness between CHM and conventional medicine such as hypoglycaemic agents remains inconclusive, CHM appears to be well tolerated by people with T2DM. Until further conclusive evidence is generated, clinical decision-making for people with T2DM should incorporate their diabetes condition, CM syndrome, treatment preferences, and previous experiences with hypoglycaemic agents and CHM.

References

1. Liu M, Liu Z, Xu B, Zhang W, Cai J. (2016) Review of systematic reviews and meta-analyses investigating traditional chinese medicine treatment for type 2 diabetes mellitus. *J Tradit Chin Med* **36**(5): 555–563.
2. Liu JP, Zhang M, Wang W, Grimsgaard S. (2009) Chinese herbal medicines for type 2 diabetes mellitus (Review). *Cochrane Database of Sys Rev* (3).
3. 杨丽娜, 龙毅, 李鸿艳, 刘娅. (2007) 中西医结合治疗2型糖尿病的 Meta 分析. 吉林大学学报(医学版) **33**(2): 241–244.
4. 张燕. (2010) 中药治疗2型糖尿病随机对照试验的系统评价. 北京中医药大学, 中国北京.
5. 马立新. (2012) 中药治疗2型糖尿病随机对照试验的系统综述及方法学评价研究. 北京中医药大学博士论文, 中国北京.
6. Ao Y, David A, David M. (2018) Chinese herbal medicine versus other interventions in the treatment of type 2 diabetes a systematic review of randomized controlled trials. *J Evid Based Integr Med* **23**: 1–10.

Study References Included in Chinese Herbal Medicine Clinical Studies

Study No.	Reference
H1	陈妍妍. (2011) '动–定序贯范氏八法' 辨证治疗新诊断 2 型糖尿病的临床研究. 广州中医药大学硕士学位论文, 中国广州.
H2	于书香,陶睿. (2013) 中西医结合治疗 II 型糖尿病湿热困脾证的临床观察. 北京中医药大学学报. 中医临床版 **20**(6): 43–45.
H3	李丽杰. (2006) 金梅消渴汤(丸)对2型糖尿病的临床研究. 湖北中医学院硕士学位论文, 中国武汉.
H4	刘贵洲, 孟玲, 夏黎明. (2014) 温阳降糖口服液治疗 2 型糖尿病临床研究. 光明中医 **29**(7): 1395–1397.
H5	刘佳. (2010) 知黄汤治疗消渴病(阴虚热盛证)临床研究. 长春中医药大学硕士学位论文, 中国长春.

(Continued)

Study No.	Reference
H6	龙邦宏, 杨春城. (2013) 连桂汤治疗 2 型糖尿病临床疗效观察. 医学信息 **26**(10): 458.
H7	骆天炯. (2012) 加减四妙颗粒改善 2 型糖尿病及前期胰岛素敏感性的临床观察与机理研究. 南京中医药大学博士学位论文, 中国南京.
H8	罗云林. (2015) 三才粉剂治疗初诊 2 型糖尿病(阴虚热盛型)的有效性及安全性观察. 成都中医药大学硕士学位论文, 中国成都.
H9	侣丽萍. (2012) '动一定序贯八法' 临证辨治消渴病. 广州中医药大学博士学位论文, 中国广州.
H10	马春玲, 阮永队, 陈红梅. (2015) 温中运脾补肾法治疗 2 型糖尿病临床研究. 云南中医学院学报 **38**(2): 65–68.
H11	庞铁良, 庞秀花. (2006) 升清降糖方对 2 型糖尿病患者胰岛素抵抗影响的临床观察. 北京中医 **25**(9): 546–548.
H12	庞宗然, 贾春华, 刘宝山, *et al.* (2003) 菩人丹胶囊治疗2型糖尿病38例疗效观察.山东中医杂志 **22**(3): 137–139.
H13	彭欣, 银浩强, 王德利, *et al.* (2014) 益气活血法对糖尿病中医证候及糖脂代谢影响的临床研究. 山东中医杂志 **33**(1): 17–19.
H14	曲丹. (2005) 参连冬胶囊治疗老年 2 型糖尿病气阴两虚兼热证的临床研究. 中国中医研究院硕士学位论文, 中国北京.
H15	全春. (2012) 消渴二仙汤治疗消渴病(气阴两虚挟瘀证)的临床研究. 长春中医药大学硕士学位论文, 中国长春.
H16	尚文斌, 程海波, 司晓晨, 滕士超. (2003) 清脂健胰胶囊改善 2 型糖尿病胰岛素抵抗的研究. 南京中医药大学学报 **19**(4): 210–212.
H17	沈坤龙. (2014) 人参白虎汤加味治疗 2 型糖尿病阴虚热盛证的临床疗效观察. 山东中医药大学, 博士学位论文, 中国济南.
H18	沈小璇, 李亚娟. (2017) 黄连降糖汤治疗 2 型糖尿病的临床疗效及对血管VEGF的影响分析. 世界中医药 **12**(10): 2318–2321.
H19	宋郁珍, 李争, 杜鸿瑶, 刘薇, *et al.* (2017) 清热益气法对初发 2 型糖尿病病人胰岛功能的保护机制研究. 中西医结合心脑血管病杂志 **15**(21): 2663–2666.
H20	孙雪. (2014) 化湿通络汤治疗糖尿病(痰湿瘀阻证)的临床研究. 长春中医药大学硕士学位论文, 中国长春.
H21	谭名媛. (2015) 清滋饮治疗新诊断阴虚热盛 2 型糖尿病的临床研究. 南京中医药大学硕士学位论文, 中国南京.

(Continued)

(Continued)

Study No.	Reference
H22	王平. (2008) 清活汤对2型糖尿病患者超敏C反应蛋白影响的临床观察. 山东中医药大学硕士学位论文, 中国济南.
H23	王帅. (2011) 苦辛运中法治疗新诊断 2 型糖尿病(湿热困脾型)的临床研究. 成都中医药大学硕士学位论文, 中国成都.
H24	王文林. (2013) 甘苦合化法治疗Ⅱ型糖尿病郁热阴伤证的研究. 南京中医药大学博士学位论文, 中国南京.
H25	肖小惠. (2016) 益气养阴活血法改善2型糖尿病胰岛素抵抗的研究. 广州中医药大学硕士学位论文, 中国广州.
H26	薛青, 谢丹红, 卫苓, *et al.* (2007) 清肝泻心汤对2型糖尿病胰岛素抵抗相关因素影响的研究. 第三军医大学学报 **29**(7): 613–616.
H27	杨殿福, 冯建文. (2009) 中西医结合治疗 2 型糖尿病63例. 中国中西医结合肾病杂志 **10**(1): 74–75.
H28	杨文军, 赵兴国. (2013) 黄连解毒汤联合二甲双胍治疗2型糖尿病的临床观察. 中国医疗前沿 **8**(9): 41–42.
H29	叶卓丁, 吴钧俊. (2009) 参芪降糖颗粒治疗 2 型糖尿病疗效分析. 实用中医药杂志 **12**(203): 788–789.
H30	Yu XT, Xu LP, Zhou Q, *et al.* (2018) The efficacy and safety of Chinese herbal formula JTTZ (jiangtangtiaozhi) for the treatment of type 2 diabetes with obesity and hyperlipidemia: A multicenter randomized, positive-controlled, open-label clinical trial. *Int J Endocrinol*. Article ID 9519231, 11 pages.
H31	苑晓烨, 温志谦, 杨圣俊, 李芳. (2011) 天麦消渴片联合格列本脲治疗2型糖尿病的临床研究. 现代中西医结合杂志 **20**(8): 926–928.
H32	张德贵, 崔晓燕, 宋学芳, 王芳. (2016) 泻肝利湿方治疗湿热型2型糖尿病早期临床观察. 山西中医 **32**(2): 43–44.
H33	张国庆, 张聚府, 赵金伟. (2011) 芩连平胃散治疗湿热困脾证2型糖尿病及对血糖和血脂的影响. 陕西中医 **32**(4): 425–426.
H34	张红红, 潘秉余. (2009) 参地生津胶囊治疗气阴两虚兼血瘀型2型糖尿病临床疗效及对血液流变学的影响. 河北中医 **31**(6): 827–828.
H35	张恒耀. (2015) 三才粉剂治疗单一口服降糖药控制不佳的 2 型糖尿病（阴虚热盛型）临床观察. 成都中医药大学硕士学位论文.
H36	张丽丽, 黄聂建. (2006) 消渴愈抗汤对 2 型糖尿病患者胰岛素抵抗的影响. 福建中医药 **37**(4): 11–12.

Study No.	Reference
H37	张睿, 田谧, 史耀勋, *et al.* (2012) 消渴脂平胶囊治疗 2 型糖尿病的临床观察. 中国中医药现代远程教育 **10**(7): 30–31.
H38	张晓立, 张洁. (2016) 益气养阴方联合西药对 2 型糖尿病患者细胞因子, 血脂的影响及疗效观察. 国际医药卫生导报 **22**(19): 3017–3019.
H39	张永忠, 匡黎明, 周杰, 王敏, *et al.* (2008) 清热解毒法治疗 2 型糖尿病 30 例. 光明中医 **23**(5): 632–634.
H40	邹毅. (2009) 益气养阴, 化痰活血方对气阴两虚兼痰瘀阻滞 2 型糖尿病患者胰岛素抵抗干预作用的临床研. 湖北中医学院硕士学位论文, 中国武汉.
H41	安小平, 崔庆荣, 康学东. (2016) 苦瓜胶囊联合二甲双胍治疗 2 型糖尿病 46 例. 西部中医药 **29**(6): 77–79.
H42	安小平, 崔庆荣, 康学东. (2017) 苦瓜胶囊治疗 2 型糖尿病胰岛素抵抗的临床观察. 西部中医药 **30**(3): 1–4.
H43	白虎明. (2006) 益气养阴活血汤治疗 2 型糖尿病 40 例. 陕西中医 **27**(10): 1237–1238.
H44	白建乐, 刘恒亮, 张书金, *et al.* (2016) 清热活血化痰法治疗 2 型糖尿病的疗效研究. 河北中医药学报 **31**(2): 11–13.
H45	白建乐, 张书金, 刘恒亮, 崔志梅. (2016) 清热活血化痰方对2型糖尿病患者胰岛素抵抗的影响. 河北医药 **38**(17): 2651–2653.
H46	蔡镇, 冷玉杰, 张跃斌, *et al.* (2015) 五味子煎剂对2型糖尿病患者血清IL–2及IL–6水平的影响. 现代生物医学进展 **12**(21): 4084–4086.
H47	曹爱梅, 张桂静, 郑杰, 单亚利. (2008) 五黄通脉汤治疗 2 型糖尿病 68 例临床观察. 北京中医药 **27**(12): 957–958.
H48	曹晶晶, 杨卫杰. (2012) 化痰祛湿行气活血法治疗痰瘀型 2 型糖尿病临床观察. 中医临床研究 **4**(1): 25–6.
H49	曹瑛, 邹碧云. (2007) 白虎人参汤加减与西药联合应用治疗 2 型糖尿病54 例临床观察. 中医药导报 **13**(11): 18–20.
H50	程平荣, 周厚地, 晋献春, *et al.* (2010) 糖脉康颗粒对 2 型糖尿病患者血糖波动影响的观察. 中医药导报 **16**(11): 34–36.
H51	陈巧玲. (2010) 李氏清暑益气汤治疗 2 型糖尿病的临床研究. 广州中医药大学硕士学位论文, 中国广州:
H52	陈艳. (2012) 健脾滋肾, 清热养阴法治疗 II 型糖尿病的临床研究. 南京中医药大学硕士学位论文, 中国南京.

(*Continued*)

Study No.	Reference
H53	陈英, 曹晶晶. (2012) 祛痰利湿化瘀法治疗痰瘀型 2 型糖尿病的临床疗效观察. 中国中医药现代远程教育 **10**(12): 133–134.
H54	崔建华, 罗会. (2006) 新中西医结合治疗2型糖尿病 40 例疗效观察. 云南中医中药杂志 **27**(4): 4–5.
H55	崔玉梅. (2011) 疏肝健脾汤治疗 2 型糖尿病肝郁脾虚证临床疗效观察. 山东中医药大学硕士学位论文, 中国济南.
H56	戴小良. (2002) 清肝泻心滋阴润燥法治疗糖尿病(心肝郁热证)的临床研究. 湖南中医学院硕士学位论文, 中国长沙.
H57	邓银泉, 范小芬, 吴国琳, 熊福林. (2006) 玉泉丸对2型糖尿病促炎细胞因子干预的影响. 中国中西医结合杂志 **26**(8): 706–709.
H58	段公, 石彩云, 陈于翠, 陈志颜. (2015) 加减抵当汤治疗痰瘀型 2 型糖尿病78例临床观察. 河北中医 **37**(11): 1667–1670.
H59	段公, 石彩云, 陈于翠, 陈志颜. (2015) 加减抵挡汤对痰瘀型糖尿病患者胰岛素抵抗的影响. 中国医药指南 **13**(23): 189–190.
H60	段金娜. (2012) 加味清心莲子饮治疗 2 型糖尿病(气阴两虚夹湿证)的临床研究. 成都中医药大学硕士学位论文, 中国成都.
H61	范英丽, 黄秀锦, 高金鸟, 陈华伟. (2014) 参芪降糖颗粒辅助治疗2型糖尿病的临床观察. 中国医学装备 **11**: 142.
H62	房露露. (2015) 醒脾除陈汤治疗湿热困脾, 痰气郁结型初发2型糖尿病的临床研究. 山东中医药大学硕士学位论文, 中国济南.
H63	傅静波. (2012) 消渴方治疗阴虚热盛型 2 型糖尿病的临床研究. 黑龙江中医药大学硕士学位论文, 中国哈尔滨.
H64	付耀华. (2016) 葛根芩连消渴方治疗湿热蕴脾型 2 型糖尿病的疗效观察. 广州中医药大学硕士学位论文, 中国广州.
H65	高蕾, 陈媛媛, 霍贵申, 万迎新. (2017) 二甲双胍联合参芪降糖胶囊治疗 2 型糖尿病的临床疗效及其对患者血糖和血脂及炎性因子的影响. 临床合理用药杂志 **10**(36): 1–2.
H66	龚丽. (2013) 黄芪消渴方治疗气阴两虚型 2 型糖尿病的疗效观察. 广州中医药大学硕士学位论文, 中国广州.
H67	郭建辉, 冯崇廉, 沈文斌, *et al.* (2012) 酸苦降气法治疗 2 型糖尿病临床研究. 吉林中医药 **32**(12): 1241–1243.
H68	郭良堂, 蒋玉燕. (2012) 二甲双胍联合玉泉颗粒治疗新发 2 型糖尿病疗效观察. 浙江临床医学 **14**(12): 1525–1526.

Study No.	Reference
H69	黄修涛, 孙慧. (2013) 中西医结合治疗 2 型糖尿病 50 例. 山东中医杂志 **32**(5): 340–341.
H70	和发新, 李庆芳, 杨继芬. (2013) 六味地黄丸联合瑞格列奈治疗 2 型糖尿病疗效观察. 基层医学论坛 **17**(13): 1735–1736.
H71	侯宇辉. (2011) 疏肝健脾法治疗 2 型糖尿病临床研究. 山东中医药大学硕士学位论文, 中国济南.
H72	黄丽慧. (2006) 加味四逆散治疗消渴病的理论与临床研究. 北京中医药大学硕士学位论文, 中国北京.
H73	蒋文静. (2012) 玉液通络汤辅治 2 型糖尿病的临床观察. 临床合理用药杂志 **5**(31): 88–89.
H74	金枝. (2017) 糖参乐丸治疗 2 型糖尿病(气阴两虚证)的临床疗效观察. 湖北中医药大学硕士学位论文, 中国武汉.
H75	雷长国, 张继华, 蔡林. (2013) 中西医结合治疗 2 型糖尿病疗效及安全性分析. 中国广州:广州中医药大学学报 **30**(5): 624–627.
H76	李金华, 肖琴. (2016) 化痰活血汤治疗老年人 2 型糖尿病临床观察. 中医临床研究 **8**(15): 64–66.
H77	李水花, 吴农田. (2012) 玉泉丸联合二甲双胍治疗 2 型糖尿病临床观察. 辽宁中医药大学学报 **14**(12): 163–164.
H78	利顺欣, 李书文, 庞景三. (2017) 渴乐宁胶囊治疗气阴两虚型糖尿病的临床效果观察. 中药药理与临床 **33**(3): 198–200.
H79	李馨兰, 范福山, 廖丽坤, 邓丽琼. (2013) 消渴方治疗 2 型糖尿病临床研究. 中医学报 **28**(8): 1215–1217.
H80	李希岭. (2014) 从肠促胰岛素作用机制探讨益气健脾法治疗 2 型糖尿病的临床研究. 山东中医药大学硕士学位论文.
H81	李振衡, 阳梅, 唐丹, 沈黎. (2011) 降糖胶囊结合西药治疗气阴两虚型 2 型糖尿病102例临床观察. 中医药导报 **17**(2): 34–36.
H82	李宗桥. (2011) 化浊益脾饮治疗痰湿内阻型 2 型糖尿病的临床研究. 黑龙江中医药大学硕士学位论文, 中国哈尔滨.
H83	林峻丞. (2011) 中药结合八段锦治疗2型糖尿病的疗效观察. 南京中医药大学硕士学位论文, 中国南京.
H84	林俊杰, 卢昉, 张间霞. (2014) 复方降糖玉液联合二甲双胍和格列美脲治疗 2 型糖尿病. 中国药师 **17**(2): 268–270.

(*Continued*)

(*Continued*)

Study No.	Reference
H85	林瑞芳, 蔡悦, 吕保阶, *et al.* (2014) 中西医结合治疗 2 型糖尿病疗效观察. 实用中西医结合临床 **14**(6): 26–27.
H86	林源, 高海燕, 郭亚菊, *et al.* (2017) 珍芪降糖胶囊联合西格列汀片治疗 2 型糖尿病. 吉林中医药 **37**(6): 560–563.
H87	林玉姣. (2016) 锦连合剂对老年 2 型糖尿病炎症因子的临床研究. 南京中医药大学硕士学位论文, 中国南京.
H88	刘畅, 葛洪, 李敏, *et al.* (2016) 益气养阴清热方对 2 型糖尿病患者血脂, 血糖及1, 25–二羟维生素d3水平影响研究. 中国生化药物杂志 **36**(2): 145–147.
H89	刘畅, 张秀媛, 马万. (2016) 千清解降糖方配合门冬胰岛素30治疗 2 型糖尿病(阴虚热盛证)的临床观察. 中医临床研究 **8**(21): 41–43.
H90	刘红樱, 胡齐鸣. (2008) 黄连素对 2 型糖尿病(湿热内蕴型)胰岛 β 细胞功能的影响. 中国中医药信息杂志 **15**(3): 12–14.
H91	刘玲, 刘德亮, 李惠林, *et al.* (2017) 活血降糖饮治疗 2 型糖尿病气阴两虚证30例. 现代中医药 **37**(5): 16–20.
H92	刘霞, 李亚. (2016) 六味地黄丸联合利拉鲁肽和二甲双胍治疗 2 型糖尿病的临床研究. 现代药物与临床 **31**(8): 1146–1150.
H93	刘小芳. (2012) 益气养阴, 化痰祛瘀法对T2DM胰岛β细胞功能影响的临床研究. 黑龙江中医药大学硕士学位论文, 中国哈尔滨.
H94	刘莹. (2010) 芪黄汤对 2 型糖尿病气阴两虚兼血瘀证的临床研究. 陕西中医学院硕士学位论文, 中国咸阳.
H95	罗学林, 赵郴. (2005) 知柏地黄汤联合二甲双胍治疗 2 型糖尿病 52 例临床观察. 中医药导报 **11**(6): 15–16.
H96	路军章. (2005) 保元活血颗粒治疗老年 2 型糖尿病气虚血瘀证的临床研究. 中国人民解放军总医院硕士学位论文, 中国北京.
H97	路军章, 唐果, 刘毅, 邓新立. (2009) 中西医结合治疗老年 2 型糖尿病临床观察. 中国中医药信息杂志 **16**(7): 8–10.
H98	罗礼达. (2009) 温脏扶正驱邪法对 2 型糖尿病T淋巴细胞免疫功能影响的临床研究. 广州中医药大学博士学位论文, 中国广州.
H99	吕予, 侯杰军, 路亚娥. (2011) 益气养阴活血法治疗 2 型糖尿病 45 例. 陕西中医 **32**(11): 1485–1486.
H100	马丹. (2016) 消渴健脾汤对 2 型糖尿病患者血糖及胰岛素影响临床研究. 新疆医科大学硕士学位论文, 中国乌鲁木齐.

Study No.	Reference
H101	马红, 王海红, 蒲小庆, 张银川. (2014) 中西医结合治疗 2 型糖尿病 68 例. 西部中医药 **27**(8): 95–96.
H102	马锐, 夏丽芳. (2016) 通心络胶囊联合津力达颗粒对 2 型糖尿病患者血糖及血管内皮功能的影响. 国际中医中药杂志 **38**(5): 411–413.
H103	马献中, 王世彪, 方玲. (2016) 黄芪乌梅汤治疗气阴两虚型 2 型糖尿病 60 例. 西部中医药 **29**(4): 92–93.
H104	毛奇. (2017) 2 型糖尿病患者应用益气育阴汤辅助治疗疗效及不良反应分析. 中国卫生标准管理 **8**(9): 96–98.
H105	孟晓嵘. (2006) 健脾化痰方治疗痰湿型 2 型糖尿病的临床研究. 福建中医学院硕士学位论文, 中国福州.
H106	欧奇伟, 李茂清. (2015) 中西医结合治疗对糖尿病患者血管内皮功能的影响. 中医学报 **30**(2): 183–185.
H107	彭苾娜, 王宏志, 郑长丰. (2009) 参芪降糖煎剂联用西药治疗 2 型糖尿病的疗效观察. 国际中医中药杂志 **31**(3): 241–242.
H108	彭利, 李忠业, 鲍宜桂. (2007) 中西医结合疗法改善 2 型糖尿病的临床观察. 中成药 **29**(8): 1112–1114.
H109	秦扬, 王勉. (2014) 加味二阴煎治疗气阴两虚型 2 型糖尿病 42 例临床观察. 中医药导报 **20**(8): 57–59.
H110	秦扬, 王勉, 邹冬吟. (2014) 加味二阴煎对 2 型糖尿病血糖波动的影响. 中国实验方剂学杂志 **20**(17): 198–201.
H111	曲波. (2003) 降糖增敏合剂对 2 型糖尿病胰岛素敏感性的影响. 山东中医药大学硕士学位论文, 中国济南.
H112	尚俊, 郑嘉泉, 苏晓兰. (2014) 中西医结合治疗对 2 型糖尿病胰岛素抵抗和胰岛β细胞功能的影响. 光明中医 **19**(6): 1197–1200.
H113	余卫吉, 吕雄. (2012) 舒正颗粒治疗消渴病 38 例临床观察. 中国社区医师: 医学专业 **14**(34): 218.
H114	石广汕, 杨静, 洪安林, 陈荣. (2008) 中西医结合治疗气阴两虚兼血瘀型 2 型糖尿病对照观察. 山西中医 **24**(2): 28–29.
H115	宋艳丽, 王秋萍. (2012) 自拟降糖方治疗 2 型糖尿病疗效观察. 当代医学 **18**(23): 44–45.
H116	唐瑛, 李劲松. (2015) 六味地黄丸加减联合二甲双胍辨治阴虚内热证 2 型糖尿病的临床研究. 湖南师范大学学报: 医学版 **12**(4): 28–31.
H117	唐艳阁, 王敏, 杨家祥. (2017) 磷酸西格列汀联合津力达颗粒对 II 型糖尿病血糖和血清炎性因子水平的影响. 内蒙古中医药 **36**(21): 108–109.

(Continued)

(Continued)

Study No.	Reference
H118	唐宗琼, 刘松. (2014) 养阴清热经验方联合西医治疗 2 型糖尿病的疗效观察. 中医药导报 **20**(10): 74–76.
H119	王彩霞, 胡曼云, 武煦峰. (2016) 参芪降糖颗粒联合西医常规疗法治疗 2 型糖尿病. 吉林中医药 **36**(5): 462–466.
H120	王德伟, 郑菊芬. (2007) 糖脂灵汤对 2 型糖尿病胰岛素抵抗的影响. 中国中医药科技 **14**(6): 465–466.
H121	王光明, 王志高. (2009) 益肾健脾法治疗 2 型糖尿病胰岛素抵抗的临床研究. 甘肃中医 **22**(4): 25–26.
H122	王国姿. (2015) 芩连降糖方联合胰岛素治疗 2 型糖尿病湿热证的临床观察. 华北理工大学硕士学位论文, 中国唐山.
H123	王亮. (2009) 降糖饮治疗气阴两虚 2 型糖尿病的临床观察. 黑龙江中医药大学硕士学位论文, 中国哈尔滨.
H124	王美玲. (2012) 糖一方治疗气阴两虚兼血瘀型2DM疗效观察. 广州中医药大学硕士学位论文, 中国广州.
H125	王明山, 马伟杰, 杜翠红. (2006) 地冬复胰胶囊配合西药治疗 2 型糖尿病临床观察. 河北中医 **28**(2): 126–127.
H126	王鸿庆. (2016) 基于甘苦合化法对阴亏热郁型 2 型糖尿病的临床研究. 山东中医药大学硕士学位论文, 中国济南.
H127	王素利. (2010) 养阴清热法对 2 型糖尿病 β 细胞功能的早期保护研究. 广州中医药大学硕士学位论文, 中国广州.
H128	王义霞, 陈晓欢, 生娣. (2010) 中西医结合治疗 2 型糖尿病疗效观察. 现代中西医结合杂志 **19**(33): 4274–4275.
H129	温立新, 陈聪水. (2010) 六昧地黄丸治疗 2 型糖尿病 58 例临床研究. 中国社区医师: 医学专业 **12**(228): 82.
H130	吴正. (2005) 健脾降糖汤治疗2型糖尿病脾虚痰瘀证的研究. 南京中医药大学硕士学位论文, 中国南京.
H131	肖燕倩, 郭美珠. (2004) 糖络饮治疗气阴两虚脉络瘀阻型糖尿病 46 例–附西药对照组35例. 辽宁中医学院学报 **6**(1): 35–37.
H132	谢谋华, 路翠棉. (2007) 地黄降糖丸治疗 2 型糖尿病疗效观察. 吉林中医药 **27**(6): 22–23.
H133	谢晓兰, 王丽娜, 姚丽翠. (2016) 津力达颗粒改善 2 型糖尿病患者胰岛功能及糖脂代谢的临床观察. 中医临床研究 **8**(31): 9–11.
H134	许成辉. (2015) 调畅枢机法治疗 2 型糖尿病临床研究. 广州中医药大学硕士学位论文, 中国广州.

Study No.	Reference
H135	徐小娟, 刘丹, 张炜宁, 王静. (2015) 参苓白术散加减对 2 型糖尿病患者胰岛素敏感指数的影响. 中医药临床杂志 **27**(7): 954–956.
H136	严余明, 杨锋, 王忆黎, 戴关海. (2008) 桑胶煎治疗 2 型糖尿病 52 例临床观察. 中华中医药杂志 **23**(2): 118–121.
H137	杨连奉. (2017) 千金文武汤联合二甲双胍治疗太阴人 2 型糖尿病的临床研究. 延边大学硕士学位论文, 中国延吉.
H138	杨威. (2011) 清热祛湿法对新诊断 2 型糖尿病湿热证的疗效观察. 辽宁中医药大学硕士学位论文, 中国沈阳.
H139	杨卫杰, 曹晶晶. (2012) 玉消汤治疗 2 型糖尿病胰岛素抵抗 33 例临床观察. 中医临床研究 **4**(1): 46–47.
H140	杨昭凤, 裴友翠. (2016) 柴胡消渴汤治疗糖尿病胰岛素抵抗疗效观察. 世界中西医结合杂志 **11**(8): 1153–1155.
H141	叶文平, 刘云雅, 张捷. (2016) 胰岛素治疗结合中医分期辨证论治 2 型糖尿病 50 例临床观察. 中国民族民间医药杂志 **25**(8): 49–51.
H142	伊善君. (2007) 降糖增敏合剂对 2 型糖尿病患者胰岛素敏感性的影响. 山东中医药大学硕士学位论文, 中国济南.
H143	虞成毕, 严东标, 张美珍, *et al*. (2013) 自制太平糖克浓缩丸治疗 2 型糖尿病临床疗效观察. 实用中西医结合临床 **13**(1): 16–17.
H144	余臣祖, 康学东, 党晓娟, 刘翠清. (2017) 加味六君子汤对脾虚痰湿证 2 型糖尿病患者胰岛β细胞功能的影响. 中国中医药信息杂志 **24**(4): 36–39.
H145	于洁. (2015) 升清降浊法合二甲双胍治疗 2 型糖尿病的临床疗效观察. 山东中医药大学硕士学位论文, 中国济南.
H146	余小红. (2017) 加服自拟参地丹杞汤治疗 2 型糖尿病气阴两虚证临床观察. 广西中医药 **40**(1): 27–9.
H147	于竹力, 周振坤, 全丰玲. (2004) 中西医结合治疗 2 型糖尿病 30 例临床观察. 现代中西医结合杂志 **13**(2): 86.
H148	曾珍. (2017) 加味桃核承气汤治疗糖尿病患者的效果及对患者血糖水平的影响. 中医临床研究 **9**(27): 48–50.
H149	张爱霞, 岳仁宋, 杨彩虹. (2012) 助脾散精法治疗 2 型糖尿病胃强脾弱证 46 例疗效观察.四川中医 **30**(10): 96–97.
H150	张博, 南征, 许崇明, *et al*. (2017) 中西医结合治疗 2 型糖尿病 30 例临床观察. 湖南中医杂志 **33**(8): 13–15.
H151	张殿鸿, 王镁. (2018) 中西医结合治疗 2 型糖尿病临床观察. 山西中医 **34**(1): 29–30.

(Continued)

(Continued)

Study No.	Reference
H152	张都全, 刘海燕. (2008) 参麦芎芍汤治疗 2 型糖尿病45例临床观察. 中医药导报 **14**(6): 45–46.
H153	章福宝, 陶怡, 宁静. (2015) 中药自拟方辅助治疗 2 型糖尿病的疗效观察. 中国中医药科技 **22**(2): 186–187.
H154	张风霞, 张铭, 孙西庆, 王新陆. (2013) 化浊行血汤治疗胰岛素抵抗及对血清炎症因子的影响. 世界中西医结合杂志 **8**(4): 393–394.
H155	张风霞. (2009) 从血浊内阻论治 2 型糖尿病的临床研究. 山东中医药大学博士学位论文, 中国济南.
H156	张国琼, 尤强, 吕蒙, 陈德磊. (2014) 益气养阴活血汤治疗2型糖尿病 36 例报告. 糖尿病新世界 **11**(22): 35–36.
H157	张光珍, 孙福庆, 郭健飞, *et al.* (2002) 中西医结合治疗 2 型糖尿病的临床研究. 现代中西医结合杂志 **11**(1): 5–7.
H158	张红, 王效非, 肖海静, *et al.* (2010) 中西医结合治疗 2 型糖尿病胰岛素抵抗临床观察. 北京中医药 **29**(10): 737–740.
H159	张红红, 潘秉余. (2009) 中西医结合治疗气阴两虚兼血瘀型 2 型糖尿病120例临床观察. 北京中医药 **28**(7): 538–540.
H160	张晶. (2012) 糖尿病脾虚证应用健脾益气法的临床疗效观察和胃肠激素研究. 山东中医药大学硕士学位论文, 中国济南.
H161	张凯婷. (2010) 益气养阴化瘀法治疗 2 型糖尿病气阴两虚夹瘀证的临床研究. 南京中医药大学硕士学位论文, 中国南京.
H162	张磊, 洪兵. (2014) 消渴康颗粒联合盐酸吡咯列酮片治疗 2 型糖尿病阴虚热盛型临床观察. 辽宁中医药大学学报 **16**(12): 117–119.
H163	张玲玲. (2015) 益气养阴降糖方治疗 2 型糖尿病的临床疗效观察. 北京中医药大学硕士学位论文, 中国北京.
H164	张利民, 谭毅, 黄伟, 张学英, *et al.* (2014) 小陷胸汤联合盐酸二甲双胍片治疗2型糖尿病痰湿蕴热型临床观察. 中国中医药信息杂志 **21**(2): 32–34.
H165	张娜. (2013) 益气养阴法治疗初发 2 型糖尿病胰岛素抵抗临床研究. 泰山医学院硕士学位论文, 中国泰安.
H166	张启发, 范丽霞. (2016) 中药复方治疗 2 型糖尿病的效果评价. 糖尿病新世界 **4**(7): 43–45.
H167	张蓉, 张华敏, 鞠萍, 李建波. (2008) 抗糖平对 2 型糖尿病胰岛素抵抗相关指标的影响. 光明中医 **23**(9): 1299–1300.
H168	张瑞方. (2009) 鹿菟饮在阳虚血瘀型 2 型糖尿病的临床疗效评价研究. 福建中医学院硕士学位论文, 中国福州.

(Continued)

Study No.	Reference
H169	张瑞方, 邱英明. (2009) 中西医结合治疗 2 型糖尿病 30 例. 福建中医药 **40**(2): 26–27.
H170	张世龙, 马登娟, 姚鹏, 范丽丽. (2015) 养阴止渴丸联合二甲双胍片治疗 2 型糖尿病60例. 中医研究 **28**(5): 10–12.
H171	张维佳. (2008) 芪连消渴方对 2 型糖尿病胰岛素抵抗及相关炎症因子的影响. 湖南中医杂志 **27**(1): 4–6.
H172	张学红, 常风云, 张炳冉, *et al.* (2007) 消糖平胶囊治疗 2 型糖尿病胰岛素抵抗患者109例临床观察. 中医杂志 **48**(9): 812–813.
H173	张晓君, 王青平, 聂晶, 吴志平. (2012) 中西医结合治疗高龄 2 型糖尿病患者30例临床观察. 中医杂志 **53**(19): 1651–1654.
H174	张晓丽. (2014) 甘露饮加减治疗湿热阴伤型 2 型糖尿病临床疗效观察. 北京中医药大学硕士学位论文, 中国北京.
H175	张新霞. (2013) 参芪复方与胰岛素联用对 2 型糖尿病患者 β 细胞功能、氧化应激及血GLP–1水平影响的临床. 成都中医药大学博士学位论文, 中国成都.
H176	Zhang XX, Liu Y, Xiong DQ, Xie CG. (2015) Insulin combined with Chinese medicine improves glycaemic outcome through multiple pathways in patients with type 2 diabetes mellitus. *J Diabetes Investig* **6**(6): 708–715.
H177	张英来, 张军, 谢富明. (2004) 中西医结合治疗继发性磺脲类失效 2 型糖尿病98例. 上海中医药杂志 **38**(7): 18–19.
H178	赵郴, 马中建, 陈玉林, 陈永忠. (2008) 玉泉丸合二甲双胍治疗 2 型糖尿病48例总结. 湖南中医杂志 **24**(3): 31–33.
H179	赵福俊, 宋静. (2009) 中药益气养阴法对治疗 2 型糖尿病的临床研究. 菏泽医学专科学校学报 **21**(1): 39–41.
H180	赵嘉晶, 范朝华. (2010) 芪灵汤治疗 2 型糖尿病气阴亏虚型30例疗效观察. 河北中医 **32**(4): 497–499.
H181	赵能江. (2007) 平糖胶囊对阴虚热盛型 2 型糖尿病患者生存质量影响的临床观察. 福建中医学院硕士学位论文, 中国福州.
H182	郑晓峰. (2009) 消渴安糖方对 2 型糖尿病患者红细胞胰岛素受体的影响. 广西中医药 **32**(1): 8–10.
H183	郑焱, 於松达. (2015) 中西医结合治疗中青年 2 型糖尿病疗效观察及对血脂水平的影响. 中华中医药学刊 **33**(6): 1530–1532.

(Continued)

Study No.	Reference
H184	周波, 黄春, 李青, 刘洁. (2015) 西洋参联合二甲双胍对糖尿病患者A1C, FPG, CRP的影响. 中医药导报 **21**(4): 88–90.
H185	周德奇, 冯平, 万鹏. (2008) 降糖合剂治疗 2 型糖尿病 50 例临床观察. 浙江中医杂志 **43**(7): 431.
H186	周建, 陈丽萍, 王宏. (2013) 天麦消渴片联合阿卡波糖治疗 2 型糖尿病的临床研究. 中国药物与临床 **13**(3): 358–359.
H187	周建军, 董勇云. (2012) 益气养阴胶囊治疗气阴两虚型消渴病 (2型糖尿病)的临床研究. 中国保健营养 **8**(8): 252–253.
H188	周家棠, 林天海, 周志昭. (2009) 糖脉康颗粒治疗 2 型糖尿病 60 例临床观察. 中国实用医药 **4**(29): 107–108.
H189	周劲勇, 沈伟. (2009) 参芪宁消汤治疗 2 型糖尿病临床观察. 中医药临床杂志 **21**(3): 204–205.
H190	周遂民, 周太民. (2007) 益气养阴降糖方治疗 2 型糖尿病 50 例疗效观察. 河南中医 **27**(11): 40–41.
H191	周永恒, 钟燕斌, 邓丽华, *et al.* (2014) 二半汤对老年 2 型糖尿病患者血糖控制的研究. 新中医 **46**(10): 90–92.
H192	朱凌波, 李靖. (2013) 降糖精颗粒对老年2型糖尿病患者血栓前状态的影响. 甘肃中医学院学报 **30**(5): 31–34.
H193	朱岚铟, 吴志伟, 成志俊. (2015) 自拟中药方联合西医治疗糖尿病的临床疗效. 辽宁中医杂志 **42**(3): 561–563.
H194	朱莎. (2008) 加味桃核承气汤治疗老年糖尿病胰岛素抵抗（气阴两虚, 瘀血阻络）的临床研究. 广州中医药大学硕士学位论文, 中国广州.
H195	朱伟嵘, 杨永华, 郑岚, 沈小珩. (2005) 金菖胶囊治疗 2 型糖尿病血瘀证患者的临床观察. 中成药 **27**(10): 1169–1173.
H196	朱震. (2007) 丹黄活血方对 2 型糖尿病血瘀证的研究. 南京中医药大学硕士学位论文, 中国南京.
H197	朱章志, 赵英英, 罗礼达. (2009) 温脏扶正祛邪方药对 2 型糖尿病虚寒证患者胰岛素抵抗的影响. 新中医 **41**(5): 19–21.
H198	周静, 高晟, 吴深涛. (2015) 补肾抗衰片对肾虚痰瘀型 2 型糖尿病临床疗效及中医证候的影响. 天津药学 **27**(4): 37–39.
H199	邹志强, 劳程强. (2016) 大黄黄连泻心汤辅助西医综合疗法治疗 2 型糖尿病(火热证)的疗效观察. 中医药导报 **22**(15): 104–106.
H200	路波, 成冬生, 沈璐, *et al.* (2006) 免热苦竹胶囊治疗 2 型糖尿病的临床观察. 陕西中医 **27**(7): 826–827.

Study No.	Reference
H201	任毅, 王彦, 杨静, 王蔚, *et al.* (2016) 小檗碱对初诊 2 型糖尿病糖脂代谢和脂联素的影响. 中西医结合心脑血管病杂志 **14**(16): 1921–1922.
H202	余晓琳, 陈军平. (2010) 黄连温胆汤治疗湿热困脾型初发 2 型糖尿病 78 例临床观察. 新中医 **42**(4): 25–26.
H203	张洁, 王立琴, 于建华. (2003) 芪黄胶囊合盐酸小檗碱治疗 2 型糖尿病临床观察. 山东中医杂志 **22**(10): 598–599.
H204	张俪潆. (2016) 清热利湿法治疗2型糖尿病湿热证的临床疗效观察. 北京中医药大学硕士学位论文, 中国北京.
H205	Chao M, Zou D, Zhang Y, *et al.* (2009) Improving insulin resistance with traditional Chinese medicine in type 2 diabetic patients. Endocrine **36**(2): 268–274.
H206	房平, 王东顺, 马国强, 徐玉芬. (2008) 绞股兰总甙胶囊治疗糖尿病 38 例临床研究. 河北医药 **30**(3): 348.
H207	苏晓燕, 施红, 吴建珊, 林心君. (2015) 石斛合剂序贯方不同剂型治疗 2 型糖尿病临床疗效比较. 中华中医药杂志 **30**(6): 2233–2235.
H208	Tong XL, Wu ST, Lian FM, *et al.* (2013) The safety and effectiveness of TM81, a Chinese herbal medicine, in the treatment of type 2 diabetes: A randomized double-blind placebo-controlled trial. Diabetes Obes Metab **15**(5): 448–454.
H209	Zhang Y, Li X, Zou D, *et al.* (2008) Treatment of type 2 diabetes and dyslipidemia with the natural plant alkaloid berberine. J Clin Endocrinol Metab **93**(7): 2559–2263.
H210	周霭. (2012) 葛根芩连汤治疗 2 型糖尿病湿热困脾证临床研究. 北京中医药大学硕士学位论文, 中国北京.
H211	李艳梅, 金徐亮. (2004) 益气滋阴丸治疗 2 型糖尿病临床观察. 山东中医杂志 **23**(9): 526–527.
H212	曾伶, 曾劲, 李颖, 刘汴生. (2005) 益糖胶囊治疗老年 2 型糖尿病的疗效观察. 中国老年学杂志 **25**(8): 987.
H213	Zhang XF. (2018) Clinical efficacy of invigorating *qi*, nourishing *yin*, and promoting blood circulation in treatment of type 2 diabetes mellitus. *Biomedical Research (India)* **29**(1): 199–202.
H214	邹冬吟. (2013) '动—定序贯八法'对早期 2 型糖尿病胰岛β细胞功能及脂联素的影响. 广州中医药大学博士学位论文, 中国广州.

(Continued)

Study No.	Reference
H215	马瑛, 温少珍. (2002) 翻白草治疗 II 型糖尿病50例疗效观察. 中草药 **33**(7): 644.
H216	冯海霞. (2012) 白虎加人参汤治疗气阴两虚型糖尿病的临床研究. 山东中医药大学硕士学位论文, 中国济南.
H217	李丽, 段爽莉. (2017) 治消滋坎饮加减联合甘精胰岛素治疗 2 型糖尿病临床分析. 四川中医 **35**(12): 128–130.
H218	路志敏, 曹清慧, 杨艳玲, 贾卫华. (2002) 消糖灵胶囊合二甲双胍治疗 2 型糖尿病150例疗效观察. 河北中医 **24**(8): 563–565.
H219	王荣欣, 马建华, 戚宏. (2003) 中西医结合治疗 2 型糖尿病 60 例. 山西中医 **19**(6): 26–27.
H220	朱云丽, 张娟, 王宝玉. (2015) 益气养阴法治疗 2 型糖尿病的临床研究. 中医临床研究**7**(3): 41–43.
H221	段颖. (2007) 糖尿病证候及柴胡疏肝散加减干预的临床研究. 北京中医药大学硕士学位论文.
H222	何威, 杨洁, 周国英. (2003) 加味增液汤对 2 型糖尿病胰岛素抵抗的影响. 中医药学刊**21**(2): 234–235.
H223	廖明波, 常桂荣, 王宏. (2006) 加用人参降糖灵治疗 2 型糖尿病 70 例. 广西中医药 **29**(5): 34.
H224	潘立文. (2009) 加味六味地黄汤治疗 2 型糖尿病的临床研究. 湖北中医学院硕士学位论文, 中国武汉.
H225	庞国明, 闫镛, 朱璞, *et al.* (2017) 纯中药治疗 2 型糖尿病(消渴病)的临床研究. 世界中西医结合杂志 **12**(1): 74–77.
H226	彭少林. (2009) 白虎加人参汤治疗初发 2 型糖尿病疗效研究. 广州中医药大学硕士学位论文, 中国广州.
H227	施红, 张学敏, 崔乙, *et al.* (2013) 糖尿病石斛合剂序贯法的初步临床观察. 中医临床研究 **5**(18): 1–3.
H228	孙霞. (2013) 克糖灵颗粒治疗2型糖尿病气阴两虚型的临床研究. 南京中医药大学硕士学位论文, 中国南京.
H229	谭漪, 谢春光. (2002) 白虎加人参汤治疗 2 型糖尿病的临床观察. 成都中医药大学学报 **25**(4): 23–24.
H230	王旭, 陈军, 周云庆, *et al.* (2015) 消渴丸治疗 2 型糖尿病患者 105 例临床疗效及安全性观察. 世界中西医结合杂志 **10**(2): 223–225.

(*Continued*)

Study No.	Reference
H231	薛莉,瞿伟,李靖,刘钧. (2005) 降糖精治疗磺脲类继发性失效 2 型糖尿病效果观察. 中国交通医学杂志 **19**(6): 611.
H232	殷国田, 崔瑞花. (2003) 益津降糖胶囊治疗 2 型糖尿病 42 例. 新乡医学院学报 **20**(5): 372–374.
H233	张振忠, 赵明君, 张喜奎, 崔春红. (2002) 消渴平胶囊治疗 2 型糖尿病的临床研究报告. 现代中医药 (6): 1–3.
H234	赵文贤, 蔡青, 潘义新, *et al.* (2000) 糖威胶囊治疗糖尿病的临床观察. 新疆中医药 **18**(4): 27–28.
H235	周素英. (2006) 疏肝调气法治疗 2 型糖尿病的临床观察. 北京中医药大学硕士学位论文, 中国北京.
H236	饶线明, 陈炳焜. (2004) 参芪降糖颗粒治疗 2 型糖尿病 32 例临床观察. 吉林中医药 **24**(1): 23–24.

6

Pharmacological Actions of Frequently Used Herbs

OVERVIEW

The available experimental evidence of herbs from the top 10 most frequently reported herbs used in randomised controlled trials of diabetes mellitus were reviewed. Many herbal extracts showed antihyperglycaemic activities in animal models of diabetes mellitus. Underlying mechanisms such as hypoglycaemic, anti-oxidant, adenosine monophosphate activated protein kinase pathway activation, peroxisome proliferator-activated receptor signalling pathways, and increased GLUT-4 expression are reported, elucidating possible mechanisms for the anti-diabetic activities of herbal extracts.

Introduction

This chapter includes the pre-clinical evidence available for the frequently used herbs identified in randomised controlled trials (RCTs) for Type 2 diabetes mellitus (T2DM). There are many experimental studies of Chinese herbal medicine (CHM) in cell and animal models of diabetes mellitus. Here we reviewed experimental data for the 10 most frequently reported herbs — *huang qi* 黄芪, *di huang* 地黄, *ge gen* 葛根, *huang lian* 黄连, *dan shen* 丹参, *mai men dong* 麦门冬, *shan yao* 山药, *fu ling* 茯苓, *tian hua fen* 天花粉 and *zhi mu* 知母 — used in randomised controlled trials, as summarised in Chapter 5.

Due to the high prevalence of T2DM worldwide, extensive research has been performed to develop new anti-diabetic agents; as a result, several diabetic animal models have been developed to mimic the human disease. Most of the models combine the two main features of T2DM — obesity-associated insulin resistance and beta-cell dysfunction with or without diminished beta-cell mass.[1] These models assist in the testing of potential anti-diabetic agents and their mechanism of action.

Among the most widely studied models for T2DM are the Lep[ob] (obese) and Lep[db] (diabetes) mice. These obese models have mutations either in the leptin gene or leptin receptor gene, respectively.[2,3] Rodent models are also used and can be classified into two broad categories: (1) genetically induced spontaneous diabetes models, and (2) experimentally induced non-spontaneous diabetes models.[4] Commonly used models include the Zucker diabetic fatty rat and Goto-Kakizaki rat.[1]

To study the effects of herbal extracts of compounds on a cellular level, peripheral tissues from diabetic animal models and related cell lines are also used. Enzymes critical to cellular energy homeostasis or glucose utilisation are studied closely to elucidate the mechanism of action of these herbal extracts and compounds.

Methods

This chapter provides a general overview of the experimental evidence relating to the pharmacology of herbs and their constituent compounds for diabetes mellitus. The constituent compounds were identified by searching herbal monographs, high-quality reviews of CHM, the herbal medicine encyclopedia,[7] Materia Medica,[8] and PubMed. To identify pre-clinical publications, a literature search of PubMed and China National Knowledge Infrastructure was undertaken. The search strategy included the terms for each herb and its constituent compounds. Relevant data was extracted, and a summary of the findings is reported here.

Experimental Studies on *huang qi* 黃芪

Huang qi 黃芪 (Astragali Radix) is the dried root of *Astragalus membranaceus* (Fisch.) Bge. or *Astragalus membranaceus* (Fisch.) Bge. var. *mongholicus* (Bge.) Hsiao.[5] *Huang qi* is a well-researched herb. To date, more than 200 compounds of *huang qi* have been identified, including flavonoids, saponins, polysaccharides and amino acids, and various biological activities of the compounds have been reported.[6] Among the identified compounds, isoflavonoids, saponins and polysaccharides are the three main types responsible for the pharmacological activities and therapeutic efficacy of *huang qi*.[7] Pharmacological activities of *huang qi* include anti-oxidant, immunomodulatory, angiogenic, erythropoietic, anti-obesity, anti-cancer activities and pain relief.[8] Pharmacological effects in relation to T2DM are reviewed below.

Huang qi compounds have shown anti-diabetic activities in various diabetic animal models. When *Huang qi* flavonoids (calycosin-7-β-D-gluocoside, ononin, calycosin and formononetin) administered to db/db diabetic mice (200 mg/kg/day) were taken daily for 12 weeks, they markedly decreased the levels of both fed and fasting glucose, reduced serum triglyceride, and also alleviated insulin resistance and glucose intolerance when compared to vehicle-treated controls.[9] In C57BKS db/db diabetic mice, the administration of *huang qi* saponins astragaloside II and isoastragaloside I (50 mg/kg/day) for six weeks significantly alleviated hyperglycaemia, glucose intolerance and insulin resistance.[10] *Huang qi* polysaccharides administration (700 mg/kg/day) for eight weeks can improve the hyperglycaemia status, insulin sensitivity, glucose update and the activation level of AMP-activated protein kinase (AMPK) in diabetic rats (high-fat diet/HFD, streptozotocin/STZ induced).[11] *Huang qi* polysaccharide admission (400 mg/kg/day) for five weeks significantly decreased body weight and plasma glucose and improved insulin sensitivity in a high-fat diet, STZ-induced rats.[12] Furthermore, *huang qi* saponin astragaloside IV could increase wound healing in STZ-induced diabetic mice by promoting collagen deposition and extracellular matrix synthesis and improving new blood vessel formation.[13]

The anti-diabetic activities of *huang qi* involve various pathways and regulators related to T2DM. The AMPK signalling pathway activation has shown to be involved in several *in vitro* studies. In the skeletal muscle of T2DM rats, *huang qi* polysaccharide alleviated glucose toxicity by the activation of AMPK.[11] In mouse 3T3-L1 adipocytes, *huang qi* polysaccharides activated the AMPK signalling pathway to promote glucose transporter 4 expression and glucose metabolism and enhanced insulin sensitivity by activating the insulin signalling pathway to promote GLUT4 from intracellular vesicles to cell membranes.[14,15]

The unfolded protein response (UPR) response pathway has also been shown to be involved. In diabetic rats, reduced insulin resistance, possibly through upregulating or maintaining the miR-203a-3p expression levels, decreasing its target GRP78 mRNA and protein expression levels, and regulating the protein expression of the UPR response pathway.[16]

Protein tyrosine phosphatase 1B (PTP1B) is a negative regulator of insulin-receptor signal transduction. In diabetic rat muscle where PTP1B levels were elevated and insulin signalling was diminished, *huang qi* polysaccharides showed insulin-sensitising and hypoglycaemic activity by reducing the elevated expression and activity of PTP1B.[12]

Experimental Studies on *sheng di huang* 生地黄

Sheng di huang 生地黄 (Rehmanniae Radix) is the dried root of *Rehmannia glutinosa* Libosch.[17] Identified chemical constituent groups of *sheng di huang* include iridoids and iridoid glycosides, other glycosides, sugars, organic acids, and amino acids.[17] *Sheng di huang* and its compounds have shown various pharmacological effects, including anti-tumour activity, liver protection and immunomodulation.[18] Pharmacological effects in relation to T2DM are reviewed below.

Iridoid compounds are the major compounds in quantity, including catalpol and dihydrocatalpol. Catalpol is an important and well-studied *sheng di huang* compound. In STZ-induced diabetic C57BL/6J mice on a high-fat diet with induced insulin resistance, catalpol administration (100 or 200 mg/kg/day) for four weeks decreased their blood glucose levels, increased their levels of serum insulin, and alleviated insulin resistance.[19] In these diabetic mice, catalpol prevented gluconeogenesis and enhanced hepatic glycogen synthesis and content.[19] Another study showed that catalpol (100 mg/kg/day for three days) could decrease a key hepatic gluconeogenesis indicator phosphoenolpyruvate carboxykinase (PEPCK) gene expression in STZ-induced rats.[20] Furthermore, in the liver, skeletal muscle, and adipose tissues of db/db mice, phosphorylation of AMPK was increased by catalpol treatment.[19,21] In diabetic mice and rats, catalpol (100 mg/kg/day) has been shown to increase protein expression of glucose transporter-4 (GLUT4) in skeletal muscle and adipose tissues.[20] In addition, catalpol has been shown to lower blood glucose and improve insulin sensitivity via activation of the phosphatidylinositol-3-Kinase (PI3K)/protein kinase B (AKT) pathway.[22]

Other *sheng di huang* compounds have shown anti-diabetic effects. Water extract stachyose (200 mg/kg/day for 15 days) reduced blood glucose levels in alloxan-induced diabetic rats.[23] *Sheng di huang* oligosaccharide (100 mg/kg/day for 15 days) showed a significant decrease in blood glucose levels and hepatic glucose-6-phosphatase activity, with an increase in hepatic glycogen content in glucose-induced hyperglycaemic and alloxan-induced diabetic rats.[24] Furthermore, *sheng di huang* oligosaccharide raised plasma insulin levels and lowered plasma corticosterone levels in diabetic rats.[24]

Experimental Studies on *ge gen* 葛根

Ge gen 葛根 (Radix Puerariae) is the dried root of *Pueraria lobata* (Willd.) Ohwi.[25] Over 70 chemical constituents of Radix Puerariae have been identified, including isoflavones, isoflavone glycosides, coumarins, puerarols, but-2-enolides and their derivatives, triterpenes and triterpenoid glycosides.[26] *Ge gen* and its compounds have shown various pharmacological activities, including cardioprotective, neuroprotective, hypocholesterolemic and anti-oxidative activities.[26] *In vitro* and *in vivo* studies have shown anti-diabetic effects of *ge gen*. These are summarised here.

Puerarin is an isoflavone from *ge gen*. In diabetic animal models, low-dose (15 mg/kg/day) and high-dose (75 mg/kg/day) puerarin can improve glucose tolerance and reduce blood glucose levels.[27–29] The hypoglycaemic effect of puerarin can be attributed to different target molecules. One study showed that it upregulated peroxisome proliferated-activated receptor gamma (*PPARγ*) and its downstream target genes, glucose transporter type 4 (*GLUT4*) and adiponectin expression, leading to increased glucose utilisation.[30] In high glucose-induced insulin-resistant rat preadipocyets, puerarin (100–150 g) promoted glucose uptake in a dose-dependent manner, possibly through the promotion of *PPARγ* expression and partly through inhibiting abnormal TNF-a-induced intracellular-free $Ca(2+)$ accumulation of endothelial cells.[31] Puerarin has been shown to increase glucose utilisation by upregulating mRNA and protein expression of the GLUT4 in diabetic rat soleus muscle cells.[28]

Supplementation of 0.2% *ge gen* root extract in normal diets for two months reduced arterial pressure, body weight, fasting plasma glucose, plasma total cholesterol, and insulin levels in stroke-prone spontaneously hypertensive rats.[32]

In db/db mice, *ge gen* compound daidzein (0.1% in the diet) reduced fasting plasma glucose, serum total cholesterol levels and the homeostasis model assessment index.[33] Reduced blood glucose and urinary glucose excretion were also observed in T2DM KKAy mice.[33] In the gastrocnemius muscle of db/db mice, daidzein supplementation markedly improved the AMPK phosphorylation, demonstrating a possible mechanism for its hypoglycaemic effects.[33]

Experimental Studies on *huang lian* 黄莲

Huang lian 黄莲 (coptidis rhizome) is the dried rhizome of *Coptis chinensis* Franch., *C. deltoidea* C. Y. Cheng et Hsiao or *C. teeta* Wall.

(Ranunculaceae).[17] It has had over 100 chemical constituents isolated and identified, including alkaloids, organic acids, coumarins, phenylpropanoids and quinones.[34] Alkaloids are the most abundant chemical component and are considered to be the main active ingredients. Berberine is considered the most representative alkaloid from *huang lian*.[34] Pharmacological effects in relation to T2DM are reviewed below.

It is reported that berberine treatment increased AMPK activity in 3T3-L1 adipocyte cells, and in turn enhanced the glucose transporter type 1 (GLUT1) expression and also stimulated the GLUT1-mediated glucose uptake by activating GLUT1.[35] A later study confirmed that berberine treatment increased the glucose uptake in L929 fibroblast cells (a cell line that expresses only GLUT1) via the activation of transport activity of GLUT1.[36]

In diabetic animal models, berberine has shown anti-diabetic activities and protective effects on pancreatic cells and tissues. Administration of berberine (100 and 200 mg/kg/day for three weeks) significantly decreased fasting plasma glucose levels, the serum content of total cholesterol (TC), triglycerides (TG) and low-density lipoprotein cholesterol (LDL-c), and effectively increased the high-density lipoprotein cholesterol (HDL-c) and nitric oxide levels in diabetic rats.[37] A histopathological study showed that berberine had restored the damage of pancreas tissues in diabetic rats, showed moderate expansion of islets, and significantly reduced the scores of the injuries of the pancreas comparable to metformin treatment.[37] Berberine (300 mg/kg/day for 12 weeks) reduced fasting plasma glucose in alloxan-induced diabetic mice, increased liver glycogen, enhanced the activity of protein kinase B and glucokinase, inhibited phosphorylation of GSL-3β, and increased glycogen synthesis in a diabetic liver.[38] Berberine also improves pancreatic β cells and promotes insulin secretion through activation of the ALT signalling pathway.[38] In normal rats, berberine enhanced glucagon-like peptide-1 secretion induced by a glucose load and promoted proglucagon mRNA expression as well as L cell proliferation in the intestine.[39] *In vitro*, berberine concentration dependently stimulated glucagon-like peptide-1 release in NCI-H716 cells.[39]

Huang lian polysaccharides too have shown anti-diabetic functions and a protective function of the pancreas and the liver. In diabetic mice, administration of *huang lian* polysaccharides (400 mg/kg/day) improved body weight and serum insulin, and decreased fasting plasma glucose and glycated serum protein concentrations. They also decreased the AGE accumulations.[40] Another study also observed reduced fasting plasma glucose in HFD with STZ T2DM rats after *huang lian* polysaccharides administration at various doses for four weeks. TG and TC levels were also reduced.[41] Compared to control diabetic mice, chronic administration of *huang lian* polysaccharides for 20 weeks in HFD-induced diabetic C57BL/6J mice showed lowered fasting plasma glucose levels and improved glucose tolerance.[42] Histological evaluation of the pancreas showed that *huang lian* polysaccharides can decrease morphological abnormalities in the pancreas and liver, recover the size of the pancreatic islets of Langerhans, and increase the secretion of insulin and glucagon in diabetic mice.[40,42]

In 3T3-L1 adipocytes from the muscles and livers of diabetic mice, *huang lian* polysaccharides increased AMPK phosphorylation and stimulated phosphoinositol-3-kinase and AMPK pathway-mediated glucose uptake in 3T3-L1 adipocytes.[42] In pancreases from diabetic mice, *huang lian* polysaccharides increased serum superoxide dismutase and catalase activities and decreased malondialdehyde content, showing antioxidant effects.[43]

Experimental Studies on *dan shen* 丹参

Active ingredients of *dan shen* 丹参 (*Salvia miltiorrhiza* Bunge) can be divided into two categories: fat-soluble diterpenoid compounds/tanshinone compounds and water-soluble phenolic acids/salvianolic acids.[44] *Dan shen* is a well-studied herb with more than 100 compounds identified, including salvianolic acid A/B/C/D/E/F/G, tanshinone I/IIA/IIB/V/VI, dihydrotanshione I, tanshindiol A, miltirone, dehydro miltirone, isotanshinone, and more.[45] The hypoglycaemic effects of *dan shen* in diabetic animal models are reviewed here.

Dan shen injection (100 mg/kg) for four weeks decreased blood glucose levels in STZ-stimulated Sprague-Dawley rats.[46]

Salvianolic acid A administration in T2DM animal models has shown hypoglycaemic effects in various studies. Blood glucose, total cholesterol, triglyceride and LDL were decreased significantly, compared with diabetic control rats (high-fat and high-sucrose fed diet STZ-induced).[47] A significant reduction in body weight and 24-hour food and water intake was observed, compared to diabetic treatment without salvianolic acid A treatment.[48,49] Reduced glycosylated haemoglobin reflecting a reduced average blood glucose level over the preceding two to three months indicated potential long-term hypoglycaemic effects.[48] In both HepG2 cells (human hepatoma cell line) and L6 (rat myoblast cell line) myotubes, salvianolic acid A increased glucose consumption and uptake in a dose-dependent manner.[48] Further analysis showed that salvianolic acid regulates glucose metabolism by increasing ATP production, decreasing mitochondrial membrane potential, and improving mitochondrial function via a Ca^{2+}/calmodulin-dependent protein kinase β/AMPK signalling pathway.[48]

Another water-soluble extract salvianolic acid B also shows hypoglycaemic effects. In HFD and STZ-induced diabetic rats, salvianolic B administration (100 and 200 mg/kg) significantly decreased blood glucose and increased the insulin sensitivity index, decreased the total cholesterol, LDL, non-esterified fatty acids, hepatic glycogen and muscle glycogen, and increased HDL.[50] A higher dose of salvianolic acid B (200 mg/kg) significantly decreased triglyceride and malondialdehyde and increased superoxide dismutase.[50] The results indicate that salvianolic acid B can inhibit symptoms of diabetes mellitus in rats.

Experimental Studies on *mai men dong* 麦门冬

Mai men dong 麦门冬 (*Radix Ophiopogonis*) is prepared from the enlarged part of the root of *Ophiopogon japonicus* Ker-Gawler (Liliaceae).[51] An Ophiopogon root contains various biologically active compounds, including steroidal saponins, homoisoflavonoids and polysaccharides, and has shown anti-oxidative, anti-cancer, anti-diabetic, immunomodulatory, anti-acute inflammatory, antitussive and antimicrobial activities.[52] Hypoglycaemic effects of *mai men dong* are reviewed below.

In pancreatic islet cell line NIT-1 cells damaged by STZ, *Radix Ophiopogonis* polysaccharides extract showed protective functions by improving the activities of NIT-1 cells, inhibited glucose absorption into intestinal brush border membrane vesicles, and reduced the activities of α-glucosidase through protection and the inhibition of carbohydrate digestion and absorption.[53]

Water-soluble β-D-fructan (MDG-1) from *mai men dong* has shown hypoglycaemic functions. In ob/ob mice, four weeks of administration of MDG-1 (300 mg/kg/day) showed improved oral glucose tolerance and reduced serum insulin levels and triglyceride content in the liver. Furthermore, a reduction in body weight gain and subcutaneous fat was observed compared to the control mice.[54] Observations in diabetic KKAy mice showed that MDG-1 (300 mg/kg/day for eight weeks) actions against diabetes might be accomplished through the absorbable monosugars and butanedioic acid via suppression of intestinal glucose absorption, enhancing liver glycogenesis, inhibiting glycogenolysis and promoting glucagon-like peptide-1 secretion.[55] In diabetic KKAy mice, MDG-1 (300 mg/kg/day for eight weeks) reduced hyperglycaemia, hyperinsulinemia and hyperlipidemia.[56] MDG-1 could ameliorate insulin resistance in the oral glucose tolerance test. MDG-1 could reduce the serum content of triglycerides and LDL-c, as well as increasing HDL-c content.[56] These observed effects were through the PI3K/Akt pathway, where MDG-1 upregulated the phosphoinositide 3-kinase p85 subunit, Akt, insulin receptor, insulin receptor substrate-1, and GLUT4 expression, but downregulated the glycogen synthase kinase 3β expression.[56]

OJP1 is a water-soluble polysaccharide extract from the roots of *mai men dong*.[57] OJP1 (300 mg/kg/day for four weeks) showed anti-diabetic effects on STZ-induced diabetic rats, causing a significant reduction in the blood glucose level when compared with the diabetic control group. Furthermore, OJP1 remediated the destruction of pancreatic islets and pancreatic β-cell damage in these diabetic rats.[57] OJP1 treatment can significantly decrease the levels of triglycerides, total cholesterol, LDL, and increase HDL levels in diabetic rats.[58] Furthermore, OJP1 significantly increased superoxide dismutase and glutathione peroxidase activity in STZ-induced diabetic rats. Biochemical and histopathological analyses also showed that OJP1 could alleviate liver and kidneys injury in diabetic rats, showing protective functions of the liver and kidneys from the diabetes injury. Circular fat droplets in the cytoplasm were significantly decreased, as too was the degeneration of the hepatocytes, and the liver cell structure was similar to normal liver architecture.[58] Renal expression of mRNA for transforming growth factor-β1 and connective tissue growth factor were both significantly increased in the diabetic group. The OJP1 treatment decreased their expression in a dose-dependent manner.[58]

Experimental Studies on *shan yao* 山药

Shan yao 山药 (Dioscoreae rhizome) is the root of *Dioscorea opposita* Thunb.[17] The major components of *shan yao* are saponins, phenolic compounds, sterols, and mucilage.[17] *Shan yao* has shown immunomodulatory and anti-inflammatory effects.[59,60] Pharmacological effects in relation to T2DM are reviewed below.

In HFD, STZ-induced TDM rats, the administration of *shan yao* polysaccharides significantly reduced fasting plasma glucose levels, increased serum insulin levels, and decreased glucagon levels, showing hypoglycaemic effects.[61,62] The hypoglycaemic effects of *shan yao* polysaccharides are comparable to metformin.[61,62]

A *Shan yao* decoction concentrate at 300 mg and 600 mg/kg for 10 consecutive days can reduce blood glucose in vehicle-controlled mice and alloxan-induced diabetic mice, significantly reducing the blood glucose level.[63] The authors also tested the preventative effect of a *shan yao* decoction on blood glucose elevation caused by adrenaline, alloxan and glucose feeding. Results showed that prior administration of a *shan yao* decoction before introducing the cause of elevated blood glucose can significantly reduce blood glucose levels compared to the control group.[63] In addition to hypoglycaemic effects, *shan yao* also has lipid lowering effects, reducing TG and TC levels in diabetic mice.[64]

Experimental Studies on *fu ling* 茯苓

Fu ling 茯苓 (Poria) is a medicinal fungus from *Poria cocos* (Schw.) Wolf.[17] It has principal constituents of triterpenes and polysaccharides, with small amounts of steroids, amino acids, choline, histidine, and potassium salts.[65] *Fu ling* compounds and their derivatives have shown various pharmacological effects, including anti-inflammatory, anti-oxidative and anti-apoptotic effects.[65,66] Pharmacological effects in relation to T2DM are reviewed below.

In C57BL/KsJ-db/db mice, a crude extract of *fu ling* at a single dose of 50 or 100 mg/kg body weight significantly reduced the blood glucose levels.[67] In STZ-treated mice whose pancreatic islet cells were destroyed, the crude extract of *fu ling* and its triterpenes, dehydrotumulosic acid and dehydrotrametenolic acid, enhanced insulin sensitivity by increasing the insulin-mediated blood glucose reduction in the same way as insulin sensitiser metformin.[67]

In db/db mice, several *fu ling* triterpenes, including pachymic acid and dihydrotrametenolic acid, induced adipose conversion, activated PPARγ, and acted as an insulin sensitiser.[68] Administration of dehydrotrametenolic acid (110 mg/kg/day for 14 days) prevented the time-dependent increase in plasma glucose concentrations and lowered plasma insulin levels in diabetic mice.[68]

In murine 3T3-L1 adipocytes, six lanostane-type *fu ling* triterpenoids 1, 2, 13, 14, 15 and 16 increased glucose uptake, GLUT4 gene expression at both mRNA and protein levels, and GLUT4 translocation but displayed no activity on GLUT1 expression.[69]

Experimental Studies on *tian hua fen* 天花粉

Tian hua fen 天花粉 (Trichosanthis Radix) is the root from *Trichosanthes Kirilowii* Maxim.[17] The major known chemical constituents include proteins, polysaccharides and amino acids,[17] while its main active ingredients include Trichosanthin/TCS, Trichosanthes kirilowii lectin (TKL) and polysaccharides.[70] Pharmacological effects in relation to T2DM are reviewed below.

Trichosans A, B, C, D and E are glycans derived from *tian hua fen*. They showed hypoglycaemic actions in normal mice.[71] Furthermore, the main glycan, trichosan A, also exhibited activity in alloxan-induced hyperglycaemic mice.[71] In HFD, STZ-induced diabetic rats, *tian hua fen* lectin (300 mg/kg/day for three weeks) significantly decreased fasting plasma glucose, glycated serum protein, and malondialdehyde, and increased superoxide dismutase and glutathione levels.[72] Compared to the diabetic control group, the TKL groups showed improved diabetic symptoms. These indicate that TKL could effectively decrease blood glucose and improve the antioxidant defence of diabetic rats.[72] *Trichosanthes Kirilowii* acqueous extract (100 mg/kg) showed hypoglycaemic abilities by reducing the blood glucose level in high-fat fed, STZ-induced diabetic mice.[73]

Experimental Studies on *zhi mu* 知母

Zhi mu 知母 (Anemarrhenae Rhizoma) is the rhizome of *Anemarrhena asphodeloides* BGE.[17] The compounds isolated from *zhi mu* mainly include steroidal saponins, flavonoids, norlignans, alkaloids, organic acids, and polysaccharides.[17,74] *Zhi mu* compounds have been studied and exhibit biological functions such as anti-inflammatory, anti-oxidation, anti-microbial, anti-viral, and immunomodulatory effects.[74] Pharmacological effects in relation to diabetes are reviewed below.

Ethanol extracts of *zhi mu* stimulated insulin secretion in the islets of normal Wistar rats and diabetic Goto-Kakizaki rats incubated both at 3.3 and 16.7 μM glucose. The mechanism involves an effect on the exocytotic machinery of the beta cell, mediated via pertussis toxin-sensitive Gi-(or Ge-) proteins.[75]

Mangiferin is a flavonoid from *zhi mu*. Mangiferin (30 or 90 mg/kg) and its glucosides (mangiferin-7-O-beta-glucoside) (30 or 90 mg/kg) showed anti-diabetic activity in KKAy mice — it lowered the blood glucose level by increasing insulin sensitivity.[76] Repeated administration of mangiferin (30 mg/kg) in KKAy diabetic mice also showed hypoglycaemic functions, most likely through decreasing insulin resistance.[77] Mangiferin and mangiferin-7-O-β-glucoside could significantly reduce blood glucose levels, and the anti-diabetic mechanism might be caused by the decrease of insulin resistance and the increase of insulin sensitivity.[78]

Another *zhi mu* compound, pseudoprototimosaponin AIII (50 mg/kg), showed hypoglycaemic bioactivity in a dose-dependently manner in STZ-diabetic mice, and the mechanism might be related to the inhibition of hepatic gluconeogenesis and/or glycogenolysis. It had no effects on glucose uptake and insulin release.[79]

Anemarans A, B, C and D at various doses from *zhi mu* displayed significant hypoglycaemic bioactivities in normal and alloxan-induced hyperglycaemic mice.[80]

Summary of Pharmacological Actions

The top 10 herbs used in CHM RCTs have shown marked anti-diabetic and hypoglycaemic activities in diabetic cell lines and animal models. A reduced blood glucose level in diabetic animal models was observed in all the listed herbs. The hypoglycaemic activities may be due to reduced insulin resistance, increased insulin sensitivity, or the inhibition of hepatic gluconeogenesis and/or glycogenolysis.

Several signalling pathways related to glucose homeostasis are involved, and different herbs have been reported to exhibit their anti-diabetic functions via different pathways. These include activation of the Akt pathway (*sheng di, huang lian, mai men dong*), activation of the AMPK pathway (*dan shen, huang qi, huang lian, mai men dong, tian hua fen*), and the UPR signalling pathway (*huang qi*). Important glucose transporters, including GLUT1 (*huang lian*) and GLUT4 (*dan shen, huang qi, huang lian, mai men dong, tian hua fen, sheng di, ge gen*), are also targeted by herbal compounds and their derivatives to correct hyperglycaemia. These mechanisms may be the underlying reason for their anti-diabetic activities.

Further to hypoglycaemic effects, protective functions of pancreatic cells have been observed in pancreatic cell lines damaged by STZ (*huang lian, mai men dong*). This suggests that CHM and compounds not only can reduce blood glucose levels after the onset of T2DM but can also have preventative functions before the disease onset. Furthermore, some herbs and their compounds have shown lipid-lowering effects in diabetic animals (*huang lian, ge gen, dan shen, mai men dong*).

Current experimental evidence suggests that an array of herbal compounds exhibit their anti-diabetic activities via multiple signalling pathways and targets. Further investigation of key compounds or compound combinations in diabetic animal models is required to further elucidate the possible mechanism of action of CHM for diabetes.

References

1. Melmed S, Polonsky KS, Larsen PR, Kronenberg HM. (2011) *Williams Textbook of Endocrinology*, 12th edition. Elsevier Sauders, Philadelphia USA, p. 1897.
2. Chung WK, Power-Kehoe L, Chua M, *et al.* (1996) Genomic structure of the human OB receptor and identification of two novel intronic microsatellites. *Genome Res* **6**(12): 1192–1199.
3. Zhang Y, Proenca R, Maffei M, *et al.* (1994) Positional cloning of the mouse obese gene and its human homologue. *Nature* **372**(6505): 425–432.
4. Islam MS, Loots du T. (2009) Experimental rodent models of Type 2 diabetes: A review. *Methods Find Exp Clin Pharmacol* **31**(4): 249–261.
5. Fu J, Wang Z, Huang L, *et al.* (2014) Review of the botanical characteristics, phytochemistry, and pharmacology of Astragalus membranaceus (Huangqi). *Phytother Res* **28**(9): 1275–1283.
6. Liu P, Zhao H, Luo Y. (2017) Anti-aging implications of astragalus membranaceus (Huangqi): A well-known chinese tonic. *Aging and Disease* **8**(6): 868–886.
7. Guo Z, Lou Y, Kong M, *et al.* (2019) A systematic review of phytochemistry, pharmacology and pharmacokinetics on Astragali Radix: Implications for Astragali Radix as a personalized medicine. *Int J Mol* **20**(6): 1463.

8. Gong AGW, Duan R, Wang HY, *et al.* (2018) Evaluation of the pharmaceutical properties and value of Astragali Radix. *Medicines (Basel, Switzerland)* **5**(2): 46.

9. Hoo RL, Wong JY, Qiao C, *et al.* (2010) The effective fraction isolated from Radix Astragali alleviates glucose intolerance, insulin resistance and hypertriglyceridemia in db/db diabetic mice through its anti-inflammatory activity. *Nutr Metab (Lond)* **7**: 67.

10. Xu A, Wang H, Hoo RLC, *et al.* (2009) Selective elevation of adiponectin production by the natural compounds derived from a medicinal herb alleviates insulin resistance and glucose intolerance in obese mice. *Endocrinology* **150**(2): 625–633.

11. Zou F, Mao X-q, Wang N, *et al.* (2009) Astragalus polysaccharides alleviates glucose toxicity and restores glucose homeostasis in diabetic states via activation of AMPK. *Acta Pharmacologica Sinica* **30**: 1607.

12. Wu Y, Ou-Yang J, Wu K, *et al.* (2005) Hypoglycemic effect of Astragalus polysaccharide and its effect on PTP1B. *Acta Pharmacologica Sinica* **26**(3): 345–352.

13. Luo X, Huang P, Yuan B, *et al.* (2016) Astragaloside IV enhances diabetic wound healing involving upregulation of alternatively activated macrophages. *Int Immunopharmacol* **35**: 22–28.

14. Zheng Y, Ley SH, Hu FB. (2018) Global aetiology and epidemiology of Type 2 diabetes mellitus and its complications. *Nat Rev Endocrinol* **14**(2): 88–98.

15. Ke B, Ke X, Wan X, *et al.* (2017) Astragalus polysaccharides attenuates TNF-alpha-induced insulin resistance via suppression of miR-721 and activation of PPAR-gamma and PI3K/AKT in 3T3-L1 adipocytes. *Am J Transl Res* **9**(5): 2195–2206.

16. Wei Z, Weng S, Wang L, Mao Z. (2018) Mechanism of Astragalus polysaccharides in attenuating insulin resistance in Rats with Type 2 diabetes mellitus via the regulation of liver microRNA203a3p. *Mol Med Rep* **17**(1): 1617–1624.

17. Bensky D, Clavey S, Stoger E. (2004) *Chinese Herbal Medicine Materia Medica*, 3rd edition. Eastland Press, Inc, Seattle, US.

18. Zhang RX, Li MX, Jia ZP. (2008) Rehmannia glutinosa: Review of botany, chemistry and pharmacology. *J Ethnopharmacol* **117**(2): 199–214.

19. Yan J, Wang C, Jin Y, *et al.* (2018) Catalpol ameliorates hepatic insulin resistance in Type 2 diabetes through acting on AMPK/NOX4/PI3K/AKT pathway. *Pharmacol Res* **130**: 466–480. doi:10.1016/j.phrs.2017.12.026

20. Shieh J-P, Cheng K-C, Chung H-H, *et al.* (2011) Plasma glucose lowering mechanisms of catalpol, an active principle from roots of Rehmannia glutinosa, in streptozotocin-induced diabetic rats. *J Agric Food Chem* **59**(8): 3747–3753.

21. Bao Q, Shen X, Qian L, *et al.* (2016) Anti-diabetic activities of catalpol in db/db mice. *Korean J Physiol Pharmacol* **20**(2): 153–160.

22. Xu D, Wang L, Jiang Z, *et al.* (2018) A new hypoglycemic mechanism of catalpol revealed by enhancing MyoD/MyoG-mediated myogenesis. *Life Sci* **203**: 313–323.

23. Zhang RX, Jia ZP, Kong LF, *et al.* (2004) Stachyose extract from Rehmannia glutinosa Libosch. to lower plasma glucose in normal and diabetic rats by oral administration. *Pharmazie* **59**(7): 552–556.

24. Zhang R, Zhou J, Jia Z, *et al.* (2004) Hypoglycemic effect of Rehmannia glutinosa oligosaccharide in hyperglycemic and alloxan-induced diabetic rats and its mechanism. *J Ethnopharmacol* **90**(1): 39–43.

25. Wong KH, Li GQ, Li KM, *et al.* (2011) Kudzu root: Traditional uses and potential medicinal benefits in diabetes and cardiovascular diseases. *J Ethnopharmacol* **134**(3): 584–607.

26. Zhang Z, Lam TN, Zuo Z. (2013) Radix Puerariae: An overview of its chemistry, pharmacology, pharmacokinetics, and clinical use. *J Clin Pharmacol* **53**(8): 787–811.

27. Chen WC, Hayakawa S, Yamamoto T, *et al.* (2004) Mediation of beta-endorphin by the isoflavone puerarin to lower plasma glucose in streptozotocin-induced diabetic rats. *Planta Med* **70**(2): 113–116.

28. Hsu FL, Liu IM, Kuo DH, *et al.* (2003) Antihyperglycemic effect of puerarin in streptozotocin-induced diabetic rats. *J Nat Prod* **66**(6): 788–792.

29. Meezan E, Meezan EM, Jones K, *et al.* (2005) Contrasting effects of puerarin and daidzin on glucose homeostasis in mice. *J Agric Food Chem* **53**(22): 8760–8767.

30. Lee OH, Seo DH, Park CS, Kim YC. (2010) Puerarin enhances adipocyte differentiation, adiponectin expression, and antioxidant response in 3T3-L1 cells. *Biofactors* **36**(6): 459–467.

31. Xu ME, Xiao SZ, Sun YH, *et al.* (2005) The study of anti-metabolic syndrome effect of puerarin in vitro. *Life Sci* **77**(25): 3183–3196.

32. Peng N, Prasain JK, Dai Y, *et al.* (2009) Chronic dietary kudzu isoflavones improve components of metabolic syndrome in stroke-prone spontaneously hypertensive rats. *J Agric Food Chem* **57**(16): 7268–7273.

33. Cheong SH, Furuhashi K, Ito K, *et al.* (2014) Daidzein promotes glucose uptake through glucose transporter 4 translocation to plasma membrane in L6 myocytes and improves glucose homeostasis in Type 2 diabetic model mice. *J Nutr Biochem* **25**(2):136–143.

34. Wang J, Wang L, Lou GH, *et al.* (2019) Coptidis Rhizoma: A comprehensive review of its traditional uses, botany, phytochemistry, pharmacology and toxicology. *Pharm Biol* **57**(1): 193–225.

35. Kim SH, Shin EJ, Kim ED, *et al.* (2007) Berberine activates GLUT1-mediated glucose uptake in 3T3-L1 adipocytes. *Biol Pharm Bull* **30**(11): 2120–2125.

36. Cok A, Plaisier C, Salie MJ, *et al.* (2011) Berberine acutely activates the glucose transport activity of GLUT1. *Biochimie* **93**(7): 1187–1192.

37. Tang LQ, Wei W, Chen LM, Liu S. (2006) Effects of berberine on diabetes induced by alloxan and a high-fat/high-cholesterol diet in rats. *J Ethnopharmacol* **108**(1): 109–115.

38. Xie X, Li W, Lan T, *et al.* (2011) Berberine ameliorates hyperglycemia in alloxan-induced diabetic C57BL/6 mice through activation of Akt signaling pathway. *Endocr J* **58**(9): 761–768.

39. Yu Y, Liu L, Wang X, *et al.* (2010) Modulation of glucagon-like peptide-1 release by berberine: In vivo and in vitro studies. *Biochem Pharmacol* **79**(7): 1000–1006.

40. Yang Y, Li Y, Yin D, *et al.* (2016) Coptis chinensis polysaccharides inhibit advanced glycation end product formation. *J Med Food* **19**(6): 593–600.

41. Jiang S, Wang Y, Ren D, *et al.* (2015) Antidiabetic mechanism of Coptis chinensis polysaccharide through its antioxidant property involving the JNK pathway. *Pharm Biol* **53**(7): 1022–1029.

42. Cui L, Liu M, Chang X, Sun K. (2016) The inhibiting effect of the Coptis chinensis polysaccharide on the type II diabetic mice. *Biomed Pharmacother* **81**: 111–119.

43. Jiang S, Du P, An L, Yuan G, Sun Z. (2013) Anti-diabetic effect of Coptis chinensis polysaccharide in high-fat diet with STZ-induced diabetic mice. *Int J Biol Macromol* **55**: 118–122.

44. Jiang Z, Gao W, Huang L. (2019) Tanshinones, critical pharmacological components in Salvia miltiorrhiza. *Front Pharmacol* **10**: 202.

45. Jia Q, Zhu R, Tian Y, *et al.* (2019) Salvia miltiorrhiza in diabetes: A review of its pharmacology, phytochemistry, and safety. *Phytomedicine* **58**: 152871.

46. Yu J, Fei J, Azad J, *et al.* (2012) Myocardial protection by Salvia miltiorrhiza Injection in streptozotocin-induced diabetic rats through

attenuation of expression of thrombospondin-1 and transforming growth factor-beta1. *J Int Med Res* **40**(3): 1016–1024.

47. Yang XY, Sun L, Xu P, *et al.* (2011) Effects of salvianolic scid A on plantar microcirculation and peripheral nerve function in diabetic rats. *Eur J Pharmacol* **665**(1–3): 40–46.

48. Qiang G, Yang X, Shi L, *et al.* (2015) Antidiabetic effect of salvianolic acid A on diabetic animal models via AMPK activation and mitochondrial regulation. *Cell Physiol Biochem* **36**(1): 395–408.

49. Wang SB, Yang XY, Tian S, *et al.* (2009) Effect of salvianolic acid A on vascular reactivity of streptozotocin-induced diabetic rats. *Life Sci* **85**(13–14): 499–504.

50. Huang M, Wang P, Xu S, *et al.* (2015) Biological activities of salvianolic acid B from Salvia miltiorrhiza on Type 2 diabetes induced by high-fat diet and streptozotocin. *Pharm Biol* **53**(7): 1058–1065.

51. Kitahiro Y, Koike A, Sonoki A, *et al.* (2018) Anti-inflammatory activities of Ophiopogonis Radix on hydrogen peroxide-induced cellular senescence of normal human dermal fibroblasts. *J Nat Med* **72**(4): 905–914.

52. Chen MH, Chen XJ, Wang M, *et al.* (2016) Ophiopogon japonicus — A phytochemical, ethnomedicinal and pharmacological review. *J Ethnopharmacol* **181**: 193–213.

53. Ding L, Li P, Lau CB, *et al.* (2012) Mechanistic studies on the antidiabetic activity of a polysaccharide-rich extract of Radix Ophiopogonis. *Phytother Res* **26**(1): 101–105.

54. Xu J, Wang Y, Xu DS, *et al.* (2011) Hypoglycemic effects of MDG-1, a polysaccharide derived from Ophiopogon japonicas, in the ob/ob mouse model of Type 2 diabetes mellitus. *Int J Biol Macromol* **49**(4): 657–662.

55. Zhu Y, Cong W, Shen L, *et al.* (2014) Fecal metabonomic study of a polysaccharide, MDG-1 from Ophiopogon japonicus on diabetic mice based on gas chromatography/time-of-flight mass spectrometry (GC TOF/MS). *Mol Biosyst* **10**(2): 304–312.

56. Wang LY, Wang Y, Xu DS, *et al.* (2012) MDG-1, a polysaccharide from Ophiopogon japonicus exerts hypoglycemic effects through the PI3K/ Akt pathway in a diabetic KKAy mouse model. *J Ethnopharmacol* **143**(1): 347–354.

57. Chen X, Jin J, Tang J, *et al.* (2011) Extraction, purification, characterization and hypoglycemic activity of a polysaccharide isolated from the root of Ophiopogon japonicus. *Carbohydr Polym* **83**(2): 749–754.

58. Chen X, Tang J, Xie W, *et al.* (2013) Protective effect of the polysaccharide from Ophiopogon japonicus on streptozotocin-induced diabetic rats. *Carbohydr Polym* **94**(1): 378–385.

59. Kim S, Shin S, Hyun B, *et al.* (2012) Immunomodulatory effects of dioscoreae rhizome against inflammation through suppressed production of cytokines via inhibition of the NF-kappaB pathway. *Immune Netw* **12**(5): 181–188.

60. Lee SC, Tsai CC, Chen JC, *et al.* (2002) The evaluation of reno- and hepatoprotective effects of huai-shan-yao (Rhizome Dioscoreae). *Am J Chin Med* **30**(4): 609–616.

61. 吕娟, 魏鹏飞, 白甫. (2017) 山药多糖对2型糖尿病大鼠血小板及酶活性的影响. 中国老年学杂志 **37**(13): 3186–3187.

62. 杨宏莉, 张宏馨, 李兰会, *et al.* (2010) 山药多糖对2型糖尿病大鼠降糖机理的研究. 河北农业大学学报 **33**(3): 100–103.

63. 郝志奇, 杭秉茜, 王瑛. (1991) 山药水煎剂对实验性小鼠的降血糖作用. 中国药科大学学报 **22**(3): 158–160.

64. 杭悦宇. (1994) 我国山药类药材对动物降血糖和降血脂的作用. 植物资源与环境 **3**(4): 59–60.

65. Rios JL. (2011) Chemical constituents and pharmacological properties of Poria cocos. *Planta Med* **77**(7): 681–691.

66. Sun Y. (2014) Biological activities and potential health benefits of polysaccharides from Poria cocos and their derivatives. *Int J Biol Macromol* **68**: 131–134.

67. Li TH, Hou CC, Chang CL, Yang WC. (2011) Anti-hyperglycemic properties of crude extract and triterpenes from Poria cocos. *Evid Based Complement Alternat Med* **2011**.

68. Sato M, Tai T, Nunoura Y, *et al.* (2002) Dehydrotrametenolic acid induces preadipocyte differentiation and sensitizes animal models of noninsulin-dependent diabetes mellitus to insulin. *Biol Pharm Bull* **25**(1): 81–86.

69. Huang YC, Chang WL, Huang SF, *et al.* (2010) Pachymic acid stimulates glucose uptake through enhanced GLUT4 expression and translocation. *Eur J Pharmacol* **648**(1–3): 39–49.

70. 丁建营, 刘春娟, 郭建军, *et al.* (2018) 天花粉化学成分的药理活性及其提取与检测方法研究进展. 中国药房 **29**(13): 1859–1863.

71. Hikino H, Yoshizawa M, Suzuki Y, *et al.* (1989) Isolation and hypoglycemic activity of trichosans A, B, C, D, and E: Glycans of Trichosanthes kirilowii roots. *Planta Med* **55**(4): 349–350.

72. 李琼, 张鹏, 郭晨, *et al.* (2015) 天花粉凝集素对糖尿病大鼠血糖及氧化应激的影响. 食品工业科技 **36**(10): 356–359.

73. Lo H-Y, Tsai-Chung L, Tse-Yen Y, *et al.* (2017) Hypoglycemic effects of Trichosanthes kirilowii and its protein constituent in diabetic mice: The involvement of insulin receptor pathway. *BMC Complementary and Alternative Medicine* **17**(1): 53.

74. Wang Y, Dan Y, Yang D, *et al.* (2014) The genus Anemarrhena Bunge: A review on ethnopharmacology, phytochemistry and pharmacology. *J Ethnopharmacol* **153**(1): 42–60.

75. Hoa NK, Phan DV, Thuan ND, Östenson CG. (2004) Insulin secretion is stimulated by ethanol extract of anemarrhena asphodeloides in isolated islet of healthy wistar and diabetic goto-kakizaki rats. *Exp Clin Endocrinol Diabetes* **112**(9): 520–525.

76. Ichiki H, Miura T, Kubo M, *et al.* (1998) New antidiabetic compounds, mangiferin and its glucoside. *Biol Pharm Bull* **21**(12): 1389–1390.

77. Miura T, Ichiki H, Hashimoto I, *et al.* (2001) Antidiabetic activity of a xanthone compound, mangiferin. *Phytomedicine* **8**(2): 85–87.

78. Miura T, Ichiki H, Iwamoto N, *et al.* (2001) Antidiabetic activity of the rhizoma of Anemarrhena asphodeloides and active components, mangiferin and its glucoside. *Biol Pharm Bull* **24**(9): 1009–1011.

79. Nakashima N, Kimura I, Kimura M, Matsuura H. (1993) Isolation of pseudoprototimosaponin AIII from rhizomes of Anemarrhena asphodeloides and its hypoglycemic activity in streptozotocin-induced diabetic mice. *J Nat Prod* **56**(3): 345–350.

80. Takahashi M, Konno C, Hikino H. (1985) Isolation and hypoglycemic activity of anemarans A, B, C and D, glycans of Anemarrhena asphodeloides rhizomes. *Planta Med* (2): 100–102.

7

Clinical Evidence for Acupuncture and Related Therapies

OVERVIEW

This chapter evaluates clinical studies investigating acupuncture and related therapies for Type 2 diabetes mellitus (T2DM). Four studies were randomised controlled trials, and 10 were non-controlled studies. Acupuncture and related therapies may improve plasma glucose measurements and lipid abnormalities associated with T2DM.

Introduction

Acupuncture is an important Chinese medicine treatment that stimulates acupuncture points to correct imbalances of energy and restore health to the body. Methods of stimulating acupuncture points include:

- Acupuncture: Insertion of an acupuncture needle into acupuncture points;
- Electro-acupuncture: After insertion of an acupuncture needle into acupuncture points, a small electric current runs between the needle pair via electrodes connected to the needles;
- Acupressure: Application of pressure to acupuncture points on the body or ears;
- Moxibustion: Burning of an herb (usually *Artemesia vulgaris, ai ye* 艾叶) close to or on the skin to induce a warming sensation.

Previous Systematic Reviews

A limited number of systematic reviews of acupuncture or related therapies are available for T2DM. Xing and colleagues evaluated the effect of acupuncture on T2DM patients; eight trials were included (740 participants).[1] Meta-analysis results showed that compared to pharmacotherapy, the acupuncture group significantly improved the levels of fasting plasma glucose (FPG) and fasting insulin (FINS), as well as the insulin resistance index and insulin sensitivity index. The results are limited by the methodological quality of the included studies.

Kim and colleagues evaluated the effectiveness of moxibustion for managing the symptoms of T2DM patients.[2] One randomised controlled trial (RCT) (335 participants) compared one-off moxibustion use with oral administration of glibenclimide and showed the significant effects of moxibustion on glycaemic control. Another RCT (60 participants) evaluated the effect of moxibustion plus conventional treatment, and the moxibustion group reported significant improvement in fasting and postprandial blood glucose (PBG) levels compared with conventional treatment. The included trials had high risk of bias. Therefore, it is difficult to conclude if moxibustion is an effective intervention for T2DM due to the small number and low methodological quality of the included trials.

Identification of Clinical Studies

A total of 66,570 citations were identified through database searches, and 3,229 full-text articles were reviewed for eligibility. Fourteen clinical studies (A1–A14) met the inclusion criteria. Four RCTs and 10 non-controlled studies (NCTs), controlled clinical trials (CCTs), were not identified (Figure 7.1). In addition, two identified studies used interventions that are not commonly practised outside of China, and they will not be presented here.[3,4]

A total of 299 people participated in the RCTs, and 1,900 people participated in the non-controlled clinical trials. The treatment duration varied from three weeks to 140 days. None of the RCT studies

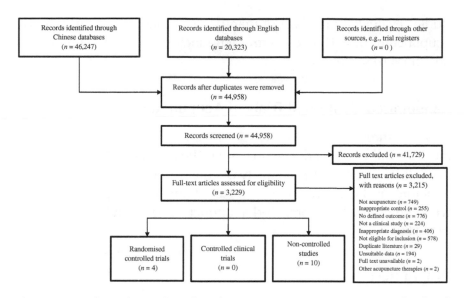

Figure 7.1. Flow chart of study selection process: Acupuncture and related therapies.

mentioned the Chinese medicine syndrome. Common syndromes that occurred in NCTs were the deficiency of both *qi* and *yin* (seven studies), Lung heat and damage to the *jin* 津 liquid (five studies), and excessive Stomach heat (four studies).

The most commonly used acupoints in the included RCT and NCTs were BL11 *Feishu* 肺俞 and SP6 *Sanyinjiao* 三阴交. Other commonly used acupoints included BL23 *Shenshu* 肾俞, EX-B3 *Yishu* 胰俞, ST36 *Zusanli* 足三里 and BL20 *Pishu* 脾俞. The most commonly used ear points were CO18 *Neifenmi* (Endocrine) 内分泌, CO4 *Wei* (Stomach) 胃 and CO13 *Pi* (Spleen) 脾.

In this chapter, the effects of acupuncture and moxa on diabetes mellitus will be presented in two separate sections.

Acupuncture

A total of 13 studies (A1–A13) were identified that used acupuncture for T2DM. The included RCTs evaluated the effect of acupuncture (*n* = 3) for T2DM. In the included non-controlled clinical studies, the studies evaluated the effect of manual acupuncture (*n* = 8), electro-acupuncture (*n* = 1), and electro-acupuncture plus ear acupuncture on T2DM (*n* = 1).

Randomised Controlled Trials of Acupuncture

A total of three acupuncture RCTs (A1–A3) and 239 participants were included; all were conducted in China. The treatment duration varied from three weeks to 140 days. Two studies (A1, A3) compared acupuncture as Integrative Medicine to pharmacotherapy (*n* = 139), while one study (A2) compared acupuncture to lifestyle intervention (*n* = 100).

Risk of Bias

All three studies were described as randomised — two studies (A1–A2) used either a random number table or permuted block randomisation and were judged as "low" risk of bias for sequence generation. One study (A3) did not provide further information on the method of randomisation and was judged as an "unclear" risk for this domain. All three studies did not provide information on allocation concealment and were therefore judged as "unclear" risk of bias. One study (A1) used sham electro-acupuncture machines for the blinding of participants and adequately described the blinding of an outcome assessor, and was judged as a "low" risk for these domains. Although the blinding of personnel (the acupuncturist) was not possible in this study, we judged that it was not possible for the acupuncturist to create a bias in the results. Therefore, we judged this domain as "low risk". The remaining studies were judged as "high" risk as the treatment and control groups were obviously different and there was no blinding attempted. All the studies provided detailed information on dropouts, and methods of data imputation where appropriate. Therefore, this domain was judged as a "low" risk of bias for all studies. No protocol could be located for the studies. A1 was judged as an "unclear" risk of bias for selective outcome reporting, while A2 and A3 were judged as "high" risk of bias because their reported outcomes did not match those that were prespecified. Overall, the judgement of the methodological quality of the included studies was limited by inadequate study details.

Acupuncture as Integrative Medicine vs. Pharmacotherapy

Pre-specified outcomes included measurements of blood glucose, body mass index (BMI), blood lipid metabolism, β-cell function assessment, quality of life, and adverse events.

Fasting Plasma Glucose

Two studies (A2–A3) of 139 participants assessed FPG. Acupuncture as Integrative Medicine did not improve on FPG more than pharmacotherapy alone (MD −1.25 [−2.77, 0.34], $I^2 = 98.1\%$).

Postprandial Blood Glucose

One study (A3) of 100 participants investigated the effect of acupuncture as Integrative Medicine compared to pharmacotherapy alone. Acupuncture plus pharmacotherapy significantly improved PBG levels compared to pharmacotherapy alone (MD −3.31 [−3.69, −2.93]).

Glycated Haemoglobin

One study (A3) of 100 participants investigated the effect of acupuncture as Integrative Medicine compared to pharmacotherapy alone. Acupuncture plus pharmacotherapy significantly improved glycated haemoglobin (A1C) levels compared to pharmacotherapy alone (MD −1.3 [−1.52, −1.08]).

Body Mass Index

One study (A2) of 39 participants investigated the effect of acupuncture as Integrative Medicine compared to pharmacotherapy alone.

Acupuncture plus pharmacotherapy significantly improved the BMI compared to pharmacotherapy alone (MD −1.5 [−2.79, −0.21]).

Triglyceride

One study (A1) of 39 participants investigated the effect of acupuncture as Integrative Medicine compared to pharmacotherapy alone. Acupuncture plus pharmacotherapy significantly improved triglyceride levels compared to pharmacotherapy alone (MD −0.41 [−0.82, −0.001]).

Low-density Lipoprotein

One study (A1) of 39 participants investigated the effect of acupuncture as Integrative Medicine compared to pharmacotherapy alone. Acupuncture plus pharmacotherapy did not significantly improve low-density lipoprotein (LDL) levels when compared to pharmacotherapy alone (MD −0.27 [−2.47, 1.93]).

High-density Lipoprotein

One study (A1) of 39 participants investigated the effect of acupuncture as Integrative Medicine compared to pharmacotherapy alone. Acupuncture plus pharmacotherapy did not significantly improve high-density lipoprotein (HDL) levels when compared to pharmacotherapy alone (MD 0.04 [−0.02, 0.10]).

Fasting Insulin

One study (A1) of 39 participants investigated the effect of acupuncture as Integrative Medicine compared to pharmacotherapy alone. Acupuncture plus pharmacotherapy significantly improved FINS levels compared to pharmacotherapy alone (MD −3.69 [−4.16, −3.22]).

Homeostasis Model Assessment-Insulin Resistance

One study (A1) of 39 participants investigated the effect of acupuncture as Integrative Medicine compared to pharmacotherapy alone. Acupuncture plus pharmacotherapy significantly improved insulin resistance compared to pharmacotherapy alone (MD −1.34 [−1.56, −1.12]).

Acupuncture Plus Lifestyle Therapy vs. Lifestyle Therapy

One study (A2) of 100 participants investigated the effect of acupuncture plus lifestyle therapy compared to lifestyle therapy alone. The addition of acupuncture significantly improved FPG (MD −1.33 [−1.78, −0.88]) and A1C levels (MD −0.5 [−0.64, −0.366]) compared to lifestyle alone.

Frequently Reported Acupuncture Points in Meta-analyses Showing Favourable Effect

In meta-analyses showing favourable effects, the most commonly used acupoints were SP6 *Sanyinjiao* 三阴交, ST36 *Zusanli* 足三里, CV12 *Zhongwan* 中脘. BL20 *Pishu* 脾俞, BL23 *Shenshu* 肾俞, BL21 *Weishu* 胃俞 and EX-B3 *Yishu* 胰俞.

Controlled Clinical Trials of Acupuncture

No non-randomised CCTs of acupuncture for T2DM were included in the analysis.

Non-controlled Studies of Acupuncture

Ten non-controlled studies (A4–A13) of acupuncture for T2DM were identified. A total of 1,900 participants were included. Various syndromes are identified in the studies; the most common syndromes were the deficiency of *qi* and *yin* (seven studies), Lung heat and damage to the *jin* 津 liquid (five studies), and excessive Stomach heat (four studies).

The most frequently used body acupoints across all studies were BL13 *Feishu* 肺俞, SP6 *Sanyinjiao* 三阴交, LU1 *Zhongfu* 中府, ST44 *Neiting* 内庭, KI3 *Taixi* 太溪, LU5 *Quchi* 曲池, BL23 *Shenshu* 肾俞, EX-B3 *Yishu* 胰俞 and ST36 *Zusanli* 足三里. The most frequently used ear acupoints across all studies were CO18 *Neifenmi* (Endocrine) 内分泌, CO14 *Fei* (Lung) 肺, CO4 *Wei* (Stomach) 胃CO11 *Yidan* (Pancreas) 胰胆, CO13 *Pi* (Spleen) 脾 and CO9 *Pangguang* (Bladder) 膀胱.

For studies that modified treatment points according to the syndrome and deficiency of both *qi* and *yin*, the most commonly used body acupoints were LU1 *Zhongfu* 中府, BL13 *Feishu* 肺俞, BL23 *Shenshu* 肾俞, SP6 *Sanyinjiao* 三阴交, GB25 *Jingmen* 京门, CV6 *Qihai* 气海 and ST36 *Zusanli* 足三里. For Lung heat and damage to the *jin* 津 fluids, the most commonly used body acupoints were LU1 *Zhongfu* 中府, BL13 *Feishu* 肺俞, ST40 *Fenglong* 丰隆, ST25 *Tianshu* 天枢, LU9 *Taiyuan* 太渊, LU5 *Chize* 尺泽 and EX-B3 *Yishu* 胰俞. For excessive Stomach heat, the most commonly used body acupoints were ST44 *Neiting* 内庭 and ST36 *Zusanli* 足三里. For studies that used ear points, for *qi* and *yin* deficiency, the most commonly used point was the Kidney. For excessive Stomach heat, it was CO4 *Wei* (Stomach) 胃, CO13 *Pi* (Spleen) 脾, CO18 *Neifenmi* (Endocrine) 内分泌 and CO11 *Yidan* (Pancreas and Gallbladder) 胰胆.

Safety of Acupuncture

The included RCTs and NCT did not report on any adverse events.

Moxibustion

One study (A14) with 60 participants examined the effect of moxa as Integrative Medicine compared to pharmacotherapy for T2DM.

The study was described as randomised but did not provide further information on the method of randomisation and was judged as an "unclear" risk for this domain. It also did not provide information on allocation concealment and was therefore judged as an "unclear" risk of bias. The study was judged as a "high" risk for the blinding of participants, personnel and outcome assessor as the treatment and control groups were obviously different, and there was no blinding attempted. There were no dropouts and the incomplete data domain was judged at a "low" risk of bias. No protocol was available for the study, and it was judged "unclear" for selective reporting.

Moxa was performed on EX-B3 *Yishu* 胰俞, BL20 *Pishu* 脾俞, BL21 *Weishu* 胃俞, BL23 *Shenshu* 肾俞 and SP6 *Sanyinjiao* 三阴交. The study showed a significant difference between groups for FPG (MD −1.63 [−2.15, −1.11]). No other included outcome measure was reported, and the study did not report on adverse events.

Summary of Clinical Evidence for Acupuncture and Related Therapies

Only a small number of studies were identified that evaluated the effect of acupuncture and related therapies for T2DM. A majority of the studies reported on fasting plasma glucose. Meta-analyses showed that acupuncture as Integrative Medicine did not improve on FPG more than pharmacotherapy alone. A meta-analysis was not possible for other comparisons and outcomes due to the very small number of included studies.

Commonly used acupoints in RCTs with a favourable effect included SP6 *Sanyinjiao* 三阴交, ST36 *Zusanli* 足三里, CV12 *Zhongwan* 中脘, BL20 *Pishu* 脾俞, BL23 *Shenshu* 肾俞, BL21 *Weishu* 胃俞 and EX-B3 *Yishu* 胰俞. The most common syndromes identified in NCTs were the deficiency of both *qi* and *yin*, Lung heat and damage to the *jin* 津 fluids, and excessive Stomach heat. The safety of acupuncture and related therapies were not reported in the included studies.

References

1. 邢春国, 孙志, 马永春, 范群. (2015) 针灸疗法对 2 型糖尿病患者胰岛功能影响的 Meta 分析. 南京中医药大学学报 **31**(4): 397–400.

2. Kim TH, Choi TY, Shin BC, Lee MS. (2011) Moxibustion for managing Type 2 diabetes mellitus: A systematic review. *Chin J Integr Med* **17**(8): 575–579.

3. 焦生林, 王彦军. (2013) 穴位埋线法治疗2型糖尿病 195 例临床观察. 实用中西医结合临床 **13**(6): 14–15.

4. 周明倩, 李婵, 韩冬宜, *et al.* (2015) 薄氏腹针埋线治疗 2 型糖尿病临床研究. 实用中医药杂志 **31**(12): 1163–1164.

References for Included Acupuncture Therapies Clinical Studies

Study No.	Reference
A1	Firouzjaei A, Li GC, Wang N, *et al.* (2016) Comparative evaluation of the therapeutic effect of metformin monotherapy with monotherapy with metformin and acupuncture combined therapy on weight loss and insulin sensitivity in diabetic patients. *Nutr Diabetes* **6**, e209.
A2	何永昌, 李秀红, 石霞萍. (2012) 针刺配合社区干预治疗社区糖尿病患者的疗效观察. 中西医结合 **20**(10): 1682–1683.
A3	唐新明, 管进. (2013) 针刺联合常规药物治疗 2 型糖尿病疗效观察.人民军医 **56**(9): 1039–1040.
A4	陈婷, 杨春, 陶涛, 樊静. (2017) 电针联合体针治疗 2 型糖尿 10 例.中国针灸 **37**(12): 1285–1286.
A5	陈万泓. (2013) 针刺 "消渴组穴"改善 2 型糖尿病特异性生命质量的临床观察研究. 北京中医药大学硕士学位论文, 中国北京.
A6	刘美君. (2015) 2 型糖尿病中医证型分布及针灸干预效应的研究. 南京中医药大学硕士学位论文, 中国南京.
A7	刘美君, 刘志诚, 徐斌. (2014) 针灸治疗气阴两虚型 2 型糖尿病的疗效分析. 中华中医药杂志 **29**(9): 3022–3024.
A8	刘美君, 刘志诚, 徐斌. (2014) 针灸治疗肺热津伤型 2 型糖尿病的疗效分析. 时珍国医国 **25**(12): 2945–2947.
A9	刘美君, 刘志诚, 徐斌. (2015) 针灸治疗 2 型糖尿病 640 例临床疗效观察. 中华中医药杂志 **30**(12): 4531–4533.

(Continued)

Study No.	Reference
A10	刘艳平. (2015) 针刺脾相关穴位治疗 2 型糖尿病的研究. 南京中医药大学, 中国南京.
A11	佟帅, 吕海波, 刘建桥, 李鑫懿. (2011) 针刺降糖即刻效应的临床观察. 中医药信息 **28**(2): 80–82.
A12	袁爱红, 魏群利, 蔡辉. (2009) 俞募配穴法为主配合耳穴贴压治疗 2 型糖尿病 35 例临床观察. 河北中医 **31**(4): 578–579.
A13	张娜. (2013) 电针联合耳针治疗 2 型糖尿病 203 例临床观察. 中医杂志 **54**(18): 1558–1561.
A14	阮志忠, 黄志兰, 董灿. (2015) 定量温和灸干预治疗 2 型糖尿病 30 例临床观察. 江苏中医药 **47**(6): 54–55.

8

Clinical Evidence for Other Chinese Medicine Therapies

OVERVIEW

Clinical evidence of other Chinese medicine therapies for Type 2 diabetes mellitus (T2DM) include *tuina* 推拿, *taichi* 太极, *qigong* 气功 and diet therapy. There was an overall lack of evidence supporting the use of other Chinese medicine therapies for T2DM. Only 11 clinical studies were identified for this chapter.

Introduction

In addition to Chinese herbal medicine and acupuncture therapies, Chinese medicine (CM) includes a range of other CM therapies to treat disease and maintain health. These include:

- *Tuina* 推拿: Chinese massage therapy.
- *Taichi* 太极: A form of mind and body exercise originating from ancient China with a long history based on ancient Chinese Taoist philosophy.
- *Baduanjin* 八段锦: A form of *qigong*. It includes a routine of eight exercises that coordinate movement and breath.
- CM diet therapy: The use of foods and herbs to regulate body functions according to individual syndrome differentiation.

Previous Systematic Reviews

Four systematic reviews were identified for other CM therapies for T2DM. He and colleagues systematically reviewed Chinese diet therapy for T2DM.[1] The review included four randomised controlled trials (RCTs) and one quasi-RCT of 408 participants. Due to the small numbers of studies and heterogeneity presented, no meta-analysis was performed, and a descriptive analysis was used instead. The authors found that compared with conventional diets, CM diet therapy was more beneficial in diabetic patients by reducing fasting plasma glucose (FPG) and glycosylated haemoglobin (AIC) values.

Another group systematically reviewed the effect of *taichi* 太极 for T2DM. It included 11 studies and results showed that compared to exercise, the *taichi* 太极 group significantly reduced levels of blood sugar, weight, triglycerides, and improved the quality of life in T2DM patients.[2] Limitations such as a low level of evidence was mentioned by the authors when drawing their conclusions. Liu and colleagues included 10 studies. Compared to regular exercise or no treatment, meta-analyses results showed that *taichi* 太极 significantly decreased FPG, A1C, improved triglyceride (TG), high-density lipoprotein (HDL) and low-density lipoprotein (LDL) levels, and the quality of life. Included studies had low methodology quality and results showed considerate heterogeneity.[3]

Yang and colleagues reviewed the effect of *baduanjin* 八段锦 for T2DM. It included seven RCTs (507 participants).[4] Compared to the control group, *baduanjin* 八段锦 reduced patients' A1C, FPG, total cholesterol levels and increased HDL cholesterol. Results show that *baduanjin* 八段锦 can decrease blood glucose and blood lipid. Yu and colleagues included 10 RCTs of 825 participants and reviewed the effect of *baduanjin* 八段锦 for T2DM. Meta-analysis results showed that the *baduanjin* 八段锦 group was superior to the control group in lowering FPG, 2-hour postprandial blood glucose (PBG) and A1C, reducing the levels of total cholesterol (TC) and TG, and increasing the level of HDL, with statistical significant differences. However, there was no statistical difference in LDL between the two groups. Due to the limitation of quantity and quality of the included studies, the conclusion should be verified by conducting large-scale high-quality RCTs.

Identification of Clinical Studies

A search of electronic databases identified 66,570 potentially relevant citations. After the removal of duplicates, the title and abstracts of citations were read and more than 41,729 irrelevant citations were excluded (Figure 8.1). The full texts of 3,229 articles were reviewed. In total, 11 clinical studies that evaluated other Chinese medicine therapies were included. Nine were RCTs and two were controlled clinical trials (CCTs). Studies are indicated by the letter "O" and then followed by a number, and their references can be found at the end of the chapter.

Based on the eligibility criteria, nine RCTs (O1–O9, Figure 8.1) and two non-controlled studies (O10–O11) were included. Evidence from the RCTs was evaluated to establish the efficacy and safety of other therapies for T2DM. A total of 356 participants were included

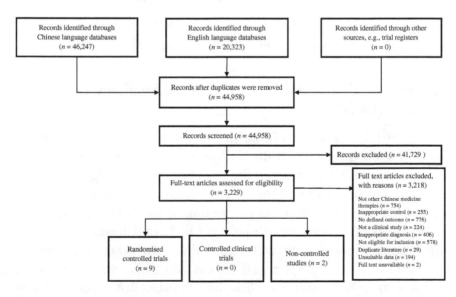

Figure 8.1. Flow chart of study selection process: Other Chinese medicine therapies.

in the RCTs. Both studies were conducted in China, with a treatment duration of equal to, or less than, six weeks. One study compared *tuina* 推拿 to fluoxetine, while the other study compared mobile cupping plus fluoxetine to fluoxetine alone. The studies did not report any CM syndromes.

Nine RCT studies were identified in our search:

- CM diet therapy (two studies) (O2, O5),
- *Baduanjin* 八段锦 (four studies) (O1, O3, O4, O9),
- *Taichi* 太极 (two studies) (O6, O8),
- *Tuina* 推拿 (one study) (O7).

Two non-controlled studies were identified in our search:

- CM diet therapy (*fu ling* 茯苓 bun) (O10),
- *Baduanjin* 八段锦 plus walking exercise (O11).

Chinese Medicine Diet Therapy 中医食疗

Three studies using CM diet therapy were identified: two were RCTs (O2, O5) and one was a non-controlled study (O10).

Randomised Controlled Trials of Chinese Medicine Diet Therapy 中医食疗

Two RCTs (O2, O5) and 170 participants were included. The studies evaluated the effect of the Chinese medicine diet therapy for T2DM. One RCT (O2) studied the effect of yam porridge for T2DM compared to no treatment for 12 weeks. One RCT (O5) compared *Yu quan san* 玉泉散 buns to no treatment for T2DM patients for eight weeks. The buns were made up of herbal formula *Yu quan san* granules mixed with water and flour. *Yu quan san* consists of *huang qin* 黄芩, *ge gen* 葛根, *shan yao* 山药, *mai dong* 麦冬, *wu wei zi* 五味子 and *tian hua fen* 天花粉. Both studies were conducted in China.

Risk of Bias

Both studies used a random number table for randomisation and were judged as a "low" risk for this domain. One study (O2) used an opaque envelope for allocation concealment and was judged as a "low" risk of bias for this domain. One study (O5) did not provide information on allocation concealment and was therefore judged as an "unclear" risk of bias. Both studies were judged as "high" risk for the blinding of participants, personnel and outcome assessors, as the treatment and control groups were obviously different, and there was no blinding attempted. All studies provided detailed information on dropouts and methods of data imputation where appropriate. Therefore, the incomplete outcome data domain was judged as a "low" risk of bias for all studies. No protocol could be located for all studies and was judged as "unclear" risk of bias for selective outcome reporting. Overall, the judgement of the methodological quality of the included studies was limited by inadequate study details.

Outcomes

The studies reported on blood glucose-related (FPG, PBG, A1C) and lipid metabolism-related outcomes (TG, TC, HDL, LDL). One study (O5) also reported on the quality of life using a Diabetes-Specific Quality of Life Scale.

Fasting Plasma Glucose

Chinese medicine diet therapy significantly improved FPG levels in 170 T2DM patients, compared to no treatment (MD −1.10 (−1.37, −0.82), $I^2 = 0\%$) (O2, O5).

Postprandial Blood Glucose

No difference was found in PBG levels when the CM diet therapy was compared to no treatment in 170 T2DM participants (MD −0.64 (−1.74, 0.46), $I^2 = 83.3\%$) (O2, O5).

Glycated Haemoglobin

One study (O5) found a significant difference in A1C levels in the *Yu quan san* buns group, compared to no treatment in 80 T2DM patients (MD −0.57 (−0.99, −0.15).

Body Mass Index

One study (O5) found a significant difference in body mass index (BMI) in the *Yu quan san* buns group, compared to no treatment in 80 T2DM patients (MD −4.07 (−5.12, −3.02).

Triglyceride

The CM diet therapy did not improve TG levels in T2DM patients, compared to no treatment (MD −0.20 (−0.51, 0.11), $I^2 = 0\%$) (O2, O5).

Total Cholesterol

The CM diet therapy significantly improved the total TC levels in T2DM patients ($n = 170$), compared to no treatment (MD −0.81 (−1.08, −0.55), $I^2 = 0\%$) (O2, O5).

Low-density Lipoprotein

The CM diet therapy did not improve LDL levels in T2DM patients ($n = 170$), compared to no treatment (MD −0.13 (−0.28, 0.02), $I^2 = 0\%$) (O2, O5).

High-density Lipoprotein

The CM diet therapy did not improve HDL levels in 90 T2DM patients, compared to no treatment (MD −0.04 (−0.18, 0.01) (O5).

Controlled Clinical Trials of Chinese Medicine Diet Therapy 中医食疗

No controlled clinical trial of CM diet therapy was identified.

Non-controlled Studies of Chinese Medicine Diet Therapy 中医食疗

One non-controlled study (O10) of CM diet therapy was identified. It included 58 participants who consumed buns made of 50 g of the Chinese herb *fu ling* daily for 14 days. The study reported on fasting plasma glucose, postprandial blood glucose, and BMI.

Safety of Chinese Medicine Diet Therapy 中医食疗

Included RCT studies did not report on the adverse events (AEs) of CM diet therapy. One study (O10) reported that there were no AEs reported during the study.

Baduanjin 八段锦

A total of five *baduanjin* 八段锦 studies were identified, consisting of four randomised clinical trials (O1, O3, O4, O9) and one non-controlled clinical trial (O11).

Randomised Controlled Trials of *Baduanjin* 八段锦

Four RCT studies (O1, O3, O4, O9) of 387 participants were identified that evaluated the effect of *baduanjin* 八段锦 on T2DM. All studies were conducted in China, and the study duration varied from 3 to 9 months. Two studies (O4, O9) were multi-arm trials and had different comparisons. These studies compared *baduanjin* 八段锦 to aerobic exercise and *baduanjin* 八段锦 to no treatment. The third study (O3) compared *baduanjin* 八段锦 to metformin (see O3 under

References for Included Other Chinese Medicine Therapies Clinical Studies), and the remaining study (O1) compared *baduanjin* 八段锦 as Integrative Medicine to pharmacotherapy alone (see O1 under References for Included Other Chinese Medicine Therapies Clinical Studies). Each *baduanjin* 八段锦 session lasted from 30 to 60 minutes and was either daily or up to four days a week.

Risk of Bias

All four studies mentioned randomised, but only one study (O3) used a random number table and was judged as a "low" risk for this domain. The rest of the studies were judged as "unclear" risk of bias. They also did not provide information on allocation concealment and were therefore judged as "unclear" risk of bias for this domain. All studies were judged as "high" risk for the blinding of participants, personnel and outcome assessors, as the treatment and control groups were obviously different and there was no blinding attempted. Three studies (O1, O3, O9) provided detailed information on dropouts and methods of data imputation where appropriate. Therefore, this domain was judged at a "low" risk of bias for these studies. One study (O4) had dropouts but there was no description of drop-outs in the Results section and therefore it was judged as an "unclear" risk of bias for this domain. No protocol could be located for all studies and was judged as an "unclear" risk of bias for selective outcome reporting for three studies (O1, O4, O9). Li (see O3 under References for Included Other Chinese Medicine Therapies Clinical Studies) did not report on all planned outcomes and was judged as a "high" risk of bias for selective reporting.

Outcomes

The studies reported on blood glucose-related (FPG, PBG, A1C), BMI and lipid metabolism-related outcomes (TG, TC, HDL, LDL).

Fasting Plasma Glucose

No significant difference was found between the two groups when *baduanjin* 八段锦 was compared to metformin in one study (O3) (86 participants) (MD −0.05 [−0.64, 0.54]), or when *baduanjin* 八段锦 was compared to aerobic exercise in 122 T2DM participants (O4, O9) (MD 0.34 [−1.13, 1.81], I^2 = 87.6%), or when *baduanjin* 八段锦 was compared to no treatment in 119 T2DM participants (MD −0.39 [−2.37, 1.59], I^2 = 90.8%) (O4, O9).

One study (60 participants) showed that *baduanjin* 八段锦 combined with sulfonylur significantly improved FPG levels, compared to sulfonylur alone (MD −0.9 [−1.71, −0.09]) (O1).

Postprandial Blood Glucose

One study (O3) compared *baduanjin* 八段锦 to metformin in 86 participants and found no significant differences between groups in PBG levels (MD 0.03 [−0.47, 0.53]). Another study (O9) compared *baduanjin* 八段锦 to walking in 24 T2DM participants and found no significant differences between the groups (MD 1.45 [−0.11, 3.01]). The same study also compared *baduanjin* 八段锦 to no treatment and found no significant difference between the groups (MD 0.25 [−1.46, 1.96]).

Glycated Haemoglobin

One study (O3) compared *baduanjin* 八段锦 to metformin in 86 participants and found no significant differences between the groups in A1C levels (MD 0.02 [−0.47, 0.52). Another study (O1) (60 participants) showed that *baduanjin* 八段锦, when combined with sulfonylur, significantly improved A1C levels, compared to sulfonylur alone (MD −0.53 [−1.05, −0.01]).

Two studies (O4, O9) found no significant difference in A1C levels in 122 T2DM participants when comparing *baduanjin* 八段锦

to a form of aerobic exercise (MD −0.26 [−0.69, 0.17], I^2 = 0%). When *baduanjin* 八段锦 was compared to no treatment in 119 T2DM patients, no significant difference was found between the groups in A1C levels (−1.02 [−2.21, 0.20], I^2 = 81.4%).

Body Mass Index

Two studies (O4, O9) of 122 participants assessed the effect of *baduanjin* 八段锦 to aerobic exercise on the BMI. No significant difference was found between the two groups (MD −0.47 [−1.46, 0.52], I^2 = 0%). The same two studies (but with 143 participants now) assessed the effect of *baduanjin* 八段锦 to aerobic exercise on BMI. No significant difference was found between the two groups (MD 0.06 [−3.74, 3.87], I^2 = 83.4%).

Triglyceride

One study (O3) (86 participants) compared *baduanjin* 八段锦 to metformin for TG and found no significant difference between the two groups (MD 0.02 [−0.08, 0.12]). Another study (O1) (60 participants) showed that *baduanjin* 八段锦 combined with sulfonylur significantly improved TG levels, compared to sulfonylur alone (MD −0.31 [−0.44, −0.18]).

Total Cholesterol

One study (O3) of 86 participants compared *baduanjin* 八段锦 to metformin for TG and found no significant difference between the two groups (MD −0.07 [−0.36, 0.22]). Another study (O1) (60 participants) showed that *baduanjin* 八段锦, when combined with sulfonylur, significantly improved TC levels, compared to sulfonylur alone (MD −0.48 [−0.76, −0.20]).

One study (O4) of 98 participants compared *baduanjin* 八段锦 to aerobic exercise and found no significant differences between the groups (MD −0.14 [−0.40, 0.12]). The same study, now with 94 participants, compared *baduanjin* 八段锦 to no treatment and found significant differences between the groups in TC levels (MD −1.11 [−1.40, −0.83]).

Low-density Lipoprotein

One study (O3) of 86 participants compared *baduanjin* 八段锦 to metformin for LDL and found no significant difference between the two groups (MD −0.07 [−0.28, 0.14]). Another study (O1) of 60 participants showed that *baduanjin* 八段锦, when combined with sulfonylur, significantly improved LDL levels compared to sulfonylur alone (MD −0.48 [−0.67, −0.29]).

High-density Lipoprotein

One study (O3) of 86 participants compared *baduanjin* 八段锦 to metformin for HDL and found no significant difference between the two groups (MD 0.03 [−0.04, 0.10]). Another study (O1) of 60 participants showed that *baduanjin* 八段锦, when combined with sulfonylur, significantly improved HDL levels compared to sulfonylur alone (MD 0.57 [0.45, 0.69]).

One study (O4) of 98 participants compared *baduanjin* 八段锦 to aerobic exercise and found no significant differences between the groups (MD 0.13 [−0.04, 0.30]). The same study (O4), compared *baduanjin* 八段锦 to no treatment (94 participants) and found significant differences between the groups in HDL levels (MD 0.26 [0.09, 0.43]).

Assessment Using Grading of Recommendations, Assessment, Development and Evaluation

An assessment of the certainty of the evidence from RCTs was made using the Grading of Recommendations, Assessment, Development and Evaluations (GRADE). Interventions, comparators and outcomes to be included were selected based on a consensus process, described in Chapter 4. The comparisons were *baduanjin* 八段锦 versus aerobic exercise. The evidence for *baduanjin* 八段锦 versus

Table 8.1. GRADE: *Baduanjin* 八段锦 vs. Aerobic Exercise for Treating Type 2 Diabetes Mellitus

Outcome Mean Treatment Duration	Estimated Absolute Effect		Relative Effect (95% CI) No. of Participants (Studies)	Certainty of the Evidence (GRADE)
	Oral Chinese Herbal Medicine	Pharmacotherapy		
FPG 6 months	**6.43** MD: 0.34 higher (95% CI: 1.13 lower to 1.81 higher)	**6.77**	**MD 0.34** (–1.13, 1.81) 122 (2 RCTs)	⊕⊕▨▨ LOW[a,b]
PBG 3 months	**7.41** MD: 0.39 lower (95% CI: 2.37 lower to 1.59 higher)	**7.8**	**MD –0.39** (–2.37, 1.59) 24 (1 RCT)	⊕⊕⊕▨ MODERATE[b]
A1C 6 months	**6.39** MD: 1.02 lower (95% CI: 2.24 lower to 0.2 higher)	**7.41**	**MD –1.02** (–2.24, 0.2) 122 (2 RCTs)	⊕⊕▨▨ LOW[a,b]
TC 9.3 weeks	**3.28** MD: 1.11 lower (95% CI: 1.39 lower to 0.83 lower)	**4.39**	**MD –1.11** (–1.39. –0.83) 98 (1 RCT)	⊕⊕⊕▨ MODERATE[b]

The risk in the intervention group (and its 95% confidence interval) is based on the assumed risk in the comparison group and the relative effect of the intervention (and its 95% CI).

Abbreviations: A1C, glycated haemoglobin; CI, confidence interval; FPG, fasting plasma glucose; GRADE, Grading of Recommendations, Assessment, Development and Evaluation; MD, mean difference; PBG, postprandial blood glucose; RCTs, randomised controlled trials; TC, total cholesterol.

Note:
[a]Considerable statistical heterogeneity.
[b]Wide confidence interval and small sample size.

References:

FPG: O4, O9
PBG: O9
A1C: O4, O9
TC: O4

aerobic exercise was of "low" to "moderate" certainty (Table 8.1). The results showed that acupuncture may reduce blood glucose and cholesterol level. The studies did not report on AEs.

Controlled Clinical Trials of *Baduanjin* 八段锦

No controlled clinical trials of *baduanjin* 八段锦 were identified.

Non-Controlled Studies of *Baduanjin* 八段锦

One non-controlled study (O11) of *baduanjin* 八段锦 was identified. The study assessed the effect of *baduanjin* and walking on the effect of fasting plasma glucose and postprandial blood glucose levels in T2DM in China. *Baduanjin* 八段锦 was practiced for one week.

Safety of *Baduanjin* 八段锦

Included studies did not report on any AEs of *baduanjin* 八段锦.

Taichi 太极

Three RCT studies (O4, O6, O8) of 257 participants evaluated the effect of *taichi* 太极 on T2DM. All studies were conducted in China, and the study duration varied from 14 weeks to nine months. Two studies (O4, O6) were multi-arm studies. The first three studies compared *baduanjin* to no treatment, while the other two studies compared *taichi* 太极 to aerobic exercise. *Taichi* 太极 was practised at different frequencies in different studies. In O4, participants practised *taichi* for 30 minutes a day for nine months. *Taichi* 太极 was practised in O6 one to three times per day, five days a week. In O8, *taichi* was practised one hour per day for 14 weeks,

Risk of Bias

One study (O4) is a multi-arm study and had been previously assessed in the *baduanjin* section; therefore, it will not be discussed here again. Another study (O6) used a patient ID order for randomisation and was judged as a "high" risk of bias for randomisation; a further study (O8) did not provide details on randomisation and was judged as an "unclear" risk of bias. Both these studies did not provide information on allocation concealment and were therefore judged as "unclear" risk of bias for this domain. They were also judged as "high" risk for the blinding of participants, personnel and outcome assessors, as the treatment and control groups were obviously different, and there was no blinding attempted. They provided detailed information on dropouts and methods of data imputation where appropriate. Therefore, this domain was judged at a "low" risk of bias for all studies. No protocol could be located for all studies and O6 and O8 were judged as "unclear" risk of bias for selective outcome reporting for both studies.

Outcomes

The studies reported on blood glucose-related (FPG, PBG, A1C), BMI and lipid metabolism-related outcomes (TG, TC, HDL, LDL).

Fasting Plasma Glucose

Two studies (O4, O6) of 147 participants compared *taichi* 太极 to aerobic exercise. The results showed that there were no significant differences between the two groups (MD −0.06 [−0.62, 0.50], I^2 = 0%). When *taichi* 太极 was compared to no treatment (*n* = 162) (O4, O6, O8), the FPG levels were significantly different between the groups (MD −1.11, [−1.73, −0.49], I^2 = 0%).

Postprandial Blood Glucose

One study (O6) of 56 participants compared *taichi* 太极 to aerobic exercise and found no significant differences between the groups for PBG levels (MD −0.32 [−1.88, 1.24]). In the same study, the no treatment group compared to *taichi* 太极 found significant differences between the groups for PBG levels (MD −2.5 [−4.56, −0.44]).

Glycated Haemoglobin

Two studies (O4, O6) of 147 participants compared *taichi* 太极 to aerobic exercise. The results showed that there were no significant differences between the two groups (MD −0.26 [−0.85, 0.32], I^2 = 62.8%). When *taichi* 太极 was compared to no treatment (*n* = 162) in the same two studies, the A1C levels were not significantly different between the groups (MD −0.60 [−1.32, 0.11], I^2 = 59.9%).

Body Mass Index

One study (O4) compared *taichi* 太极 to aerobic exercise in 91 T2DM participants and found no significant difference between the groups in the BMI (MD 0.23 [−0.93, 1.39]). When *taichi* 太极 was compared to no treatment (*n* = 87) in the same study, no significant difference was found between the groups (MD −0.8 [−3.00, 0.70]).

Triglyceride

One study (O8) compared *taichi* 太极 to no treatment in 19 participants. There was no significant difference between the groups (MD −0.13 [−0.60, 0.34]).

Total Cholesterol

One study (O4) compared *taichi* 太极 to aerobic exercise in 91 T2DM participants and found no significant difference between the groups in TC (MD 0.23 [−0.08, 0.54]). When *taichi* 太极 was compared to no treatment (*n* = 106) (O4, O8), no significant difference was found between the groups (MD −0.45 [−1.08, 0.18], I^2 = 76.2%).

Low-density Lipoprotein

One study (O8) compared *taichi* 太极 to no treatment in 19 T2DM participants and found no significant difference between the groups in LDL (MD −0.04 [−0.46, 0.38]).

High-density Lipoprotein

One study (O4) compared *taichi* 太极 to aerobic exercise in 91 T2DM participants and found no significant difference between the groups in LDL (MD 0.09 [−0.10, 0.28]). When *taichi* 太极 was compared to no treatment ($n = 106$) (O4, O8), no significant difference was found between the groups (MD 0.2 [0.02, 0.38], $I^2 = 0\%$).

Assessment using Grading of Recommendations, Assessment, Development and Evaluation

An assessment of the quality of the evidence from RCTs was made using GRADE. Interventions, comparators and outcomes to be included were selected based on a consensus process, described in Chapter 4. The comparison was *taichi* 太极 versus aerobic exercise, and the evidence was of "low" to "moderate" certainty (Table 8.2). The results showed that *taichi* 太极 may reduce blood glucose and cholesterol levels. The studies did not report on any AEs.

Safety of *Taichi* 太极

The included studies did not report on any AEs.

Tuina 推拿

One randomised controlled study (O7) was identified. The study included 45 participants and compared the treatment effect of *tuina* plus metformin to metformin alone. The treatment duration was eight weeks. *Tuina* was performed on BL17 *Geshu* 膈俞, EX-B3 *Yishu* 胰俞, BL18 *Ganshu* 肝俞, BL19 *Danshu* 胆俞, BL20 *Pishu* 脾俞, BL21 *Weishu* 胃俞, BL23 *Shenshu* 肾俞, BL22 *Sanjiaoshu* 三焦俞, CV13 *Shangwan* 上脘, CV12 *Zhongwan* 中脘, CV6 *Qihai* 气海 and CV4 *Guanyuan* 关元 for one minute each. Other acupoints included SP10 *Xuehai* 血海, ST36 *Zusanli* 足三里 and SP6 *Sanyinjiao* 三阴交.

Risk of Bias

The RCT (O7) did not provide detailed information on the method of randomisation and allocation concealment and was judged as an "unclear" risk of bias in both domains. The study was judged as

Table 8.2.   GRADE: *Taichi* 太极 **vs. Aerobic Exercise for Treating Type 2 Diabetes Mellitus**

Outcome Mean Treatment Duration	Estimated Absolute Effect		Relative Effect (95% CI) No. of Participants (Studies)	Certainty of the Evidence (GRADE)
	Oral Chinese Herbal Medicine	Pharmacotherapy		
FPG 7.5 months	**7.03** MD: 0.06 higher (95% CI: 0.62 lower to 0.5 higher)	**7.09**	**MD 0.06** (−0.62, 0.5) 147 (2 RCTs)	⊕⊕⊕⊡ MODERATE[a]
PBG 6 months	**8.22** MD: 0.32 lower (95% CI: 1.88 higher to 1.24 higher)	**8.54**	**MD −0.32** (1.88, 1.24) 56 (1 RCTs)	⊕⊕⊕⊡ MODERATE[a]
A1C 7.5 months	**7.44** MD: 0.26 lower (95% CI: 0.85 lower to 0.32 higher)	**7.7**	**MD −0.26** (−0.85, 0.32) 147 (2 RCTs)	⊕⊕⊕⊡ MODERATE[a]
TC 9 months	**4.16** MD: 0.23 lower (95% CI: 0.08 lower to 0.54 lower)	**4.39**	**MD −0.23** (−0.08. 0.54) 91 (1 RCT)	⊕⊕⊕⊡ MODERATE[a]

The risk in the intervention group (and its 95% confidence interval) is based on the assumed risk in the comparison group and the relative effect of the intervention (and its 95% CI).

Abbreviations: A1C, glycated haemoglobin; CI, confidence interval; FPG, fasting plasma glucose; GRADE, Grading of Recommendations, Assessment, Development and Evaluation; MD, mean difference; PBG, postprandial blood glucose; RCTs, randomised controlled trials; TC, total cholesterol.

Note:
[a]Wide confidence interval and small sample size.
[b]Considerable statistical heterogeneity.

References:

FPG: O4, O6
PBG: O6
A1C: O4, O6
TC: O4

"high" risk for the blinding of participants, personnel and outcome assessors, as the treatment and control groups were obviously different and there was no blinding attempted. The studies provided detailed information on dropouts and methods of data imputation where appropriate. Therefore, this domain was judged as a "low" risk of bias. The study reported on outcomes that were not included in the Methods section and was therefore judged as a "high" risk of bias for selective outcome reporting.

Outcomes

The studies reported on blood glucose-related outcomes FPG and PBG.

Fasting Plasma Glucose

After eight weeks of treatment, a significant difference was found between the groups for FPG (MD −1.5 [−2.64, −0.36]).

Postprandial Blood Glucose

After eight weeks of treatment, a significant difference was found between the groups for PBG (MD −1.5 [−2.44, −0.56]).

Safety of *Tuina* 推拿

The study did not report on any AEs.

Summary of Other Chinese Medicine Clinical Evidence

There is limited clinical evidence for other CM therapies treatments for diabetes mellitus, thus further research is to be carried out. *Baduanjin* 八段锦 was the most frequently evaluated intervention as it was tested in five clinical studies. The combination of *baduanjin* 八段锦 and sulfonylur significantly improved aspects of glucose metabolism (FPG, A1C levels) and lipid metabolism (TG, TC, LDL and HDL levels). When comparing *baduanjin* 八段锦 to no treatment, metformin or aerobic exercise, improvements for glucose and lipid metabolism are seen, but there are no significant differences between the treatment groups. Taken together, the body of evidence is small, and future research is required to further elucidate the role of *baduanjin* 八段锦 in the treatment of diabetes mellitus. *Taichi* 太极 was another type of CM physical exercise tested in the included studies. *Taichi* 太极 showed a benefit in improving FPG levels as compared to no treatment, but no benefit was seen in PBG levels. Although there was an improvement trend, no significant difference was found for glucose or lipid metabolism when *taichi* 太极 and aerobic exercise were compared; however, the certainty of the evidence was moderate. The *baduanjin* 八段锦 and *taichi* 太极 studies did not report on any AEs.

CM diet therapy is recommended in the clinical guidelines and textbooks described in Chapter 2. Conflicting evidence was found in controlled trials. Two RCTs found significant improvement in FPG levels, but not PBG, TG, TC, LDL or HDL levels. There was no reporting of any AEs in the two RCTs; one non-controlled study reported that there were no AEs during the study.

Tuina 推拿 is a recommended therapy in the clinical guidelines and textbooks described in Chapter 2. However, only one RCT met the inclusion criteria for this review. Reasons for the lack of eligible controlled trials is not clear.

Due to the small number of included studies and methodological limitations, there is currently only limited evidence for the efficacy and safety of other CM therapies for diabetes.

References

1. 何方敏, 孟繁洁, 靳英辉. (2012) 中医食疗治疗糖尿病的系统评价. 护理实践与研究 **9**(21): 1–3.
2. 唐青, 郭瑜洁, 李萍, *et al*. (2017) 太极拳在2型糖尿病患者中应用效果的Meta分析. 现代预防医学 **44**(14): 2516–2521.
3. 刘永进, 杜博, 黄博威, *et al*. (2017) 太极拳锻炼对2型糖尿病患者糖脂代谢和生活质量影响的系统评价. 康复学报 **27**(4): 55–59.
4. 杨继鹏, 刘琛莹, 吕纹良, *et al*. (2015) 健身气功八段锦治疗2型糖尿病疗效的Meta分析. 中华中医药杂志 **30**(4): 1307–1309.

References for Included Other Chinese Medicine Therapies Clinical Studies

Study No.	Reference
O1	黄荣春, 邓新但. (2011) 八段锦治疗 2 型糖尿病. 河北中医 **33**(12): 1828–1829.
O2	李婉婷. (2016) 薯蓣粥对 2 型糖尿病患者血糖, 血脂的影响. 福建中医药大学硕士学位论文., 中国福州.
O3	李岳. (2017) 八段锦运动干预对新发 2 型糖尿病患者临床疗效研究. 辽宁中医药大学学报 **19**(8).
O4	李智滨, 齐丽丽, 赵磊, 刘恒亮. (2013) 八段锦在 2 型糖尿病患者有氧运动治疗中的优势. 辽宁中医杂志 **40**(9): 1858–1860.
O5	林丰兰, 叶彬华, 陈桂铭, 兰花兰. (2014) 玉泉散馒头辅助治疗气阴两虚型 2 型糖尿病 40 例. 福建中医药 **45**(4): 9–10.
O6	唐渊博. (2014) 太极拳辅助治疗 2 型糖尿病的量效关系研究. 南京中医药大学硕士学位论文, 中国南京.
O7	张世勤. (2008) 推拿配合药物治疗 2 型糖尿病 24 例临床观察.吉林中医药 **28**(3): 177–178.
O8	Zhan, Y, Fu FH. (2008) Effects of 14-week Tai Ji Quan exercise on metabolic control in women with Type 2 diabetes. *Am J Chinese Med* **36**(4): 647–654.
O9	周嘉琪. (2012) 健身气功八段锦辅助治疗 2 型糖尿病患者的临床观察性研究. 南京中医药大学硕士学位论文, 中国南京.
O10	蔡缨, 沈忠松. (2006) 茯苓对老年 2 型糖尿病降糖效果观察.解放军预防医学杂志 **24**(3): 198–199.
O11	胡源, 何珂, 朱丽华, *et al.* (2017) 八段锦及步行运动对 2 型糖尿病患者餐后血糖的影响. 浙江中西医结合杂志 **27**(11): 963–965.

9

Clinical Evidence for Combination Therapies

OVERVIEW

Clinical practice of Chinese medicine (CM) often sees several therapy types used in combination, such as Chinese herbal medicine (CHM) plus acupuncture. Twelve studies including eight randomised controlled trials, two controlled clinical trials, and two non-controlled studies were reviewed in this chapter. The most common combination was CHM with acupuncture therapies. The combination of CM therapies showed beneficial effects for type 2 diabetes mellitus (T2DM) by improving blood glucose metabolism and lipid metabolism.

Introduction

Combination CM Therapies are defined as two or more CM interventions from different categories administered together, for example, herbal medicine plus acupuncture, herbal medicine plus *qigong* 气功, or herbal medicine plus *tuina* 推拿. This is a common approach in clinical practice. No previous systematic review of combination therapies was identified.

Identification of Clinical Studies

A search of electronic databases identified 66,570 potentially relevant citations. After the removal of duplicates, the title and abstracts of citations were read, and more than 41,729 irrelevant citations

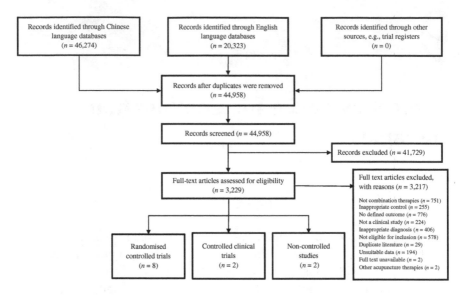

Figure 9.1. Flow chart of study selection process: Combination therapies.

were excluded (Figure 9.1). The full texts of 3,229 articles were reviewed. In total, 12 clinical studies that evaluated combinations of CM therapy were included. Eight were randomised controlled trials (RCTs), two were controlled clinical trials (CCTs), and two were non-controlled case series. Studies are indicated by the letter "C" and then followed by a number, and references for these studies can be found at the end of the chapter.

Randomised Controlled Trials of Combination Therapies

Eight studies (C1–C8) were identified as RCTs of combinations therapies. A total of 916 participants were included in the studies. The most common syndrome reported was phlegm-dampness with Blood stasis 痰湿血瘀, *yin* deficiency with excessive heat 阴虚热盛, and Kidney deficiency 肾虚. Included therapies were:

- CHM plus acupuncture (C4, C5),
- CHM plus acupuncture plus metformin (C7),

- CHM plus *tuina* 推拿 plus pioglitazone (C1, C6),
- CHM plus *baduanjin* 八段锦 plus metformin (C2),
- CHM plus moxibustion plus sulfonylureas and α-Glucosidase inhibitors (C8), and
- CHM plus acupuncture, massage, CM diet therapy and metformin (C3).

Risk of Bias

One study (C3) used a random number table for sequence generation and was assessed as a "low" risk of bias. Two studies (C1, C6) used a patient ID number for sequence generation and were judged as "high" risk for this domain. None of the studies described methods of allocation concealment and were assessed as an "unclear" risk. All studies were judged as "high" risk for blinding due to the nature of the interventions and comparators. Where applicable, reasons for dropping out were reported and dropout numbers were balanced between the groups. These studies were assessed as a "low" risk of bias for incomplete outcome data. One study (C5) did not report on the reasons for drop-outs and was judged as an "unclear" risk of bias for this domain. Two studies (C7, C3) either did not report on all planned outcomes or only reported on outcomes that were not planned, and therefore were judged as "high" risk of bias for selective reporting. No protocols were identified for the remaining studies and these studies were assessed as "unclear" risk of bias for selective reporting.

Clinical Evidence for Combination Therapies from Randomised Controlled Trials

Chinese Herbal Medicine Plus Acupuncture

Two studies (C4, C5) of 350 participants compared the effect of CHM plus acupuncture to hypoglycaemic agents. Meta-analysis results showed significant improvement in fasting plasma glucose (FPG) levels (MD −1.12 [−1.50, −0.73], I^2 = 0%) and postprandial blood glucose (PBG) levels (MD −2.76 [−3.44, −2.09], I^2 = 0%). One study

(C4) with 70 participants reported on glycated haemoglobin (A1C) levels but did not find significant differences between the two groups (MD −0.2 [−0.84, 0.44]). The studies did not report on any adverse events (AEs).

Chinese Herbal Medicine Plus Acupuncture Plus Metformin

One study (C7) with 64 participants evaluated the effect of CHM plus acupuncture as integrative medicine compared to metformin alone. The mean PBG levels were significantly different between the groups (MD −1.52 [−2.48, −0.56]), but there was no significant difference between the groups for FPG levels (MD −0.09 [−1.09, 0.91]) and A1C levels (MD −0.98 [−2.07, 0.11]). The study reported that there were no AEs.

Chinese Herbal Medicine Plus Tuina 推拿 Plus Pioglitazone

Two studies (C1, C6) of 280 participants compared the effect of CHM plus *tuina* 推拿 and pioglitazone to pioglitazone alone. Meta-analysis results showed significant improvement in FPG, PBG, triglyceride (TG), total cholesterol (TC), low-density lipoprotein (LDL), and high-density lipoprotein (HDL) levels. The results are presented in Table 9.1. CHM plus *tuina* 推拿 and pioglitazone (160 participants) significantly improved A1C levels (MD −0.83 [−1.25, −0.41]) (C1). The studies did not report on any AEs.

Chinese Herbal Medicine Plus *Baduanjin* 八段锦 Plus Metformin

One RCT (C2) assessed CHM plus *baduanjin* 八段锦 and metformin with metformin alone. Combination Therapies as Integrative Medicine in 40 participants after two months of treatment showed significant improvement in FPG levels (MD −1.22 [−1.64, −0.80]), PBG levels (MD −2.15, [−2.72, −1.60]) and A1C levels (MD −1.03 [−1.51, −0.55]). The study did not report on any AEs.

Table 9.1.   Evidence for Combination Therapies from Randomised Controlled Trials

Outcome	No. of Studies (Participants)	Effect Estimate (MD, 95% CI, I²%)	Included Studies
CHM plus acupuncture vs. hypoglycaemic agents			
FPG	2(350)	MD −1.12 [−1.50, −0.73]*, 0.0%	C4, C5
PBG	2(350)	MD −2.76 [−3.44, −2.09]*, 0.0%	C4, C5
A1C	1(70)	MD −0.2 [−0.84, 0.44]	C4
CHM plus acupuncture plus metformin vs. metformin			
FPG	1(64)	MD −0.09 [−1.09, 0.91]*	C7
PBG	1(64)	MD −1.52 [−2.48, −0.56]*	C7
A1C	1(64)	MD −0.98 [−2.07, 0.11]	C7
CHM plus tuina 推拿 plus pioglitazone vs. pioglitazone			
FPG	2(280)	MD −1.12 [−1.45, −0.78]*, 0.0%	C1, C6
PBG	2(280)	MD −0.84 [−1.13, −0.54]*, 0.0%	C1, C6
A1C	1(160)	MD −0.83 [−1.25, −0.41]*	C1
TG	2(280)	MD −0.46 [−0.65, −0.27]*, 0.0%	C1, C6
TC	2(280)	MD −0.44 [−0.72, −0.16]*, 0.0%	C1, C6
LDL	2(280)	MD −0.44, [−0.61, −0.28]*, 0.0%	C1, C6
HDL	2(280)	MD 0.34 [0.25, 0.43]*, 0.0%	C1, C6
CHM plus baduanjin 八段锦 plus metformin vs. metformin			
FPG	1(40)	MD −1.22 [−1.64, −0.80]*	C2
PBG	1(40)	MD −2.15, [−2.72, −1.60]*	C2
A1C	1(40)	MD −1.03 [−1.51, −0.55]*	C2
CHM plus moxibustion plus sulfonylureas and α-glucosidase inhibitors vs. sulfonylureas and α-glucosidase inhibitors			
FPG	1(48)	MD −1.91 [−3.10, −0.72]	C8
PBG	1(48)	MD −2.92 [−4.27, −1.57]*	C8
A1C	1(48)	MD −1.25 [−2.16, −0.34]*	C8
TG	1(48)	MD −1.05 [−1.29, −0.81]*	C8
TC	1(48)	MD −1.63 [−2.17, −1.09]*	C8
LDL	1(48)	MD −1.16 [−1.52, −0.8]*	C8
HDL	1(48)	MD −0.06 [−0.20, 0.08]	C8

Table 9.1. (*Continued*)

Outcome	No. of Studies (Participants)	Effect Estimate (MD, 95% CI, I²%)	Included Studies
CHM plus acupuncture, Chinese medicine diet therapy and metformin vs. metformin			
FPG	1(128)	MD −0.8 [−1.37, −0.23]	C3
PBG	1(128)	MD −1.28 [−2.21, −0.36]*	C3
A1C	1(128)	MD −0.49 [−0.91, −0.07]*	C3
TG	1(128)	MD −0.58 [−1.14, −0.02]*	C3
TC	1(128)	MD −0.68 [−1.11, −0.26]*	C3
LDL	1(128)	MD −0.49 [−0.85, −0.13]*	C3
HDL	1(128)	MD 0.62 [0.34, 0.90]*	C3
BMI	1(128)	MD −1.61 [−3.27, 0.05]	C3

* Statistically significant, see Chapter 4, Statistical Analysis.

Abbreviations: A1C, glycated haemoglobin; BMI, body mass index; CHM, Chinese herbal medicine; CI, confidence interval; CM, Chinese medicine; FPG, fasting plasma glucose; HDL, high-density lipoprotein; LDL, low-density lipoprotein; MD, mean difference; PBG, postprandial blood glucose; TC, total cholesterol; TG, total glycerol.

Chinese Herbal Medicine Plus Moxibustion Plus Sulfonylureas and α-Glucosidase Inhibitors

One RCT (C8) assessed CHM plus moxibustion and hypoglycaemic agents to hypoglycaemic agents alone. The combination therapies as integrative medicine in 48 participants after eight weeks of treatment found significant differences between the groups in FPG, PBG, A1C, TG, TC, LDL levels, but not HDL levels. The results are presented in Table 9.1. The study did not report on any AEs.

Chinese Herbal Medicine Plus Acupuncture, Massage, Chinese Medicine Diet Therapy and Metformin

One RCT (C3) assessed various CM therapies, including CHM, acupuncture, massage, Chinese medicine diet therapy, and metformin. The combination therapy was combined with hypoglycaemic agents and compared to hypoglycaemic agents alone. The results highlighted that combination therapies as integrative medicine in 48 participants after eight weeks of treatment showed significant improvement in FPG, PBG, A1C, TG, TC, LDL and HDL levels (Table 9.1). The combined therapies did not show significant improvement in body mass index (BMI) (MD −1.61 [−3.27, 0.05]). The study reported that there were no AEs.

Controlled Clinical Trials of Combination Therapies

Two non-randomised CCTs were included. One study (C3) compared CM treatment and diet therapy to no treatments. This study did not include syndrome differentiation. In 584 participants, six months of treatment showed significant difference between groups for FPG (MD −0.6 [−0.9, −0.3]), PBG (MD −1.5 [−2.07, −0.93]) and A1C (MD −0.4 [−0.66, −0.14]) levels.

Another study (C10) included 30 patients, where treatment involved 12 weeks of ear acupressure plus Chinese medicine diet therapy, compared to guideline-recommended hypoglycaemic agents. The results showed significant differences between groups for FPG (MD −0.83 [−1.61, −0.05]) and A1C levels (MD −0.99 [−1.12, −0.56]), but not TG (MD −0.48 [−1.19, 0.23]) or TC levels (MD −0.62 [−1.57, 0.33]). The included CCT studies did not report on any AEs.

Non-Controlled Studies of Combination Therapies

Two non-controlled studies of Combination Therapies were identified. A total of 92 participants were included in the studies. One study (C11) assessed the effect of CHM, acupuncture and *taichi* 太极, and aerobic exercise for T2DM for six months in 52 participants. The authors reported that combination therapies improved BMI. They also reported AEs — eight cases reported local bruising, and five cases reported abdominal pain and sweating after exercising within 20 minutes of food consumption, but they could continue with treatments once this was corrected.

One study (C12) assessed *baduanjian* 八段锦 and *taichi* 太极. The study included 40 participants for 12 weeks. Significant improvements in FPG and A1C levels were observed in the participants. No AEs were reported.

Summary of Clinical Evidence for Combination Therapies

This chapter evaluated the combination of two or more CM therapies used in the management of diabetes mellitus. Diversity was seen in the CM combinations in the included studies ($n = 12$), and the most common combination of CM therapies was CHM plus acupuncture ($n = 4$). The combination of CHM and acupuncture therapies showed beneficial effects for T2DM by improving blood glucose metabolism and lipid metabolism. When the duo was used as integrative therapy with metformin, conflicting results showed a benefit in improving PBG levels but not FPG or A1C levels.

When Combination Therapies were used as integrative therapy with hypoglycaemic agents, the combination of CHM plus *tuina* 推拿 and CHM plus *baduanjin* 八段锦 significantly improved the levels of FPG, PBG and A1C.

Oral CHM was used in eight out of 12 studies. The CHM formulae of the studies investigated were diverse, with no overlap across studies. The most frequently used herbs were *huang qi* 黄芪, *ze xie* 泽泻, *sheng di huang* 生地黄, *shan yao* 山药, *zhi mu* 知母 and *bai zhu* 白术. Based on the actions of these herbs, the key aim of the CHM treatment was to nourish *yin*, nourish *qi*, remove dampness, strengthen the Spleen and generate fluids. For studies that used acupuncture therapy (including moxibustion), the most frequently used points across studies were ST36 *Zusanli* 足三里 and SP6 *Sanyinjiao* 三阴交, mainly to strengthen the Spleen and Stomach. The ear point Pancreas was used in two studies. Different combinations of herbs and acupoints were used across studies, so there is no indication of a beneficial combination from the included studies.

Two included RCTs (C7, C3), two CCTs (C9, C10), and one non-controlled clinical trial (C12) reported that there were no AEs. Acupuncture-related local bruising was reported in one study assessing the combination of CHM, acupuncture and *taichi* 太极 for T2DM. The remaining six studies did not report on the safety of CM Combination Therapies.

Clinical studies in this review did not include studies comparing two or more CM therapies to only one of the therapies (e.g., CHM plus acupuncture vs. CHM). Therefore, it is unclear whether combining CM therapies is more beneficial than the use of CM interventions individually.

Overall, there is insufficient evidence for the efficacy and safety of combination therapies of CM for the treatment of T2DM. Results from the included studies do not provide sufficient evidence for clinical guideline recommendations. Further research is needed to evaluate CM combination therapies for the management of T2DM.

References for Included Combination Therapies Clinical Studies

Study No.	Reference
C1	曹晶晶, 杨卫杰. (2015) 自拟祛痰化瘀汤合推拿治疗痰瘀型 2 型糖尿病临床观. 光明中医 **30**(4): 762–763.
C2	林峻丞. (2011) 中药结合八段锦治疗 2 型糖尿病的疗效观. 南京中医药大学硕士学位论文, 中国南京.
C3	林玉平. (2015) "动—定序贯八法" 2 型糖尿病养生方案的构建及临床研究. 广州中医药大学博士学位论文, 中国广州.
C4	石艳凌, 李丽, 王庆杰. (2014) 参芪降糖片结合针刺治疗 2 型糖尿病临床观察. 内蒙古中医药 **10**: 41–42.
C5	汪凤祥. (2012) 葛根降糖汤合针刺治疗 2 型糖尿病临床观察. 中国保健营养 1653.
C6	汪建平, 曹晶晶, 杨卫杰, 陈英. (2013) 中西医结合治疗 2 型糖尿病胰岛素抵抗 60 例. 中国中医药现代远程教育 **11**(19): 58–59.
C7	杨继英. (2015) 针药结合治疗痰湿型 2 型糖尿病 32 例疗效观察. 中国民间疗法 **23**(6): 65–66.
C8	袁艳娟. (2015) 益肾化瘀汤联合穴位艾灸治疗老年 2 型糖尿病临床研究. 亚太传统医药 **11**(20): 70–71.

(Continued)

(Continued)

Study No.	Reference
C9	马桂芳, 朱秀英, 张莹, *et al.* (2017) 中医体质干预在 2 型糖尿病患者中的应用及效果评价. 重庆医学 **46**: 2–3.
C10	季春艳. (2014) 耳穴埋籽联合辨证饮食指导护理对 2 型糖尿病患者糖脂代谢影响的临床研究. 江苏中医药 **46**(11): 60–61.
C11	潘虹霞, 陈志明, 李军. (2010) 多种中医方法治疗新诊断 2 型糖尿病 52 例. 现代中西医结合杂志 **19**(6): 670–671.
C12	张函菲. (2015) 中医特色运动处方治疗 2 型糖尿病的临床观察. 北京中医药大学硕士学位论文, 中国北京.

10

Summary and Conclusions

OVERVIEW

This chapter summarises the main findings of previous chapters, including those from classical literature, clinical trial evidence, and experimental evidence. Chinese medicine therapies, including herbal medicine and acupuncture, are discussed regarding the clinical management of type 2 diabetes mellitus. Limitations of the available evidence are reported, and future directions identified for clinical and experimental research.

Introduction

Chinese medicine (CM) therapies, often in combination with pharmacotherapies, are used as a part of the management of type 2 diabetes mellitus (T2DM). Current conventional management of T2DM includes prevention, pharmacological and non-pharmacological interventions with a goal to achieve a target glycaemic level in the individual. Prevention of T2DM occurs when individuals identified at a high risk of developing T2DM are screened and take lifestyle interventions, pharmacologic agents and diabetes self-management education and support programs to prevent the progression of diabetes development.

Metformin is considered the first-line therapy for T2DM; it has been shown to be effective, safe, cost-effective and is even used as a preventative therapy for diabetes in pre-diabetic patients.[1,2] For most patients, metformin will be used in combination with lifestyle modifications. Lifestyle management is a fundamental part of managing

T2DM. Diabetes self-management education and support, nutrition therapy, prescribed physical activity, and psychosocial care are all part of lifestyle management for diabetes. Each therapy plays a crucial role in reaching the glycaemic goal and maintaining it. However, current therapies do not slow the loss of beta cells. Clinically, T2DM is a lifelong and progressive disease and requires lifelong management.

This monograph includes a "whole-evidence" analysis of CM for the management of T2DM. A review of clinical guidelines and text-books has identified the main syndromes for T2DM and recommended CM treatments, including oral Chinese herbal medicine (CHM) and acupuncture (Chapter 2). A review of the classical literature identified the traditional use of herbal medicine (Chapter 3). Many clinical trials reveal the promising benefits of oral CHM for T2DM (Chapter 5). Current available pre-clinical evidence has also been reviewed to explain the probable mechanisms of action of the commonly used herbs (Chapter 6). There are a limited number of acupuncture studies for T2DM, and the available evidence did not suggest that adding acupuncture to pharmacotherapy adds benefit to fasting glucose level (Chapter 7). The evaluation of other CM therapies such as *baduanjin* 八段锦, *taichi* 太极, *tuina* 推拿 and diet therapy for T2DM in clinical studies are limited, and further research is warranted (Chapter 8). The combination of CHM plus other CM therapies was evaluated in a limited number of studies with some evidence of benefit (Chapter 9).

Chinese Medicine Syndrome Differentiation

Current clinical guidelines and textbooks categorise T2DM into 10 syndromes according to the presenting signs and symptoms.[3–6] For each syndrome, formulae with modifications according to a different symptom are suggested as a guide for clinical practice (Chapter 2). In classical literature (Chapter 3), there was an emphasis on T2DM being caused by heat and the deficiency of *zang fu* 脏腑, which are the two main factors that cause diabetes. Ancient citations also recognise that overeating could be another main cause of diabetes.

Most CHM clinical studies did not specify the use of CM syndromes for the selection of CHM interventions in people with T2DM, but a few studies did use syndrome differentiation as inclusion criteria or as criteria for selecting the formula used. The most common syndromes were generally consistent with those mentioned in the clinical practice guidelines (Chapter 2), although there were some differences. In studies that described CM syndromes, the common syndromes included *qi* and *yin* deficiency 气阴两虚, *yin* deficiency and excessive heat 阴虚热盛, damp heat obstructing the Spleen 湿热困脾, phlegm-dampness and Blood stasis 痰湿血瘀.

In the acupuncture RCTs, no studies mentioned syndrome differentiation. In the non-controlled acupuncture studies, the most commonly reported syndrome was a deficiency of both *qi* and *yin* 气阴两虚, Lung heat and damage to the *jin* liquid 肺热伤津, and excessive Stomach heat 胃热. Studies assessing other CM therapies did not mention syndrome differentiation. In the nine combination CM therapy RCTs, the most common syndrome was phlegm-dampness and Blood stasis 痰湿血瘀, *yin* deficiency with excessive heat 阴虚热盛, and Kidney deficiency 肾虚证.

For CHM studies, syndrome differentiation was used as a classifying factor to pool studies and analyse whether a particular syndrome was more or less effective in producing a positive effect in the clinical studies. Mixed results were produced with statistical heterogeneity, so no firm conclusion could be drawn.

Chinese Herbal Medicine

In total, 236 clinical studies evaluated CHM for T2DM. Most studies were randomised controlled trials (RCTs) and compared CHM to hypoglycaemic drugs, or administered a combination of CHM and hypoglycaemic drugs, compared to hypoglycaemic drugs alone. All the CHM interventions were orally administered. Of the hypoglycaemic drugs, biguanides were the most frequently used.

The outcomes with sufficient data suitable for pooling were the blood glucose measurements, such as fasting plasma glucose (FPG), postprandial blood glucose (PBG), glycated haemoglobin (A1C);

plasma lipids (triglycerides [TG], cholesterol [TC], low-density lipo-protein [LDL], high-density lipoprotein [HDL]); and β-cell function (fasting insulin [FINS], Homeostasis Model Assessment-Insulin Resistance [HOMO-IR], Homeostasis Model Assessment-Insulin Sensitivity [HOMO-IS]). Other outcomes like body mass index (BMI), quality of life, and fasting Oh C-peptide (CP) were not commonly used. Most studies provided data at the end of the treatment period (after two to 24 weeks of treatment).

Compared to hypoglycaemic agents, CHM reduced PBG and plasma lipids (TG, TC, LDL), increased HDL, and improved the β-cell function as indicated by FINS and the insulin resistance index. However, the meta-analysis results showed moderate-to-high statistical heterogeneity, and the source of heterogeneity could not be identified by subgroup analysis. Baseline FBG levels, age of patients, disease history, and different CHM interventions in terms of treatment duration, ingredients, dosage and medication compliance may be the cause of heterogeneity.

Meta-analysis also showed that CHM reduced blood glucose (FBG, PBG, HbA$_{1c}$), improved plasma lipids (TG, TC, LDL, HDL) and FINS, compared with placebo and lifestyle intervention. Despite the positive results, there were a limited number of studies with small sample sizes.

When CHM was combined with hypoglycaemic drugs (Integrative Medicine), the pooled results showed more benefits than hypogly-caemic drugs alone in terms of reducing the value of blood glucose (included FBG, PBG, HbA$_{1c}$), BMI and improving blood lipids (TG, TC, LDL, HDL) and β-cell function (FINS, IR, IS). Despite the positive results, there was considerable heterogeneity, which might be due to inconsistency across studies in terms of the patient's condition, compliance, CHM used, study protocols, treatment duration, and outcome measurement.

In terms of safety of CHM, the total adverse events (AEs) in the CHM groups, either CHM alone or integrative CHM, was less than that in the control groups.

Chinese Herbal Medicine Formulae in Key Clinical Guidelines and Textbooks, Classical Literature and Clinical Studies

This section summarises the evidence from Chapters 2, 3 and 5. Overall, the CHM used for T2DM is different between classical literature, contemporary clinical practice guidelines, and clinical trials, but there were also consistent formulae (see Table 10.1).

Table 10.1. Summary of Chinese Herbal Medicine Formulae

| Formula Name | Included in Clinical Guidelines and Textbooks (Chapter 2) | Included in Classical Literature (No. of Citations) | Included in Clinical Studies (Chapter 5) | | | Included in Combination Therapies (Chapter 9) |
			RCTs (No. of Studies)	CCTs (No. of Studies)	Non-controlled Studies (No. of Studies)	
Oral formulae						
Bai hu jia ren shen tang 白虎加人参汤	Yes	18	2	0	0	1
Bu yang huanwu tang 补阳还五汤	Yes	0	0	0	0	0
Da chai hu tang 大柴胡汤	Yes	0	0	0	0	0
Gen gen qin lian tang 葛根芩连汤	Yes	0	1	0	0	0
Liu wei di huang wan 六味地黄丸	Yes	32	5	0	0	0
Modified *Dang gui bu xue tang* 当归补血汤	Yes	0	0	0	0	0
Modified *Huo pu xia ling tang* 藿朴夏苓汤加减	Yes	0	0	0	0	0

(Continued)

Table 10.1. (Continued)

Formula Name	Included in Clinical Guidelines and Textbooks (Chapter 2)	Included in Classical Literature (No. of Citations)	Included in Clinical Studies (Chapter 5)			Included in Combination Therapies (Chapter 9)
			RCTs (No. of Studies)	CCTs (No. of Studies)	Non-controlled Studies (No. of Studies)	
Modified *Si miao san* 四妙散	Yes	0	0	0	0	0
Modified *Si ni san* 四逆散加减	Yes	0	0	0	0	0
Modified *Tao hong si wu tan* 桃红四物汤	Yes	0	0	0	0	0
Modified *Wu ling san* 五苓散	Yes	0	0	0	0	0
Modified *Yin chen hao tang* 茵陈蒿汤	Yes	0	0	0	0	0
Modified *Zuo gui wan* 左归丸	Yes	0	0	0	0	0
Shen qi wan 肾气丸	Yes	31	0	0	0	0
Xiao ke fang 消渴方	Yes	0	3	0	0	0
Xiao xian xiong tang 小陷胸汤	Yes	0	0	0	0	0
Yu nv jian 玉女煎	No	3	2	0	0	0
Yu quan wan 玉泉丸	Yes	0	3	0	0	0
Yu ye tang 玉液汤	Yes	0	0	0	0	0
Manufactured products						
Huang lian su pian 黄连素片	No	0	4	0	0	0
Jin li da ke li 津力达颗粒	Yes	0	4	0	0	0
Shen qi jiang tang ke li/pian 参芪降糖颗粒/片	Yes	0	4	1	0	0

Abbreviations: CCTs, controlled clinical trials; RCTs, randomised controlled trials.

Fifteen formulae were specified in Chapter 2 based on CM syndrome differentiation. These are generally consistent with the most frequently used formulae in the classic literature, including *Liu wei di huang wan* 六味地黄丸, *Shen qi wan* 肾气丸 and *Ren shen bai hu tang* 人参白虎汤.

Out of these, *Shen qi wan* 肾气丸, which is used for deficiency of Kidney *yang*, was recommended in guidelines but not researched in clinical trials. This is likely to be because *Shen qi wan* 肾气丸 is composed of *Liu wei di huang wan* 六味地黄丸 plus *gui zhi* 桂枝 and *fu zi* 附子. *Shen qi wan* is mainly used for the treatment of insufficient Kidney *yang*, weakness in the lower back and knees, cold limbs, difficulty or frequent urination. However, there are few diabetic patients with a single deficiency of Kidney *yang*, which is often combined with the deficiency of Kidney *yin* or Blood stasis. Therefore, treatment is to supplement *yang* or invigorate Blood stasis on the basis of *Liu wei di huang wan* 六味地黄丸. The common formulae in the clinical trials were *Shen qi jiang tang ke li* 参芪降糖颗粒, *Jin li da ke li* 津力达颗粒, *Huang lian su pian* 黄连素片, *Xiao ke fang* 消渴方, *Yu quan wan* 玉泉丸, *Shen di sheng jin jiao nang* 参地生津胶囊, *Tian mai xiao ke pian* 天麦消渴片, *Da huang huang lian xie xin tang* 大黄黄连泻心汤 and *Yu nv jian* 玉女煎.

A few formulae found in Chinese clinical guidelines have not been investigated in clinical studies and classical literature; these include *Xiao xian xiong tang* 小陷胸汤 and *Yu ye tang* 玉液汤. This may be because *Xiao xian xiong tang* 小陷胸汤 has a focus on removing phlegm, dampness and heat. It is used for diabetic patients who are obese, suffer from thirst, prefer cold drinks, drink lots of water, have abdominal distension, possess a bigger appetite and get hungry easily, feel irritable, experience a bitter taste in the mouth, and have dry stool and yellow urine. At present, many doctors will choose another famous CM formula — *Ge gen qin lian tang* 葛根芩连汤 for T2DM, the clinical efficacy of this formula is similar to *Xiao xian xiong tang* 小陷胸汤. *Ge gen qin lian tang* 葛根芩连汤 has four herbs and shows hypoglycaemic effects. It was also recommended in the clinical guidelines of conventional medicine for the treatment of T2DM. On another note, *Yu ye tang* 玉液汤 and *Yu quan wan* 玉泉丸 are both used for treating the deficiency of both *qi* and *yin* in

T2DM. The herbal ingredients of the formulae are the same, and the pills are convenient to take. This may have been why Yu quan wan 玉泉丸 is used more in clinical trials instead of Yu ye tang 玉液汤.

The most commonly used formula in clinical trials was *Liu wei di huang wan* 六味地黄丸, which appeared in five RCTs. *Liu wei di huang wan* 六味地黄丸, combined with conventional therapy, showed benefits in terms of reducing the value of blood glucose (FBG, PBG, A1C), improving blood lipids (TG, TC, LDL, HDL), and β-cell function (FINS, IR, CP). The total number of AEs in integrative medicine groups was less than that in the control groups. *Liu wei di huang wan* 六味地黄丸 was also recommended in textbooks and professional books for Kidney *yin* deficiency syndrome for T2DM. *Liu wei di huang wan* 六味地黄丸 was the most cited formula in classical literature citations and is also recommended in contemporary clinical practice guidelines and textbooks.

Another frequently researched formula in clinical trials was *Shen qi jiang tang ke li* 参芪降糖颗粒. It is a formula in the form of granules, which appeared in four RCTs and one non-controlled study. The granule ingredients include ginsenoside 人参皂甙, *wu wei zi* 五味子, *huang qi* 黄芪, *shan yao* 山药, *sheng di huang* 生地黄, *fu pen zi* 覆盆子, *mai men dong* 麦门冬, *fu ling* 茯苓, *tian hua fen* 天花粉, *ze xie* 泽泻 and *gou qi zi* 枸杞子. When used in combination with conventional treatment, *Shen qi jiang tang ke li* 参芪降糖颗粒 showed benefits in reducing the value of blood glucose (FBG, PBG, A1C), improving blood lipids (TG, TC, LDL, HDL), and β-cell function (FINS, IR).

Other patent products that were researched were *Jin li da ke li* 津力达颗粒 and *Huang lian su pian* 黄连素片, which appeared in four RCTs separately.

Jin li da ke li 津力达颗粒 is a compound preparation of modern Chinese medicine, which consists of *ren shen* 人参, *huang jing* 黄精, *cang zhu* 苍术, *ku shen* 苦参, *mai men dong* 麦门冬, *di huang* 地黄, *he shou wu* 何首乌, *shan zhu yu* 山茱萸, *fu ling* 茯苓, *pei lan* 佩兰, *huang lian* 黄连, *zhi mu* 知母, *yin yang huo* 淫羊藿, *dan shen* 丹参, *ge gen* 葛根, *li zhi he* 荔枝核 and *di gu pi* 地骨皮. It is recommended for the treatment of deficiency of both *qi* and *yin* in T2DM in the *Guidelines for Prevention and Treatment of* Type 2 Diabetes Mellitus, published by the Chinese Diabetes Society.[5]

Jin li da ke li 津力达颗粒, added to conventional treatments (metformin, insulin, sitagliptin), compared to conventional treatments, showed benefits in terms of reducing the value of blood glucose (FBG, PBG, A1C), improving blood lipids (TG, TC) and β-cell function (included FINS, IR).

Huang lian su pian 黄连素片 mainly consisted of berberine hydrochloride. When compared to lifestyle intervention, *Huang lian su pian* 黄连素片 showed benefits in terms of reducing the value of blood glucose (included FBG, PBG, A1C) and improving β-cell function (FINS). Compared to a placebo, *Huang lian su pian* 黄连素片 reduced the value of FBG, PBG, A1C, TG, TC and LDL. *Huang lian su pian* 黄连素片 alone or combined with metformin reduced the value of FBG, A1C, TG, TC and LDL.

Ge gen qin lian tang 葛根芩连汤 is a classical formula that was also found in clinical studies and is recommended in clinical guidelines of the Chinese Diabetes Society. Despite current clinical trial research, more high-quality RCTs are needed to further confirm their efficacy and safety.

Experts in T2DM and CM were consulted to identify important clinical questions. Grading of Recommendations, Assessment, Development and Evaluation (GRADE) assessments were used to assess the quality of evidence (Chapter 5, Tables 5.27 and 5.28). When oral CHM was compared to hypoglycaemic agents, moderate certainty evidence showed the benefit of oral CHM in reducing levels of FPG and TC (Chapter 5, Table 5.27). No difference was seen between groups for FPG. Moderate certainty evidence favoured oral CHM at reducing TC levels. Low certainty evidence favoured oral CHM at reducing levels of PBG, TG and FINS (Chapter 5, Table 5.27).

When comparing oral CHM plus hypoglycaemic agents to hypoglycaemic agents alone, moderate certainty evidence favoured oral CHM as integrative medicine in reducing levels of TC (Chapter 5, Table 5.28). Oral CHM as integrative medicine significantly improved levels of FPG, PBG, A1C, TG and FINS; however, the evidence was found to be of low certainty (Chapter 5, Table 5.28).

Overall, CHM showed promising effects on glycaemic levels, lipid profiles and β-cell function in T2DM patients and was safe for them. Nevertheless, interpretation of the results should consider the poor methodological quality of the studies, including a general lack of blinding of participants and personnel, small sample sizes, and considerable heterogeneity. These study aspects reduce the reliability of the results and lead to the downgrading of the quality of the evidence in GRADE.

Acupuncture and Related Therapies

This section summarises the evidence from Chapters 2, 3 and 7. The clinical guidelines and CM textbooks (Chapter 2) recommend manual acupuncture using a few main acupuncture points based on syndrome differentiation. Ten citations in the classical literature reported acupuncture and moxibustion for diabetes (Chapter 3). In modern literature, three RCTs on acupuncture for T2DM were identified. More clinical studies evaluated the effects of acupuncture for T2DM in a non-controlled setting. There were no CCTs. The acupuncture therapies recommended in Chapter 2, and found in Chapter 3, have also been studied in clinical trials and are listed in Table 10.2. Several CM syndromes have been reported in clinical studies, which overlap with syndromes recommended in guidelines and textbooks and classical literature. Deficiency of Kidney *qi* and *yin*, Lung heat and damage to the *jin* 津 liquid were common across all types of literature.

Acupoints ST36 *Zusanli* 足三里 and BL20 *Pishu* 脾俞 were points described across the classical, contemporary and clinical study literature. SP6 *Sanyinjiao* 三阴交 is commonly used in clinical trials and recommended in guidelines but not found in classical literature texts for the use of T2DM. Commonly used acupoints in clinical trials include BL13 *Feishu* 肺俞, SP6 *Sanyinjiao* 三阴交, BL23 *Shenshu* 肾俞, EX-B3 *Yishu* 胰俞, ST36 *Zusanli* 足三里 and BL20 *Pishu* 脾俞.

Table 10.2. Summary of Acupuncture and Related Therapies

Intervention	Included in Clinical Guidelines and Textbooks (Chapter 2)	Included in Classical Literature (Chapter 3) (No. of Citations)	Included in Clinical Studies (Chapter 7)			Included in Combination Therapies (Chapter 9) (No. of studies)
			RCTs (No. of Studies)	CCTs (No. of Studies)	Non-controlled Studies* (No. of Studies)	
Acupuncture	Yes	8	3	0	10	4
Electro-acupuncture	No	0	0	0	1	0
Ear-acupuncture	Yes	0	0	0	1	1
Moxibustion	Yes	2	1	0	0	1
Acupuncture Points						
BL13 Feishu 肺俞	Yes	0	2	0	10	0
SP6 Sanyinjiao 三阴交	Yes	0	4	0	8	1
BL23 Shenshu 肾俞	Yes	0	3	0	8	2
EX-B3 Yishu 胰俞	Yes	0	3	0	7	0
ST36 Zusanli 足三里	Yes	3	3	0	7	4
BL20 Pishu 脾俞	Yes	2	0	0	6	2
CV12 Zhongwan 中脘	Yes	3	2	0	6	1
LI11 Quchi 曲池	Yes	0	0	0	8	1
CV6 Qihai 气海	Yes	0	0	0	6	0
KI3 Taixi 太溪	No	7	0	0	8	1

(Continued)

Table 10.2. *(Continued)*

Intervention	Included in Clinical Guidelines and Textbooks (Chapter 2)	Included in Classical Literature (Chapter 3) (No. of Citations)	Included in Clinical Studies (Chapter 7)			Included in Combination Therapies (Chapter 9) (No. of studies)
			RCTs (No. of Studies)	CCTs (No. of Studies)	Non-controlled Studies* (No. of Studies)	
Ear Acupuncture Points						
CO11 *Yidan* (Pancreas and Gallbladder)胰胆	Yes	0	0	0	4	1
CO18 *Neifenmi* (Endocrine) 内分泌	Yes	0	0	0	4	2
CO4 *Wei* (Stomach) 胃	Yes	0	0	0	4	0
CO13 *Pi* (Spleen) 脾	No	0	0	0	4	1
CO14 *Fei* (Lung) 肺	Yes	0	0	0	2	0
CO10 *Shen* (Kidney)肾	Yes	0	0	0	3	0
CO17 *Sanjiao* 三焦	Yes	0	0	0	0	1

*Some studies used more than one intervention, e.g., acupuncture plus moxibustion. They are counted separately in this table.

Abbreviations: CCTs, controlled clinical trials; RCTs, Randomised controlled trials.

Guidelines also recommend ear acupuncture for T2DM. The commonly used ear points in clinical trials were CO11 *Yidan* (Endocrine) 胰胆, CO4 *Wei* (Stomach) 胃 and CO13 *Pi* (Spleen) 脾, which are also recommended in guidelines. The use of ear points was not documented in classical literature.

In clinical studies that used moxibustion, acupoints ST36 *Zusanli* 足三里 and BL23 *Shenshu* 肾俞 were commonly used. These points are also recommended in the guidelines.

There are a limited number of studies available for acupuncture and moxa for T2DM ($n = 3$). Evidence from acupuncture RCTs showed that acupuncture as integrative medicine did not improve on FBG more than pharmacotherapy alone. For other outcomes, evidence is only available from single studies. Meta-analysis was not possible for other comparisons and outcomes due to the very small number of included studies. The safety of acupuncture was not reported in the included RCT and non-controlled studies of acupuncture and moxa studies. Therefore, it is difficult to draw a reliable conclusion on the efficacy and safety of acupuncture and moxa for T2DM.

Other Chinese Medicine Therapies

This section summarises the evidence from Chapters 2, 3 and 8. Limited clinical trial evidence on other CM therapies was presented for diet therapy, *tuina* 推拿, *taichi* 太极 and *baduanjin* 八段锦 for T2DM (Table 10.3). The guidelines recommended diet therapy for T2DM, where recipes using foods that have *yin* and *qi* tonifying properties are recommended. Limited evidence was available for diet therapy in the clinical studies, though benefits were observed in FBG and PBG levels using the diet therapy. However, there was no mention of diet therapy in classical literature. *Tuina* 推拿 was performed along the back *shu* 腧 points along the Bladder meridian and acupoints ST36 *Zusanli* 足三里 and SP6 *Sanyinjiao* 三阴交. Points used in the *tuina* 推拿 study overlapped with the most frequently used acupuncture points in acupuncture clinical studies (Table 10.2).

Table 10.3. Summary of Other Chinese Medicine Therapies

| Intervention | Clinical Guidelines and Textbooks (Chapter 2) | Classical Literature (Chapter 3) (No. of Citations) | Clinical Studies (Chapter 8) | | | |
			RCTs (No. of Studies)	CCTs (No. of Studies)	Non-controlled Studies (No. of Studies)	Combination Therapies (Chapter 9)
Diet therapy	Yes	0	1	0	0	1
Tuina 推拿	Yes	0	1	0	0	2
Taichi 太极	No	0	3	0	0	2
Baduanjin 八段锦	No	0	4	0	1	1

Abbreviations: CCTs, controlled clinical trials; RCTs, randomised controlled trials.

The *tuina* 推拿 study showed a significant difference between the groups for FBG and PBG.

The *taichi* 太极 studies used different frequencies of practice and length and showed the benefits in FBG compared to aerobic exercise, but not other blood glucose or lipid profile outcome measures. *Baduanjin* 八段锦 combined with pharmacotherapy significantly improved FBG levels compared to pharmacotherapy alone, but not other blood glucose or lipid profile outcome measures.

Overall, there were nine RCTs and two non-controlled studies of other CM therapies for T2DM. The available studies were not blinded, and there were inadequacies in the reporting of study methods. These included studies did not report information on AEs. Due to the small number of studies and poor methodological quality, it was not possible to conclude the effectiveness and safety of these therapies.

Limitations of Evidence

Significant effort was made to collect and analyse data from a range of sources, yet omissions from each of the data sets are possible. The overview of current CM clinical practices in Chapter 2 is taken from authoritative clinical practice guidelines and CM textbooks. However, this is not a comprehensive list, and some syndromes and treatments that are not widely used are not included in Chapter 2. Thus, recommendations for practice may change in the future.

The classical literature in Chapter 3 is a comprehensive summary of the treatment of diabetes mellitus in ancient times. However, the literature was only from one source, the *Encyclopedia of Chinese Medicine* (*Zhong Hua Yi Dian* 中华医典, ZHYD). The ZHYD is the largest searchable resource, but it does not contain every historical CM text, and some classical books may have been missed. Nineteen search terms were used to find the diabetes mellitus citations, yet a search for more terms may have found more citations. In terms of the search results, there were only a very small number of acupuncture citations, and it is unknown if acupuncture was seldom used in ancient times or whether relevant citations were inadvertently omitted from the search.

Clinical trial evidence presented in Chapters 5 and 7 to 9 includes literature from a comprehensive search of Chinese and English scientific databases. However, errors or misclassification may have occurred during the screening process. When appropriate, meta-analysis was conducted to provide aggregate data from multiple studies. The evidence for CM interventions, compared to placebos or conventional treatments such as hypoglycaemic agents and lifestyle management, showed consistent results in favour of CHM/acupuncture or integrative medicine (CHM/acupuncture plus hypoglycaemic agents). Of studies included in meta-analyses, variations such as demographic features and outcome measurements were considerable. Consequently, substantial statistical heterogeneity was observed in pooled results that could not be explained by subgroup analysis. To account for the heterogeneity, a random effects model was used to provide conservative estimations of effect sizes.

In addition, most studies had methodological shortfalls, including insufficient random allocation procedures, a lack of blinding of participants and personnel, and small sample sizes. These methodological shortfalls and insufficient reporting in the published manuscripts compromised the results, leading to a downgrading of the evidence quality. Furthermore, AEs were insufficiently reported.

Limited clinical evidence of other CM therapies, such as CM diet therapy, *baduanjin* 八段锦, *taichi* 太极 and *tuina* 推拿, was available for synthesis. CHM and acupuncture, given together were assessed in a small number of clinical studies, and different herbs and acupuncture points were used in the studies. Therefore, it was difficult to draw a firm conclusion on their efficacy for diabetes mellitus. The limitations discussed above should be taken into consideration when interpreting the results in this monograph.

Implications for Practice

T2DM is a complicated disease with many CM syndromes presented. A summary of information from clinical guidelines and CM textbooks (Chapter 2) provides important guidance for syndrome differentiation and the selection of appropriate CM treatments for people with T2DM. Constitutional deficiencies, overeating, obesity and emotional disorders are all closely related to diabetes mellitus. The main organs involved are the Lung, Spleen and Kidney.

Qi and *yin* deficiency have been described across contemporary, classical and clinical trial evidence, and should be considered the main syndrome for diabetes mellitus. To develop a beneficial treatment plan that is suitable for the individual, clinicians need to consider the complexity of the disease and use the presenting symptoms and signs of patients and treat the manifestation syndromes with the root cause of diabetes mellitus in mind.

Chinese herbal medicine or acupuncture alone, or combined with a hypoglycaemic agent, improves blood glucose levels, lipid profiles, and β-cell function. Other CM therapies such as *taichi* 太极 and *baduanjin* 八段锦 are not found in contemporary or classical literature and have limited clinical evidence.

Overeating and an improper diet have been recognised as the main cause of diabetes in classical texts. Chinese medicine diet therapy has been recommended in contemporary guidelines and recommends foods to nourish *yin* (e.g., *bai he* 百合, *gou qi zi*

枸杞子), clear heat (e.g., bitter melon) and tonify *qi* (e.g., *shan yao* 山药).[7]

The most frequently used herbal formula in classical texts, *Liu wei di huang wan* 六味地黄丸, is also recommended in textbooks and guidelines for the syndrome of Kidney *yin* deficiency for diabetes mellitus. In clinical studies, using *Liu wei di huang wan* 六味地黄丸 as an adjunct to hypoglycaemic agents results in greater improvements in glucose and lipid metabolism in diabetic patients.

Included clinical studies evaluated CHM formulas that are recommended in textbooks and guidelines. The actions of these formulae include clearing heat and generating body fluids (*Xiao ke fang* 消渴方, *Bai hu jia ren shen tang* 白虎加人参汤), clearing damp heat from the Lower-*jiao* 下焦 (*Ge gen qin lian tang* 葛根芩连汤) and nourishing the *yin* 阴 (*Liu wei di huang wan* 六味地黄丸).

The most commonly studied herbs with a favourable effect for T2DM are *huang qi* 黄芪, *sheng di huang* 生地黄, *ge gen* 葛根, *huang lian* 黄连 and *dan shen* 丹参. The most commonly studied acupuncture points with a favourable effect are SP6 *Sanyinjiao* 三阴交, ST36 *Zusanli* 足三里, CV12 *Zhongwan* 中脘. BL20 *Pishu* 脾俞, BL23 *Shenshu* 肾俞, BL21 *Weishu* 胃俞 and EX-B3 *Yishu* 胰俞. These acupuncture points can be used to tonify the Spleen, Stomach and Kidney functions.

Implications for Research

Many clinical studies evaluated the effect and safety of CM therapies for T2DM. Encouraging evidence is available for CHM and acupuncture therapies, but the evidence is lacking for other CM therapies. Further research will increase knowledge and help to improve the management of T2DM. Despite the common use of several herbs in clinical studies, pre-clinical studies relevant to diabetes were limited, especially for *shan yao* 山药, *fu ling* 茯苓 and *tian hua fen* 天花粉. Future experimental studies will improve the understanding of their mechanisms of action and may lead to new therapeutic agents.

Clinical Trial Design

Rigorous methodology is needed when designing future clinical trials of CM therapies for T2DM. Methods of sequence generation and allocation concealment should be clearly stated. Future RCTs should have their protocols published and be registered to minimise reporting bias and increase transparency in the reporting of the results.

Blood glucose, lipid profile and β-cell function readings at baseline, and the disease course should be taken into consideration when designing trials; more comparable and reliable results will be produced if similar participants are recruited. Outcome measures directly related to blood glucose, lipid profiles, and β-cell function were reported as the main outcome measures. Other clinically important outcomes such as quality of life would provide another aspect in understanding the effect of CM therapies for T2DM.

The majority of clinical trials included treatment for four to 12 weeks and only a few reported follow-up data. T2DM is a progressive and lifelong disease and a follow-up assessment would provide long-term evidence of CM therapies and further strengthen the evidence. Most studies did not specify the use of CM syndromes for the selection of CHM or acupuncture interventions. Where possible, CM treatments should be given based on syndrome differentiation. This will validate the CM theory and improve the translation of results into clinical practice.

The majority of RCTs included in this monograph were assessed as "unclear" risk of bias for many domains due to insufficiency of the details provided. Future clinical studies should follow the items required by the Consolidated Standards of Reporting Trials (CONSORT)[8] and its extensions for herbal medicine, traditional CM and acupuncture.[9–12] Informative reporting of trial participants, the reason for intervention selection, comparator, and results of validated outcome measures will provide high-level clinical evidence and benefit practitioners, researchers and patients.

References

1. American Diabetes Association. (2019) 9. Pharmacologic approaches to glycemic treatment: Standards of medical care in diabetes — 2019. *Diabetes Care* **42**(1): S90.

2. Holman RR, Paul SK, Bethel MA, *et al.* (2008) 10-year follow-up of intensive glucose control in Type 2 diabetes. *N Engl J Med* **359**(15): 1577–1589.

3. 国家中医药管理局. (1994) 中医病证诊断疗效标准. 南京大学出版社, 南京.

4. 吴勉华, 王新月. (2012) 全国中医药行业高等教育"十二五"规划教材, 中医内科学. 中国中医药出版社, 北京.

5. 中华医学会糖尿病学分会. (2018) 中国2型糖尿病防治指南(2017年版). 中华糖尿病杂志 **10**(1): 4–67.

6. 中华中医药学会. 中医内科常见病诊疗指南: 中医病证部分. 中国中医药出版社, 北京.

7. 范冠杰, 邓兆智. (2013) 专科专病中医临床诊治丛书—内分泌科专病与风湿病中医临床诊治. 人民卫生出版社, 北京.

8. Schulz KF, Altman DG, Moher D. (2010) CONSORT 2010 statement: Updated guidelines for reporting parallel group randomised trials. *Trials* **11**: 32.

9. Bian Z, Liu B, Moher D, *et al.* (2011) Consolidated standards of reporting trials (CONSORT) for traditional Chinese medicine: Current situation and future development. *Front Med* **5**(2): 171–177.

10. Gagnier JJ, Boon H, Rochon P, *et al.* (2006) Reporting randomized, controlled trials of herbal interventions: An elaborated CONSORT statement. *Ann Intern Med* **144**(5): 364–367.

11. MacPherson H, Altman DG, Hammerschlag R, *et al.* (2010) Revised Standards for Reporting Interventions in Clinical Trials of Acupuncture (STRICTA): Extending the CONSORT statement. *J Evid Based Med* **3**(3): 140–155.

12. MacPherson H, White A, Cummings M, *et al.* (2002) Standards for reporting interventions in controlled trials of acupuncture: The STRICTA recommendations. Standards for Reporting Interventions in Controlled Trails of Acupuncture. *Acupunct Med* **20**(1): 22–25.

Glossary

Terms	Acronym	Definition	Reference
95% confidence interval	95% CI	A measure of the uncertainty around the main finding of a statistical analysis. Estimates of unknown quantities, such as the odds ratio comparing an experimental intervention with a control, are usually presented as a point estimate and a 95% confidence interval. This means that if someone were to keep repeating a study in other samples from the same population, 95% of the confidence intervals from those studies would contain the true value of the unknown quantity. Alternatives to 95%, such as 90% and 99% confidence intervals, are sometimes used. Wider intervals indicate lower precision; narrow intervals, greater precision.	https://training. cochrane.org/ handbook
Acupuncture	—	The insertion of needles into humans or animals for remedial purposes.	*WHO International Standard Terminologies of Traditional Medicine in the Western Pacific Region*, World Health Organization, 2007.

(Continued)

(Continued)

Terms	Acronym	Definition	Reference
Allied and Complementary Medicine Database	AMED	Alternative medicine bibliographic database.	https://www.ebsco.com/products/research-databases/allied-and-complementary-medicine-database-amed
Antihyperglycaemic agents	—	Drugs that can reduce the blood glucose level to reach a target glucose level.	—
Australian New Zealand Clinical Trial Registry	ANZCTR	Clinical trial registry based in Australia.	www.anzctr.org.au/
Body mass index	BMI	Measurement of body fat to classify underweight, overweight and obesity in adults. Defined as weight in kilograms divided by the square of the height in meters (kg/m^2).	—
C-peptide	—	Produced in equal amounts to insulin and can be used to assess insulin secretion.	—
China National Knowledge Infrastructure	CNKI	Chinese language bibliographic database.	http://www.cnki.net
Chinese Biomedical Literature Database	CBM	Chinese language bibliographic database.	www.imicams.ac.cn
Chinese Clinical Trial Registry	ChiCTR	Chinese clinical trial registry.	http://www.chictr.org.cn/
Chinese herbal medicine	CHM	Chinese herbal medicine.	—
Chinese medicine	CM	Chinese medicine.	—
Chongqing VIP Information Company	CQVIP	Chinese language bibliographic database.	http://www.cqvip.com
ClinicalTrials.gov	—	Clinical trial registry based in the United States of America.	https://clinicaltrials.gov/

Terms	Acronym	Definition	Reference
Cochrane Central Register of Controlled Trials	CENTRAL	Bibliographic database that provides a highly concentrated source of reports of controlled trials.	https://community.cochrane.org/editorial-and-publishing-policy-resource/overview-cochrane-library-and-related-content/databases-included-cochrane-library/cochrane-central-register-controlled-trials-central
Combination therapies	—	Two or more Chinese medicines from different therapy groups (e.g., Chinese herbal medicine, acupuncture therapies or other Chinese medicine therapies) are administered together.	—
Controlled clinical trials	CCT	A study in which people are allocated to different interventions using methods that are not random.	https://training.cochrane.org/handbook
Convention on International Trade in Endangered Species of Wild Fauna and Flora	CITES	International convention aimed at preventing or regulating trade in threatened and endangered species of plants and animals.	https://www.cites.org/eng/disc/text.php
Cumulative Index of Nursing and Allied Health Literature	CINAHL	Bibliographic database.	https://www.ebscohost.com/nursing/products/cinahl-databases
Cupping therapy	—	Suction by using a vaccumised cup or jar.	*WHO International Standard Terminologies of Traditional Medicine in the Western Pacific Region*, World Health Organisation, 2007.

(*Continued*)

(*Continued*)

Terms	Acronym	Definition	Reference
Disability adjusted life years	DALY	DALYs are a measurement of disease expressed in units. Years lived with disability are added to the number of years of life lost for a certain disease.	https://www.nimh.nih.gov/health/statistics/disability/what-are-ylds.shtml
Effect size	—	A generic term for the estimate of the effect of a treatment in a study.	http://handbook.cochrane.org/
Electroacupuncture	—	Electric stimulation of the acupuncture needle following insertion.	*WHO International Standard Terminologies of Traditional Medicine in the Western Pacific Region*, World Health Organization, 2007.
EU Clinical Trials Register	EU-CTR	European clinical trial registry.	https://www.clinicaltrialsregister.eu
Excerpta Medica database	Embase	Bibliographic database.	http://www.elsevier.com/solutions/embase
Fasting insulin	FINS	Used to assess insulin sensitivity; impaired insulin sensitivity precedes glucose intolerance.	—
Fasting plasma glucose	FPG	Diagnostic test for diabetes mellitus; a blood sample is taken after at least eight hours of no caloric intake.	https://www.diabetes.org/
Grading of Recommendations, Assessment, Development and Evaluation	GRADE	Approach used to grade quality of evidence and strength of recommendations.	http://www.gradeworkinggroup.org/
Haemoglobin A1c	A1C	Diagnostic test for diabetes mellitus.	—

Terms	Acronym	Definition	Reference
Heterogeneity	—	Used in a general sense to describe the variation in, or diversity of, participants, interventions and measurement of outcomes across a set of studies, or the variation in internal validity of those studies. Used specifically, as statistical heterogeneity, to describe the degree of variation in the effect estimates from a set of studies. Also used to indicate the presence of variability among studies beyond the amount expected due solely to the play of chance.	https://training. cochrane.org/ handbook
High-density lipoprotein	HDL	Absorbs cholesterol from the body and carries it back to the liver.	—
Homogeneity	—	Used in a general sense to mean that the participants, interventions and measurement of outcomes are similar across a set of studies. Used specifically to describe the effect estimates from a set of studies where they do not vary more than would be expected by chance.	https://training. cochrane.org/ handbook
Hyperglycaemia	—	High level of glucose in the blood, a hallmark metabolic abnormality associated with Type 2 diabetes mellitus.	World Health Organization, Definition, diagnosis and classification of diabetes mellitus and its complications: Report of a WHO consultation.

(*Continued*)

(*Continued*)

Terms	Acronym	Definition	Reference
			Part 1, Diagnosis and classification of diabetes mellitus. Geneva, Switzerland, 1999.
I^2	—	A measure of study heterogeneity that indicates the percentage of variance in a meta-analysis.	https://training. cochrane.org/ handbook
Insulin	—	Hormone made by the pancreas to allow blood glucose passage into the body's systems. It maintains a normal blood glucose level by facilitating cellular glucose uptake, carbohydrate, lipid and protein metabolism.	—
Insulin sensitivity	—	The ability of insulin to stimulate glucose uptake, promote peripheral glucose disposal, and suppress hepatic glucose production.	—
Insulin resistance	—	Reduced responsiveness to normal levels of insulin by target tissues, mainly liver and skeletal muscle, to insulin action.	—
Integrative medicine	—	CM combined with pharmacotherapy or other conventional therapy.	—
Low-density lipoprotein	LDL	Transports cholesterol from the liver to the tissues and cells of the body.	—
Mean difference	MD	In meta-analysis: A method used to combine measures on continuous scales, where the mean, standard deviation and sample size in each group are known.	https://training. cochrane.org/ handbook

Terms	Acronym	Definition	Reference
		The weight given to the difference in means from each study (e.g., how much influence each study has on the overall results of the meta-analysis) is determined by the precision of its estimate of effect; mathematically, this is equal to the inverse of the variance. This method assumes that all of the trials have measured the outcome on the same scale.	
Meta-analysis	—	The use of statistical techniques in a systematic review to integrate the results of included studies. Sometimes misused as a synonym for systematic reviews, where the review includes a meta-analysis.	—
Non-controlled studies	—	Observations made on individuals, usually receiving the same intervention, before and after an intervention but with no control group.	https://training.cochrane.org/handbook
Other Chinese medicine therapies	—	Other Chinese medicine therapies include all traditional therapies except Chinese herbal medicine and acupuncture, such as *taichi* 太极, *qigong* 气功, *tuina* 推拿 and cupping.	—
Postprandial blood glucose	PBG	Blood glucose level two hours after an oral glucose tolerance test.	https://www.diabetes.org/
PubMed	PubMed	Bibliographic database.	http://www.ncbi.nlm.nih.gov/pubmed

(*Continued*)

(*Continued*)

Terms	Acronym	Definition	Reference
Randomised con-trolled trial	RCT	Clinical trial that uses a random method to allocate participants to treatment and control groups.	—
Risk of bias	—	Assessment of clinical trials to indicate if the results may overestimate or underestimate the true effect because of a bias in study design or reporting.	https://training.cochrane.org/handbook
Risk ratio (relative risk)	RR	The ratio of risks in two groups. In intervention studies, it is the ratio of the risk in the intervention group to the risk in the control group. A risk ratio of one indicates no difference between comparison groups. For undesirable outcomes, a risk ratio that is less than one indicates that the intervention was effective in reducing the risk of that outcome.	https://training.cochrane.org/handbook
Standardised mean difference	SMD	In meta-analysis: A method used to combine results for continuous scales that measure the same outcome but in different ways (e.g., with different scales). The results of studies are standardised to a uniform scale to allow data to be combined.	https://training.cochrane.org/handbook
Summary of findings	—	Presentation of results and rating the quality of evidence based on the GRADE approach.	http://www.gradeworkinggroup.org/
Thiazolidinedione	—	Insulin sensitisers with predominant action in peripheral insulin-sensitive tissues.	—

Terms	Acronym	Definition	Reference
Tuina 推拿	—	Chinese massage: Rubbing, kneading, or percussion of the soft tissues and joints of the body with the hands, usually performed by one person on another, especially to relieve tension or pain.	*WHO International Standard Terminologies of Traditional Medicine in the Western Pacific Region*, World Health Organization, 2007.
Triglyceride	TG	Esters of glycerol and fatty acid in a stoichiometric molar ratio of 1:3. It is the most common form of fat in the body.	—
Wangfang database	Wanfang	Chinese language bibliographic database.	www.wanfangdata.com
World Health Organization	WHO	WHO is the directing and coordinating authority for health within the United Nations system. It is responsible for providing leadership on global health matters, shaping the health research agenda, setting norms and standards, articulating evidence-based policy options, providing technical support to countries, and monitoring and assessing health trends.	http://www.who.int/about/en/
Zhong Hua Yi Dian 中华医典	ZHYD	The Zhong Hua Yi Dian (ZHYD) "Encyclopaedia of Traditional Chinese Medicine" is a comprehensive series of electronic books on a compact disc. The collection was put together by the Hunan electronic and audio-visual publishing house. It is the largest collection of Chinese	Hu R, ed. (2000) *Zhong Hua Yi Dian [Encyclopaedia of Traditional Chinese Medicine]*. 4th ed. Hunan Electronic and Audio-Visual Publishing House, Chengsha.

(*Continued*)

(Continued)

Terms	Acronym	Definition	Reference
		electronic books and includes the major Chinese ancient works, many of which are from rare manuscripts and are the only existing copies. These books cover the period from ancient times up to the period of the Republic of China (1911–1948).	

Index

Evidence-based Clinical Chinese Medicine

(*Continued from page ii*)